CLINICAL RESEARCH in COMPLEMENTARY THERAPIES

Commissioning Editor: Claire Wilson
Development Editor: Natalie Meylan, Louisa Welch
Project Manager: Sruthi Viswam
Designer: Kirsteen Wright
Illustration Manager: Merlyn Harvey
Illustrator: Ethan Danielson

CLINICAL RESEARCH in COMPLEMENTARY THERAPIES

PRINCIPLES, PROBLEMS AND SOLUTIONS

SECOND EDITION

Edited by

George T. Lewith MA DM FRCP MRCGP
Professor of Health Research
Complementary and Integrated Medicine Research Unit
University of Southampton
Southampton, UK

Wayne B. Jonas MD
President and CEO
Samueli Institute;
Professor of Family Medicine, Georgetown University
Alexandria, VA, USA

Harald Walach Dip Psych PhD
Professor, European University Viadrina
Institute for Transcultural Health Studies & Samueli Institute
European Office
Frankfurt, Germany

Foreword by

Harold Sox MD MACP

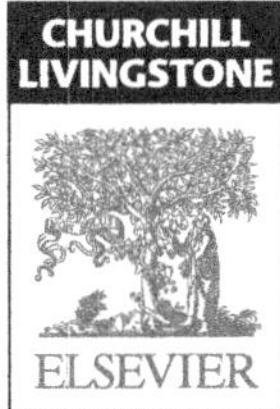

EDINBURGH LONDON NEW YORK OXFORD PHILADELPHIA ST LOUIS
SYDNEY TORONTO 2011

CHURCHILL
LIVINGSTONE
ELSEVIER

First edition 2002
Second edition 2011

ISBN 978-0-443-06956-7

British Library Cataloguing in Publication Data
A catalogue record for this book is available from the British Library

Library of Congress Cataloging in Publication Data
A catalog record for this book is available from the Library of Congress

Notices

Knowledge and best practice in this field are constantly changing. As new research and experience broaden our understanding, changes in research methods, professional practices, or medical treatment may become necessary.

Practitioners and researchers must always rely on their own experience and knowledge in evaluating and using any information, methods, compounds, or experiments described herein. In using such information or methods they should be mindful of their own safety and the safety of others, including parties for whom they have a professional responsibility.

With respect to any drug or pharmaceutical products identified, readers are advised to check the most current information provided (i) on procedures featured or (ii) by the manufacturer of each product to be administered, to verify the recommended dose or formula, the method and duration of administration, and contraindications. It is the responsibility of practitioners, relying on their own experience and knowledge of their patients, to make diagnoses, to determine dosages and the best treatment for each individual patient, and to take all appropriate safety precautions.

To the fullest extent of the law, neither the Publisher nor the authors, contributors, or editors assume any liability for any injury and/or damage to persons or property as a matter of products liability, negligence or otherwise, or from any use or operation of any methods, products, instructions, or ideas contained in the material herein.

Printed in China

CONTENTS

*Deceased

CONTRIBUTORS

Mones Abu-Asab PhD
Senior Research Biologist, Laboratory of Pathology, National Cancer Institute, National Institutes of Health, Bethesda, MD, USA

Mikel Aickin PhD
Department of Family and Community Medicine, University of Arizona, Tucson, AZ, USA

Hakima Amri PhD
Assistant Professor, Director of the Complementary and Alternative Medicine Master's of Science Program in Physiology, Department of Physiology & Biophysics, Georgetown University Medical Center, Washington, DC, USA

Enrique Auba MD PhD
Department of Psychiatry and Medical Psychology, Clinica Universidad de Navarra, Pamplona, Navarra, Spain

William 'Mac' Beckner MIS
Vice President, Operations and Technology, Samueli Institute, Alexandria, VA, USA

Herbert Benson MD
Benson-Henry Institute for Mind Body Medicine at Massachusetts General Hospital, Boston, MA, USA

Heather S. Boon BScPhM PhD
Leslie Dan Faculty of Pharmacy, University of Toronto, Toronto, ON, Canada

John Brazier BA MSc PhD
Professor of Health Economics, The University of Sheffield, Sheffield, UK

Alan Breen DC PhD
Anglo-European College of Chiropractic, Bournemouth, UK

Ian D. Coulter PhD
RAND/Samueli Chair for Integrative Medicine, RAND Corporation, Santa Monica; Professor, School of Dentistry, UCLA, Los Angeles, CA, USA

Jeffery A. Dusek PhD
Director of Research, Penny George Institute for Health and Healing at Abbott Northwestern Hospital, Minneapolis, MN, USA

Elisabetta Fenu MSc
National Clinical Guideline Centre, Royal College of Physicians, London, UK

Tiffany Field
Director, Touch Research Institute, University of Miami Medical School and Fielding Graduate University, Miami, Florida, USA

Peter Fisher MD
Clinical Director, Royal London Homoeopathic Hospital, London, UK

Gregory L. Fricchione MD
Benson-Henry Institute for Mind Body Medicine at Massachusetts General Hospital, Boston, MA, USA

John Gabbay MB ChB MSc FFPH
Emeritus Professor, University of Southampton, Lymington, UK

Corina Güthlin PhD
Institute for General Practice, Johann-Wolfgang Goethe-University, Frankfurt, Germany

William Harlan MD
Retired, National Institutes of Health, Chevy Chase, MD, USA

Pedro Huertas MD PhD
Benson-Henry Institute for Mind Body Medicine at Massachusetts General Hospital, Boston, MA, USA

John A. Ives PhD
Director, Brain, Mind & Healing, Samueli Institute, Alexandria, VA, USA

Wayne B. Jonas MD
Samueli Institute, Alexandria, VA, USA

Raheleh Khorsan MA
Research Associate, Military Medical Research and Integrative Medicine, Samueli Institute, Corona del Mar, CA, USA

Niko Kohls PhD
Samueli Scholar, Generation Research Program, Human Science Center, University of Munich & Peter-Schilffarth Institute, Bad Tolz, Germany; Samueli Institute, Washington, USA

Andrée le May BSc Hons PhD RGN PGCE(A)
Retired Professor of Nursing University of Southampton, Lymington, UK

George T. Lewith MA DM FRCP MRCGP
Complementary and Integrated Medicine Research Unit, University of Southampton, UK

Klaus Linde MD
Institute of General Practice, Technische Universität München, München, Germany

Robert T. Mathie BSc (Hons) PhD
Research Development Adviser, British Homeopathic Association, Luton, UK

Simon Y. Mills MA FNIMH MCPP
Project Lead, Integrated Self Care in Family Practice, Culm Valley Integrated Centre for Health, Cullompton, UK

Anne Morgan
Health Services Research, Walkley, Sheffield, UK

Elisabeth Targ MD†
Director, Complementary Medical Research Institute, California Pacific Medical Center, San Francisco, CA, USA

Lene Vase PhD
Department of Psychology, Aarhus University, Denmark

Marja J. Verhoef MSc PhD
Department of Community Health Sciences, University of Calgary, AB, Canada

Andrew J. Vickers DPhil
Associate Attending Research Methodologist, Department of Epidemiology and Biostatistics, Memorial Sloan-Kettering Cancer Center, New York, NY, USA

Harald Walach Dip Psych PhD
Professor, European University Viadrina Institute for Transcultural Health Studies & Samueli Institute, European Office Germany

Adrian White MA MD BM BCh DRCOG DipMedAc
Clinical Research Fellow, Peninsula Medical School, Plymouth, UK

Claudia M. Witt MD MBA
Vice Director, Institute for Social Medicine, Epidemiology and Health Economics, Charité University Medical Center Berlin, Germany

David Wonderling MSc
National Clinical Guideline Centre, Royal College of Physicians, London, UK

Albert Yeung MD ScD
Massachusetts General Hospital, Boston, MA, USA

†Deceased

FOREWORD

As I see it, the name "complementary and alternative medicine" (CAM) is destined for the history books. As suggested by a 2005 Institute of Medicine Committee report[1], the advent of high quality research about the effectiveness of CAM will dissolve the dichotomy between conventional medicine and CAM and replace it with the more universal distinction between proven and unproven therapies. *Clinical Research in Complementary Therapies – Principles, Problems and Solutions* should contribute importantly to this evolution.

The field of CAM research has grown rapidly in less than two decades. Unlike the authors of this book, I am an observer rather than a participant, and my history of its growth may seem idiosyncratic to some. I would begin with the 1993 survey that described the widespread use of CAM interventions by the American public[2]. The next key step was the establishment in 1998 of the National Center for Complementary and Alternative Medicine (NCCAM) in the National Institutes of Health. The 2010 budget of the Center is $129 million. This level of year-to-year funding is enough to ensure testing of important CAM interventions in large-scale comparative trials. Patients will find out if they are effective and in whom. Research in CAM began before NCCAM, and *Annals of Internal Medicine* (the journal that I edited from 2001 to 2009) summarized this evidence in a series of review articles about specific CAM interventions. This amount of attention from a high impact, high circulation journal was another milestone for CAM. In 2003-2005, the aforementioned IOM committee on the Use of Complementary and Alternative Medicine by the American Public addressed the role of CAM. Its most important recommendation stated that:

> "The committee recommends that the same principles and standards of evidence of treatment effectiveness apply to all treatments, whether currently labeled as conventional medicine or CAM. Implementing this recommendation requires that investigators use and develop as necessary common methods, measures, and standards for the generation and interpretation of evidence necessary for making decisions about the use of CAM and conventional therapies."[1]

I was a member of this committee, and I agreed that this perspective forecasts a future in which CAM would be compared to conventional medical practices, in effect putting these two forms of health care on the same playing field.

In just a few years, the emergence of comparative effectiveness research (CER) has begun to change the landscape of clinical research. The 2010

Patient Protection and Affordable Care Act (U.S. health reform) establishes a new public-private Institute that will fund CER. In describing the purpose of the Institute, the language of the legislation effectively defines the purpose of CER:

> "The purpose of the Institute is to assist patients, clinicians, purchasers, and policy-makers in making informed health decisions …"

To achieve this purpose, CER will, according to a recent Institute of Medicine report, have three key characteristics[(3)]. Each has implications for research comparing CAM and conventional medical services. First, CER shall directly compare active treatments, which means fewer explanatory trials that test whether an intervention is more effective than placebo. Second, the study populations shall be typical of daily practice, rather than carefully selected to maximize the likelihood of seeing an effect. Third, researchers shall plan their research to uncover evidence that will help individualize treatment. To respond to this requirement, they will search systematically for clinical findings that predict a response to one or the other of the compared treatments.

As I look at its Table of Contents, I wonder if *Clinical Research in Complementary Therapies – Principles, Problems and Solutions* will prepare researchers for the particular requirements of CER. But, I am not concerned. CAM researchers are resourceful, and they will find a way to succeed in this changing environment of clinical research. Meanwhile, this second edition will help a new generation of researchers to do first-class comparative clinical research.

Harold C. Sox, MD, MACP
Professor of Medicine and of the Dartmouth Institute (emeritus, active)
Dartmouth Medical School, UK

REFERENCES

1. Institute of Medicine (U.S.) Committee on the Use of Complementary and Alternative Medicine by the American Public, 2005. *Complementary and Alternative Medicine in the United States*. The National Academy Press, Washington, DC.
2. Eisenberg, D.M, Kessler, R.K, Foster, C., et al., 1993. Unconventional medicine in the United States: prevalence, costs, and patterns of use. New Engl. J Med. 328, 246–252.
3. IOM (Institute of Medicine), 2009. *Initial National Priorities for Comparative Effectiveness Research*. The National Academies Press, Washington, DC.

PREFACE

Since publishing the first edition of this research textbook in 2002 there have been substantial advances within the field of integrated and complementary medical research. In many of the western industrialized nations a process of thoughtful evidence-based integration has been occurring at pace; many of the major cancer centres in the USA now offer integrative medical programmes as an essential part of their patient management and the use of acupuncture is now widely seen as evidence-based in the management of pain, largely as a consequence of the German and American investment in acupuncture research. Acupuncture is now accepted by the German health insurance companies as well as the National Health Service (NHS) as a cost-effective and safe treatment for some common conditions. This represents thoughtful, scientific progress based on sound and rigorous evidence with the primary therapeutic aim of safely improving the care and well-being of patients.

We've also seen substantial advances in how we think about complementary medicine; research funders are beginning to understand that the range of complementary and alternative medicines (CAM) on offer are not simply 'alternative medications' but in themselves complex whole systems of diagnosis and treatment. The mixed qualitative and quantitative research methods beginning to unravel this complex therapeutic interaction may not only allow us to understand how complementary medicines themselves may be offering benefit, but should also give us remarkable insights into the management (and self-management) of a variety of different chronic problems. It will guide and inform us as to how we can enable our patients, particularly those with chronic illness, to improve their own well-being. We have begun to understand that simple placebo-controlled randomized clinical trials offer us a very limited evidence base and that we need to expand our research methodology and its interpretation, taking into account a whole variety of different types of evidence so that we can begin to understand how best to manage illness within the community. These approaches are beginning to filter into the way we consider and manage NHS and US health service policy within conventional medicine for a range of interventions.

The more we understand about chronic illness, the more we understand how limited some of our evidence base appears to be and the more we need to understand about illness and its societal personal and environmental impact. The more we understand that the human organism is a complex system that creates health on a continuous basis, the more we can see that there are multiple roads of teasing a diseased system back into optimal balance. This is what has become known as the self-healing response and complementary therapies can be conceptualized as methods of making use of this self-healing response of the organism. Investigating CAM provides us with these important methodological insights and understandings.

The scientific breadth of research within complementary medicine has expanded substantially over the last decade and we hope that the new chapters in our second edition reflect this expansion along with our increasing expertise and maturity as a research discipline. As a consequence this edition of our book has been substantially restructured. Our initial chapter begins with a broadly based summary looking at how we interpret evidence and the kinds of methodological approaches that we might use to obtain evidence. The importance of mixed-methods approaches demands that we include detailed chapters on qualitative research, laboratory research and, importantly, pragmatically based health services research. These approaches are essential for us to be able to understand why people may seek a particular medical approach and what its comparative impact may be on the whole person as well as within the laboratory.

We have also included some specific and rather controversial areas in relation to particular therapies. The study of prayer and spiritual healing along with mind–body therapies presents us with challenges but also important methodological issues such as the use and value of various control interventions. Many of these areas are simply not amenable to placebo-controlled trials but are popular and important parts of complementary medical practice. Our approach has been to consider them carefully to try and understand what the therapists are attempting to achieve with their interventions and then design a reasonable research agenda around their approach. This will enable the development of a relevant and coherent research that we believe will continue to progress over the next decade.

The third section allows us to think creatively about statistical design and analysis and also begins to help us understand and 'interpret data' and exactly what we mean by the placebo or meaning and context response. Importantly, we look at how evidence-based medicine is applied to clinical practice within primary care which provides us with important understanding of how to apply evidence-based medicine in all of health care.

We hope this new edition of our textbook will excite thoughtful debate in this developing area. There is no doubt that the quality of CAM research has increased enormously since our first edition some 18 years ago. Our current methodological approaches map the increasingly sophisticated understanding of CAM research and its development and how illness management integrates conventional and complementary approaches to disease.

George T. Lewith

Wayne B. Jonas

Harald Walach

2010

SECTION I
STANDARDS OF QUALITY IN CAM RESEARCH

SECTION CONTENTS

Toward standards of evidence for CAM research and practice

1

Wayne B. Jonas • George T. Lewith

CHAPTER CONTENTS

DOI: 10.1016/B978-0-443-06956-7.00001-X

KEY POINTS

- Health care is complex and requires several types of evidence
- Evidence-based medicine (EBM) in complementary and alternative medicine (CAM) is necessarily pluralistic
- The translation of evidence (EBM) into clinical practice (evidence-based practice: EBP) is not fundamentally hierarchical – it operates through a mixed-method or circular strategy
- EBP needs to balance specificity and utility for both the individual and groups of patients – the evidence house strategy
- Standards and quality issues exist in medicine and can be applied to CAM; we don't need to reinvent them
- The integrity of individual CAM practice, therapies and principles needs to be respected within a rigorous EBM framework – this is called model validity
- Improving the application of EBM in CAM practice is desirable, possible and practical

INTRODUCTION

Complementary and alternative medicine (CAM) forms a significant subset of the world's health care practices that are not integral to conventional western care but are used by a substantial minority (and in some countries substantial majority) of patients when they make their health care decisions. The World Health Organization (WHO) has estimated that 80% of the developing world's population also use these medical practices (World Health Organization 2003). In developing countries, numerous surveys have documented CAM use by the public ranging from 10% to over 60%, depending on the population and practices included in the samples (Fisher & Ward 1994; Eisenberg et al. 1998; Ernst 2000; Barnes et al. 2002; Graham et al. 2005; Tindle et al. 2005).

CAM encompasses a number of diverse health care and medical practices, ranging from dietary and behavioural interventions to high-dose vitamin supplements and herbs, and includes ancient systems of medicine such as Ayurvedic medicine and traditional Chinese medicine (TCM). CAM has been defined slightly differently in the USA (http://nccam.nih.gov/health/camcancer/#what) than the UK (House of Lords Select Committee on Science and Technology 2000). In a recent history of alternative medicine, historian Roberta Bivins documents that, while competing forms of health care have often been part of every culture and time, the concept of a collective group of practices that are complementary or alternative to a dominant 'biomedicine' has occurred only in the last 100 years (Bivins 2007). Furthermore patients may view CAM in a variety of ways. For example, they may see manipulative therapies as conventionally based, with biomechanical mechanisms and whole systems such as Ayurveda and homeopathy as alternative medical systems while potentially perceiving acupuncture for pain as complementary to conventional medical interventions (Bishop et al. 2008). Consequently the definition of CAM is fundamentally politically defined and ultimately depends very much on 'who you are asking' (Clouser et al. 1996). By almost any definition, however, the use of CAM has been steadily growing for decades, so reliable information on its safety and effectiveness is needed by both patients and health care providers.

What then is evidence and how shall it be applied to CAM? The application of science to medicine is a relatively recent phenomenon manifesting itself mainly over the last 100 years. Current methods such as blinded human experiments were first used by homeopaths in 1835 and this methodology has become increasingly dominant within conventional medical (clinical) research over the last 60 years (Stolberg 1996; Jadad 1998; Kaptchuk 1998a). In this chapter and book we hold the assumption that research into alternative medical practices should use the same meticulous methods as those developed for conventional medicine, but researchers will necessarily need to apply them pragmatically so they are relevant to the various stakeholders within CAM clinical practice. We also assume that full knowledge and evidence about CAM practices require a plurality of methods, each designed to provide a part of the complex picture of what CAM is and its value and impact within health care. In this chapter, we aim to describe that plurality, review the research standards that apply to all evidence-based medicine (EBM) and explore the special issues required for application of those methods to the diverse practices encompassed in CAM. In subsequent chapters each author will describe in more detail the application of research to specific CAM practices.

SCIENCE AND VALUES

One cannot reasonably discuss the appropriate application of science to health care without addressing the issue of human values and the goals of medicine (Cassell 1991). Bradford Hill (1971), who developed the modern randomized controlled trial (RCT), often emphasized the importance of human ethical issues in its application. Scientific research is not simply a matter of applying a pre-set group of methods for all kinds of research problems. It involves selecting research designs that are ethical and appropriate to the questions, goals and circumstances addressed by the researchers while being relevant to the research commissioners and the research audience (Jonas 2002a).

Two crucial issues arise in developing appropriate (and ethically grounded) evidence: the rigour and the relevance of the information. Rigour refers to the minimization of bias that threatens the validity of conclusions and interpretation of data. It is an attempt to make sure we are not fooled by our observations and approach truth. Relevance addresses the value to which the information will be put by a specific audience and involves the values placed on different types of information by the research audience. Failure to consider different values when designing and conducting research risks 'methodological tyranny' in which we become slaves to rigid, preordained and potentially misleading assumptions (Schaffner 2002).

It would, for instance, be very important for both clinicians and patients to have a substantial amount of rigorous evidence when thinking of prescribing a potentially life-saving but new and possibly lethal chemotherapeutic agent for malignant melanoma. There might be a different set of arguments and evidence for the prescription of a safe new agent for rhinitis; we do need to consider context alongside risk and benefit and this frequently occurs within medicine practised in the community for benign, chronic or transient conditions.

Research strategies must start with specific questions, goals and purposes before we decide which information to collect and how to collect it. Questions of importance for determining relevance relate mostly to whom and for what purpose evidence will be used (the audience). For example: How do the values of the patient, practitioner, scientist and provider infuse the research and how will the data be used? What is the context of the research, and what do we already know about the field? Has the practice been in use for a long time, and hence is there implicit knowledge available, or are we dealing with a completely new intervention? It is mostly at this initial level that implicit paradigmatic incompatibilities arise between conventional and complementary medicine but we believe that evidence-based practice (EBP) must start with the values of the audience it purports to serve (Jonas 2002b).

THE AUDIENCE AND THE EVIDENCE

One of the striking features of the current interest in CAM is that it is a publicly driven trend (Fonnebo et al. 2007). The audience for CAM use is primarily the public. Surveys of unconventional medicine use in the USA have shown that CAM use increased by 45% between 1990 and 1997. Visits to CAM practitioners in the USA exceed 600 million per year, more than to all primary care physicians. The amount spent on these practices, out of pocket, is $34 billion, on a par with conventional medicine out-of-pocket costs (Barnes 2007). Two-thirds of the US and UK medical schools teach about CAM practices (Rampes et al. 1997; Wetzel et al. 1998) and many hospitals are developing complementary and integrated medicine familiarization programmes and more and more health management organizations include alternative practitioners (Pelletier et al. 1997).

The mainstream is also putting research money into these practices. For example, the budget of the Office of Alternative Medicine at the US National Institutes of Health rose from $5 million to $89 million in 7 years, and it then became the National Center for Complementary and Alternative Medicine (NCCAM) (Marwick 1998). Despite resistance to NCCAM's formation, its budget is now nearly $125 million annually, a far larger investment than in any of the other western industrialized nations. The public has been at the forefront of the CAM movement and driven this change in perception (Jonas 2002). The audience for CAM and CAM research is therefore both diverse and critical. Its various audiences will often want exactly the same information but will have different emphases in how they understand and interpret the data available (Jonas 2002). Social science studies of applied knowledge show that interpretation and application of evidence can be quite complex and vary by prior experience and training, individual and cultural beliefs and percieved and real needs (Friedson 1998; Kaptchuk 1998a). Some of these factors are briefly summarized below.

PATIENTS

Patients who are ill (and their family members) often want to hear details about other individuals with similar illnesses who have used a treatment and recovered. If the treatment appears to be safe and there is little risk of harm, evidence from these stories frequently appears to be sufficient for them to decide to use the treatment. Patients may interpret this as a sign that the treatment is effective, and to them this evidence is important and relevant for both CAM and conventional medicine. The skilled and informed clinician will need to place this type of evidence into an individual and patient-centred context with respect for all the evidence available from both qualitative and quantitative investigations.

HEALTH PRACTITIONERS

Health care practitioners (conventional doctors, CAM practitioners, nurses, physical therapists) also want to know what the likelihood or probability is that a patient will recover or be harmed based on a series of similar patients who have received that treatment in clinical practice. Such information may come from case series or clinical outcomes studies or RCTs (Guthlin et al. 2004; Witt et al. 2005a,b). They also want to know about the safety, complications, complexity and cost of using the therapy, and this information comes from the collection of careful safety data and health economic analyses.

CLINICAL INVESTIGATORS

Clinical scientists will value the same type of evidence as clinicians but will often look at the data differently because of their research training and skills. They often want to know how much improvement occurred in a group who received the treatment compared to another group who did not receive it or a group that received a placebo. If 80% of patients who received a treatment got better, do 60% of similar patients get better just from coming to the doctor? This type of comparative evidence can only come from RCTs, which is the major area of interest for most clinical researchers. These types of studies can include a placebo control but sometimes are pragmatic studies, which compare two treatments or have a non-treatment arm or other types of controls.

LABORATORY SCIENTISTS

Laboratory scientists focus on discovering mechanisms of action. Basic science facilitates understanding of underlying mechanisms and allows for greater precision testing in more highly controlled, (and artificial) environments.

PURCHASERS OF HEALTH CARE

Those in charge of determining public policy often need aggregate 'proof' that a practice is safe, effective and cost-effective. This usually involves a health economic perspective within a complex process of treatment evaluation. Systematic reviews, meta-analyses and health services research including randomized trials and outcome studies provide this type of evidence. Health services research also provides data that evaluates the cost, feasibility, utility and safety of delivering treatments within existing delivery systems.

While day-to-day decision-making is more complex than the brief summaries above, the point is that different audiences have legimate evidence needs that cannot be accommodated by a 'one size fits all' strategy. The CAM researcher must keep in mind the need for quality research in a variety of domains and attend carefully to the audience and use of the results of their research once collected and interpreted (Callahan 2002; Jonas & Callahan 2002). As stated by Ian Coulter, there is a difference between the academic creation of information in EBM and the clinical application of knowledge in EBP and investigators should keep EBP and the patient perspective in mind when designing and interpreting research (Coulter & Khorsan 2008). In addition, more social science research is needed on models, applications and dynamics of EBM to help guide that interpretation (Mykhalovskiy & Weir 2004).

HOW IS EVIDENCE ACTUALLY USED IN PRACTICE?

The two main audiences that make day-to-day decisions in health care are practitioners and patients. The differing information preferences of these two audiences are exhibited in their pragmatic decision-making. Gabbay & le May (2004) demonstrate that, while much health policy is based on RCTs, and indeed these are vital for family physicians (general practitioners: GPs), they may not employ a linear model of decision-making on an individual clinical basis. The GPs they worked with commented that they would look through guidelines at their leisure, either in preparation for a practice meeting or to ensure that their own practice was generally up to standard. Most practitioners used their 'networks' to acquire information that they thought would be the best evidence base from sources that they trusted, such as popular free medical magazines, word of mouth through other doctors they trusted and pharmaceutical representatives; in effect they operated in a circular decision-making model. Thus, clinicians relied on what Gabbay & le May call 'mindliness' – collectively reinforced, internalized tacit guidelines that include RCTs but are not solely dependent on them – which were informed by brief reading, but mainly guided by their interactions with each other and with opinion leaders, patients and through other sources of knowledge built on their early training and their own colleagues' experience. The practical application of clinical decision-making in conventional primary care demonstrates that a hierarchical model of EBM is interpreted cautiously by clinicians in managed health care environments.

Patients who use CAM report that one of the reasons for CAM use is that the criteria for defining healing and illness and in defining valid knowledge about health care are dominated by licensed health care professionals and are not patient-centred (O'Connor 2002). Many accept 'human experience as a valid way of knowing' and regard 'the body as a source of reliable knowledge', rejecting the assumption that 'personal experiences must be secondary to professional judgment'. This 'matter of fact' lay empiricism often stands in sharp contrast to our scientific insistence that in the absence of technical expertise and controlled conditions our untrained observations are untrustworthy and potentially misleading (Sirois & Purc-Stephenson 2008). Most patients accept basic biological knowledge and theory but find biology insufficient to explain their own complex health and illness experiences and so do not restrict their understanding to strictly biological concepts. Many assert their recognition of the cultural authority of science and seek to recruit it to the cause of complementary medicine – both as a means to its validation and legitimization and as a source of reliable information to facilitate public decision-making about CAM.

KNOWLEDGE DOMAINS AND RESEARCH METHODS

STRATEGIES BASED ON EVIDENCE-BASED MEDICINE

What are the elements of a research strategy that matches this pluralistic reality? How can we build an evidence base that has both rigour and relevance? In the diverse areas that CAM (or indeed conventional primary care) encompasses, at least six major knowledge domains are relevant. Within these domains are variations that allow for precise exploration of differing aspects of both CAM and conventional health care practice.

THE HIERARCHY STRATEGY

In conventional medicine, knowledge domains often follow a hierarchical strategy with sophisticated evidence-based synthesis at its acme (Sackett et al. 1991) (www.cochrane.org). The hierarchical strategy can be graphically depicted by a pyramid (Figure 1.1). At the base of this hierarchy are case series and observational studies. This is then followed by cohort studies in which

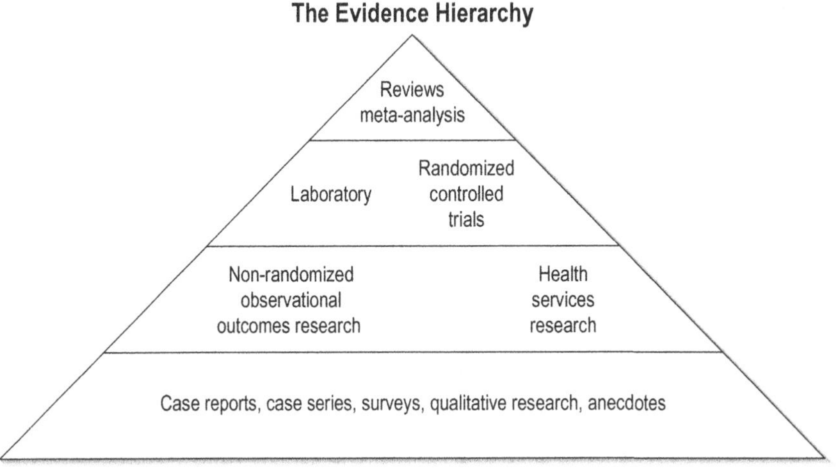

FIGURE 1.1 The evidence hierarchy. *Adapted with permission from Jonas (2001).*

groups of patients or treatments are observed over time in a natural way, often without any inclusion or exclusion criteria. Randomized studies come next. Here, the decision about which treatments an individual receives is generated by a random allocation algorithm. This usually involves the comparison of two or more treatments with or without a sham or placebo treatment. If several of those studies are then pooled they produce a meta-analysis. This is a summary of the true effect size of an intervention against control.

Internal validity and randomization

The hierarchical model has as its basis the goal of establishing internal validity, defined as the likelihood that observed effects in the trial are due to the independent variable. The greater the internal validity, the more certain we are that the result is likely to be valid as a consequence of the methodological rigour of a study. The threat to the internal validity of a research study is bias. Bias is introduced if factors that are not associated with the intervention produce shifts or changes in the results (outcomes) that appear to be due to the intervention but are in fact due to other spurious factors (confounders). For instance, we may compare two naturally occurring groups with the same illness, one that has chosen a CAM intervention (*x*) and the other that has chosen a conventional medical interventional (*c*). If we suppose that *x* produces better results than *c*, the uncritical observer might suggest that CAM is better than conventional care. It may also be that those choosing treatment *x* have less severe disease or fewer additional risk factors because they were better educated, didn't smoke and drank less alcohol.

Randomization and stratification allow us to create groups that are equal in all the known and, presumably, most of the unknown confounding factors so that we can safely attribute changes we see in outcomes to the interventions rather than to any confounding variable. Randomization creates homogeneous and comparable groups by allocating patients into groups without bias.

External validity

A complexity arises with the hierarchical strategy when there is a trade-off between internal and external validity (Cook & Campbell 1979). External validity is the likelihood that the observed effects will occur consistently in a range of appropriate clinical environments. As internal validity increases we develop security about attributing an observed difference to a known intervention. However, we often lose external validity because the population under study becomes highly selected. External validity represents the usefulness of the results and their generalizability to the wider population of people with the illness. If we want to strengthen internal validity (a fastidious trial) we define the study population very specifically and restrict the study to specific types of patients by adjusting the inclusion and exclusion criteria.

Pragmatic studies represent the opposite of fastidious studies. Here volunteers are entered, often with little exclusion. The study design may ask: 'If we add treatment *Q* to the current best guidelines available, will this improve our outcomes and will it be cost-effective?' Good examples of these pragmatic trials come from acupuncture and include those by Vickers et al. (2004) and Thomas et al. (2006) as well as their associated health economic analyses (Wonderling et al. 2004). The disadvantage of pragmatic studies is that we have no placebo control group and the heterogeneity of study groups may create wide variability in outcome. These studies then, even when carried out very competently, do not answer the question as to whether the treatment is better than placebo and may provide poor discrimination between treatments. This, however, is the basis for comparative effectiveness research.

The main danger with a rigid hierarchical strategy is the emphasis on internal validity at the risk of external validity and its consequences. We may produce methodologically sound results that are of little general value because they do not reflect the real-world situation (Travers et al. 2007).

ALTERNATIVE STRATEGIES TO THE HIERARCHY

Given the complexities of clinical decision-making and the various types of evidence just described, it is now becoming clear that EBM approaches that focus exclusively on the hierarchy strategy are inadequate in the context of clinical practice (Sackett & Rennie 1992; Gabbay & le May 2004). They are too simplistic and there is almost always not enough evidence to place the many treatments for most chronic illnesses at the top of any evidence hierarchy; there is and has to be much more powerful and exacting evidence when the risk to patients is high, for instance in the treatment of cancer. It is not surprising then that most physicians don't completely rely on these approaches for all their clinical decision-making (Gabbay & le May 2004) so the need for alternative strategies is self-evident.

THE EVIDENCE HOUSE

There are several alternative strategies to the evidence hierarchy that attempt to balance the risk of the poor relevance it produces. One of these is called the 'evidence house' and seeks to lateralize the main knowledge domains in science in order to highlight their purposes. It does this by aligning methodologies that isolate specific effects (those with high internal validity potential) and those that seek to explore utility of practices in real clinical settings (those with high external validity potential) (Figure 1.2). For example, mechanisms, attribution and research synthesis each seeks to isolate specific effects whereas utility is investigated though methods that assess meaning, association and cost (both financial cost and safety). Each of these knowledge domains has its own goals, methodology and quality criteria. The corresponding methods for each of the six domains are: for isolating effects, laboratory techniques, RCTs, meta-analysis; and for utility testing, qualitative research methods, observational methods, health services (including economic) research. Of course, variations in these methods can often be mixed in single studies, producing 'mixed-methods' research (such as qualitative studies nested inside RCTs) that seek to address dual goals. This strategy can be conceptualized in what has been called an 'evidence house' (Jonas 2001; Jonas, 2005). In this strategy the knowledge domains are placed in relationship to each other and the primary audience they serve. The evidence house helps balance the misalignment

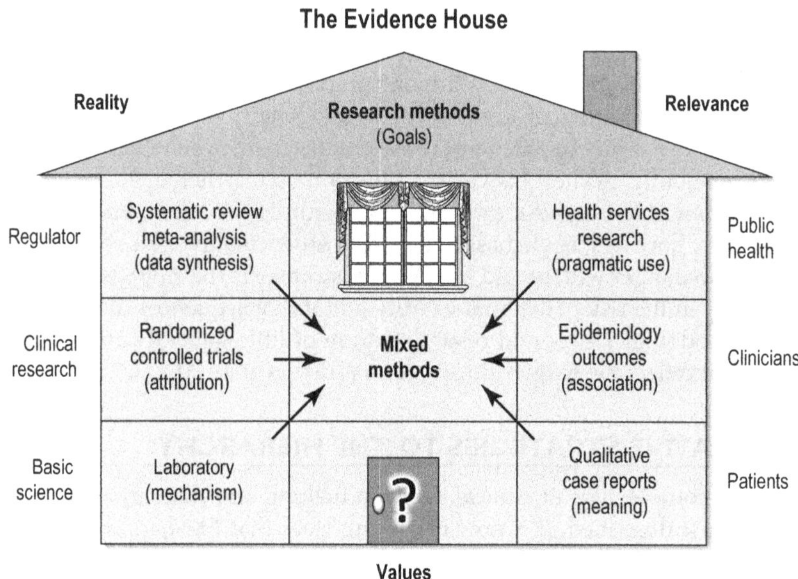

FIGURE 1.2 The evidence house. *Adapted with permission from Jonas (2001).*

produced by the evidence hierarchy, by linking the method to the goal to the primary audience. The six major knowledge domains of the evidence house are briefly described below.

Mechanisms and laboratory methods

This asks the questions: 'what happens and why?' Laboratory and basic science approaches examine the mechanisms that underly interventions thought to be effective. Basic research can provide us with explanations for biological processes that are required to refine and advance our knowledge in any therapeutic field. For the development of new substances such research into potential mechanisms is at the beginning of the research chain, while for complex interventions that are already widely available and in clinical practice, such as homeopathy, acupuncture, TCM or physiotherapy interventions, this type of research is normally preceded by safety and clinical effectiveness studies (Fonnebo et al. 2007).

Attribution and randomized controlled trials

'Attribution' refers to the capacity to attribute effects to a certain cause. In clinical research, attributional knowledge is termed 'efficacy' and is best obtained through research methods such as the RCT. Efficacy is usually thought of as the effect size that differentiates between the overall effect of the specific intervention and the effect of placebo in an exactly comparable group of patients. In the sort of chronic illness frequently treated by CAM it is usual to find efficacy-based effect sizes of the order of 5–15% for both CAM and conventional medicine. These are often four times less than the overall treatment effect, suggesting the rest (75%) of the effect is generated by non-specific factors, such as the meaning and context (MAC) and the generic healing potential: 'having treatment is what works' (White et al. 2004).

Confidence and research summaries

Evidence synthesis is the basis of the knowledge domain that seeks to reduce uncertainty. It is important to be explicit about the processes involved in evidence synthesis. Meta-analysis, systematic reviews and expert review and evaluation are methods for judging the accuracy and precision of research. Methods of expert review and summary of research have evolved in the last decade by using protocol-driven approaches and statistical techniques. These are used along with subjective reviews to improve confidence that the reported effects of clinical research are accurate and robust (Haynes et al. 2006).

These three areas and their corresponding methods are listed on the left side of Figure 1.2. These information domains often build on themselves. On the right-hand side of the evidence house are three knowledge domains that focus on obtaining information on utility or relevance. Those are described now.

Meaning and qualitative methods

Given the contribution of MAC to clinical outcomes, research that explores these areas is important. Meaning provides information about whether our research incorporates patient-centred outcomes and patient preferences. This knowledge reduces the risk of substituting irrelevant outcomes when a therapy is tested. Context research examines the effect of communication, cultural and physical processes and environments of practice delivery. Qualitative methods are important here and include detailed case studies and interviews that systematically describe medical approaches and investigate patient preferences and the meaning they find in their illness and in treatments. Qualitative research has rigorous application standards and is not the same as a story or anecdote (Miller & Crabtree 1994; Crabtree & Miller 1999; Malterud 2001). Sometimes it is necessary to start the cycle of research with qualitative methods if a field is comparatively unknown, to enable our understanding of some basic parameters. Who are the agents in a therapeutic setting? Why are they doing what they do? What do patients experience? Why do they use CAM and pay money? Some examples of qualitative research in CAM show that patients' and researchers' perceptions are often radically different (Warkentin 2000). Some proponents of qualitative methods argue that they are radically different from the quantitative positivist one employed by mainstream medical research. While in theory this might be true, research has shown that both methods can complement each other well.

Indirect association and observational methods

A main goal of scientific research is linking causes to effects. Experimental research methods such as laboratory experiments or randomized controlled studies are designed to produce this knowledge. However, in many cases, it is impractical, impossible or unethical to employ such methods so we have to resort to substitutes. For example, adverse effects are often not investigated directly, although good clinical practice guidelines may alter this. Adverse reactions are normally only discovered through long-term observations or serendipity. Post hoc reasoning is then used to establish whether an adverse reaction was due to a medical intervention by observing event rates in those receiving the intervention. Although this post hoc reasoning stems from observational research and is not direct experimental proof, it is often sufficient evidence.

Often, retrospective case series or institutional audits will be able to give us initial suggestions that can be used to justify clinical experiments. However, we need to consider that in some cases such experiments will not be feasible. This may occur whenever there is too much a priori knowledge or bias among patients and providers towards an intervention. It may also occur where patients are enthusiastic about a treatment and choose it for themselves. Sometimes it is unethical to gather experimental evidence when an intervention is harmful and without the hope of personal benefit to the patient (http://bioethics.od.nih.gov/internationalresthics.html). The majority of the initial evidence base that relates to the harm caused by smoking is not based on clinical experiments but on large epidemiological outcomes studies and animal experiments; someone cannot be randomized to be a convict, or an outdoor athlete or religious. It is also unnecessary to convince ourselves of the obvious: parachutes prevent death from falling out of airplanes (Smith & Pell 2003) and penicillin treats bacterial infection – neither needs a RCT.

Observational research is excellent at obtaining local information about the effects of interventions in individual practices. Sometimes called quality assurance or clinical audit, such data can help improve care at the point of delivery (Rees 2002).

Generalizability and health services research

Efficacy established in experimental research may not always translate into clinical practice. If we want to see whether a set of interventions works in clinical practice, we have to engage in a more pragmatic approach, called 'evaluation research' or 'health services research' (Coulter & Khorsan 2008). Most of these evaluations are quite complex and another modern term for this type of research is 'whole-systems research' (Verhoef et al. 2006) or, as the Medical Research Council suggests, 'evaluating complex interventions' (Campbell et al. 2007). All these involve evaluation of a practice in action and produce knowledge about effects in the pragmatic practice environment and emphasize external validity (Jonas 2005). These methods evaluate factors like access, feasibility, costs, practitioner competence, patient compliance and their interaction with proven or unproven treatments. They also study an intervention in the context of delivery, together with other elements of care and long-term application and safety (Figure 1.2). These approaches may be used to evaluate quite specific interventions both within and outside CAM. Alternatively these approaches can be used in a substantially different strategic order to evaluate a whole-systems-based approach (Verhoef et al. 2004). In these situations we may need to understand the overall effect of the whole system. To do that one would start with direct observation of practices and a general uncontrolled outcomes study evaluating the delivery of the intervention and its qualitative impact on the targeted population (Coulter & Khorsan 2008).

A CIRCULAR MODEL

The circular model explores the relationship of the clinical methods used in the middle two domains of the evidence house. It assumes that there is no such thing as 'an entirely true effect size' but that the effect sizes vary based on patient recruitment, specific therapists (Kim et al. 2006) and the environment (context) in which that therapy is provided (Hyland et al. 2007). This suggests that we may have difficulty in completely controlling for bias and confounding when we have no real understanding of the underlying mechanisms of the treatments being delivered. In these circumstances further development of a circular model may allow us to arrive at an approximate estimate of reality as it relates to complex pictures of chronic disease within the community (Walach et al. 2006) (Figure 1.3).

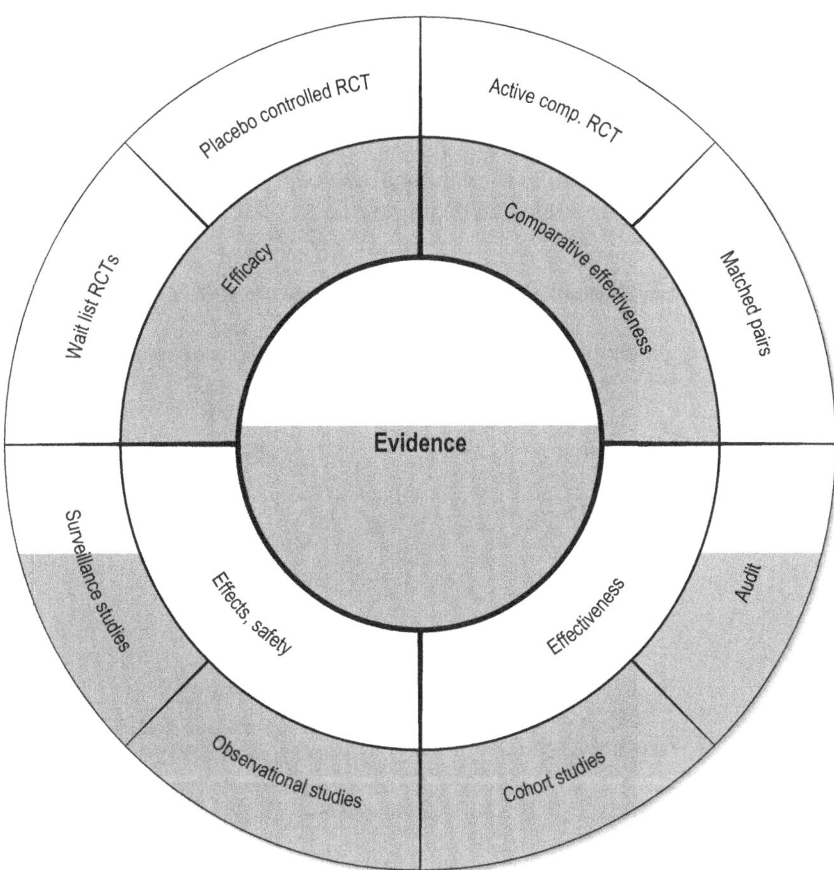

FIGURE 1.3 Circular model. RCT, randomized controlled trial. *Adapted with permission from Walach et al. (2006).*

In a circular strategy the principle is that information from all sources is used to establish consensus around the most appropriate therapeutic approaches in a particular therapeutic environment. This allows development of best practices even when there is little RCT evidence. We have to bear in mind that clinicians are obliged to treat people even when they present with conditions for which the treatment is not supported by a substantial body of research (Flower & Lewith 2007). The circular strategy also actively involves patients in the decision-making process, which could be important since there is evidence that empowering patient decisions has an impact on outcome (Kalauokalani et al. 2001; Bausell et al. 2005; Linde et al. 2007a). Acupuncture, as practised within a western European medical environment, is a prime example of this, as the debate about the evidence from both the German Acupuncture Trials (GERAC) and Acupuncture Research Trial (ART) studies illustrates (Linde et al. 2005; Melchart et al. 2005; Witt et al. 2005a, c, 2006; Brinkhaus et al. 2006; Scharf et al. 2006).

THE REVERSE-PHASES MODEL

By and large most complementary treatments are widely available, have often been in use for a long time and in some countries even have a special legal status. Consequently we may wish (for reasons of public health and pragmatism) to evaluate the safety of the intervention and the quality of the practitioners providing that intervention, before conducting research on theoretical or specific biochemical mechanisms that may be triggered by a particular product or practice. These strategic differences between the research approaches that may need to be applied to conventional and complementary medicine are summarized by Fonnebo et al. (2007) (Figure 1.4).

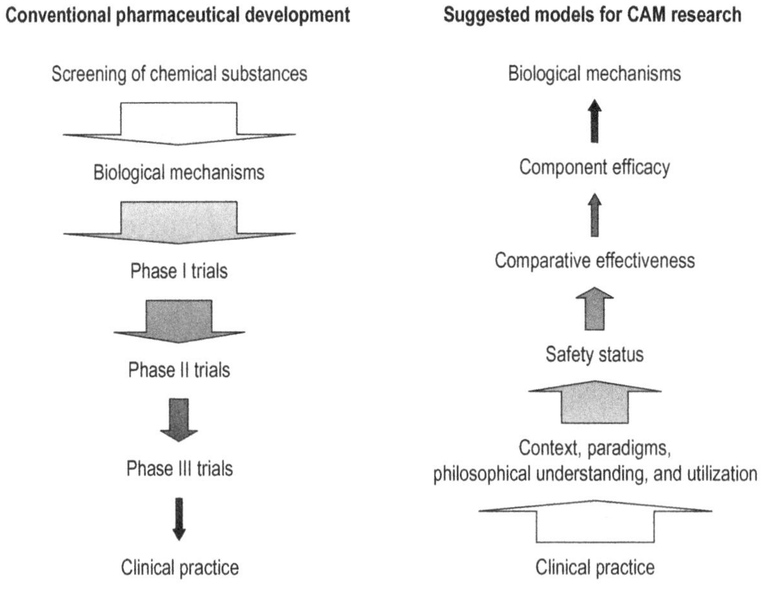

FIGURE 1.4 The gatekeeper. CAM, complementary and alternative medicine. *Adapted from Fonnebo et al. (2007).*

For example, a large pharmaceutical company will develop a new pharmaceutical through a phased approach that will involve both in vivo and in vitro laboratory experiments before preliminary human evaluation of a new chemical agent. This contrasts dramatically with the evaluation of a complementary medical intervention such as homeopathy and acupuncture, where opinions and beliefs about its veracity, effect and safety are widely debated and diverse. Inevitably this influences the public's expectation and opinion about a particular intervention which may have an impact on any systematic evaluation of the therapy and its equipoise within a clinical trial.

ADDITIONAL STRATEGIES

New, more sophisticated and pluralistic approaches to EBM incorporating the full spectrum of the information needed for making clinical decisions are being developed for all medical interventions; examples include the RAND 'appropriateness' approaches (Coulter et al. 1995), the Agency for Health Care Research and Quality's (AHRQ) efforts on consumer or patient-centred evidence evaluations (Clancy & Cronin 2005; Nilsen et al. 2006), decision models and new 'synthesis' approaches (Haynes 2006) and 'care pathway' applications of EBM (Astin et al. 2006), as well as the comparative effectiveness research by the Institute of Medicine (Sox 2009). All of these approaches have their own strengths and weaknesses and call for systematic incorporation of concepts such as goals, problem formulation and values into the formulation of consistent and customized EBM decisions that account for the complexity of information needed in the clinical setting. Taken together, it might be worthwhile distinguishing some of the more academic debates around EBM from the practical applications by defining EBP (Coulter & Khorsan 2008). We believe that EBP requires, at a minimum, the establishment of quality standards for each of the information domains described in Figures 1.2 and 1.3 and may be thought of as 'best research guidelines'.

QUALITY CRITERIA FOR CLINICAL RESEARCH

The above discussion speaks to the importance of defining standards of quality for each of the evidence domains described. Uniform criteria should be used to define 'quality' within each evidence domain (Sackett et al. 1991). For example, experimental, observational and research summaries are three designs with published quality criteria (Begg et al. 1996; Moher 1998; Egger & Davey 2000; Stroup et al. 2000). The evaluation of research quality in CAM uses the same approach as that in conventional medicine but there are additional items relevant to specific CAM areas (MacPherson et al. 2001; Dean et al. 2006). The Consolidated Standards of Reporting Trials (CONSORT) group has produced a widely adopted set of quality reporting guidelines for RCTs (Begg et al. 1996; Moher 1998). These criteria focus on the importance of allocation concealment, randomization method, blinding, proper statistical methods, attention to drop-outs and several other factors. They include internal and some external validity criteria.

Table 1.1 lists some of the published quality criteria in each of these evidence domains. These quality criteria serve as the best published standards

Table 1.1 ***Published Quality Reporting Criteria of Evidence***

Type of research	Quality scoring system	Where to go to	Description
Systematic Reviews/ Meta-Analysis	QUOROM guidelines	http://www.consort-statement.org/mod_product/uploads/QUOROM%20checklist%20and%20flow%20diagram%201999.pdf	Part of CONSORT, this checklist describes the preferred way to present the abstract, introduction, methods, results and discussion sections of a report of a meta-analysis
	SIGN 50	http://www.sign.ac.uk/guidelines/fulltext/50/checklist1.html	Checklist used by chiropractic best practices guidelines committee for their reviews
	AMSTAR	Shea *et al. BMC Medical Research Methodology* 2007 7:10 doi:10.1186/1471-2288-7-10	Measurement tool for the 'assessment of multiple systematic reviews' (AMSTAR) consisting of 11 items and has good face and content validity for measuring the methodological quality of systematic reviews
	OXMAN	Oxman AD et al. J Clin Epidemiol 1991; 44(1): 91–98	Used to assess the scientific quality or research overviews
	QUADAS	Whiting P et al. BMC Medical Research Methodology 2003; 3:25 http://www.biomedcentral.com/1471-2288/3/25	A tool for the quality assessment of studies of diagnostic accuracy included in systematic reviews consisting of 14 items.
Randomized Controlled Trials	CONSORT	www.consort-statement.org	An evidence-based, minimum set of recommendations for reporting RCTs and offers a standard way for authors to prepare reports of trial findings, facilitating their complete and transparent reporting, and aiding their critical appraisal and interpretation
	Cochrane	www.cochrane.org	Four key factors that are considered to influence the methodological quality of the trial: generation of allocation sequence, allocation concealment, blinding, and inclusion of all randomized participants. Cochrane advises against using scoring systems and checklists and uses these above to comment on in the analysis
	LOVE	Jonas WB and Linde K 2000.	Provides a convenient form for applying the four major categories of validity most applicable to complex systems as found in CAM (internal validity, external validity, model validity and quality reporting)

	SIGN 50	http://www.sign.ac.uk/guidelines/fulltext/50/checklist2.html	Checklist used by chiropractic best practices guidelines committee for assessing the quality of RCTs
	Bronfort	Bronfort G et al. Efficacy of spinal manipulation and mobilization for low back pain and neck pain: a systematic review and best evidence synthesis. Spine J 2004; 4: 335–356	Contains eight items with three choices, yes, partial and no on categories on baseline characteristics, concealment of treatment allocation, blinding of patients, of provider/attention bias, of assessor/unbiased outcome assessment, dropouts reported and accounted for, missing data reported and accounted for, and intention to treat analysis done.
	JADAD	Jadad AR, Moore RA, Carrol D *et al.* Assessing the quality of reports of randomized clinical trials: is blinding necessary? *Controlled Clin* Trials 1996;17:1–12	Widely used to assess the quality of clinical trials and composed of the following questions: 1) Is the study randomized? 2) Is the study double blinded? 3) Is there a description of withdrawals? 4) Is the randomization adequately described? 5) Is the blindness adequately described?
Laboratory Research	Modified LOVE	Sparber AG, Crawford CC, Jonas WB. 2003 Laboratory research on bioenergy. In: Jonas WB, Crawford CC Healing, Intention and Energy Medicine. Churchill Livingstone London Pg. 142	Modification of standard LOVE scale developed by Jonas WB et al to focus specifically on laboratory studies
	Quality Evaluation Score	Linde, K., Jonas, W.B., Melchart, D., Worku, F., Wagner, H., and Eitel, F. Critical review and meta-analysis of serial agitated dilutions in experimental toxicology. *Human & Experimental Toxicology*. 1994; 13: 481–492	Quality evaluation criteria for assessing animal studies in homeopathy
Health Services Research: Utilization Studies		Born PH. Center for Health Policy Research American Medical Association 1996 http://www.ama-assn.org/ama/upload/mm/363/dp963.pdf	There is no widely accepted measure of quality for health care utilization studies. Because of this differences across plans in proxy measures, such as outcomes or patient satisfaction are used as evidence of a managed care-quality link

(Continued)

Table 1.1 ***Published Quality Reporting Criteria of Evidence—Cont'd***

Type of research	Quality scoring system	Where to go to	Description
Health Services Research: Quality of Life Studies		Smeenk FW BMJ 1998; 316(7149): 1939–44	Much like other scales assessing quality criteria but with the addition of addressing quality of life outcomes
		Testa MA. Diabetes Spectrum 2000; 13: 29	Brief checklist of critical questions particularly relevant to quality-of-life measurement and study design
Health Services Research: Cost-Effectiveness Studies	SIGN 50	http://www.sign.ac.uk/guidelines/fulltext/50/notes6.html for economic evaluations only	Checklist used by chiropractic best practices guidelines committee for assessing the quality of economic studies
		Ch 13: How to read reviews and economic analyses In: Sackett DL et al Clinical Epidemiology. Little, Brown and Co. Boston 1991	Guides for assessing an economic analysis of health care
Epidemiology Outcomes: Cohort Studies	SIGN 50	http://www.sign.ac.uk/guidelines/fulltext/50/checklist3.html	Checklist used by chiropractic best practices guidelines committee for assessing the quality of cohort studies
	STROBE	http://www.strobe-statement.org/Checklist.html	Provides guidance on how to report observational research well
	New Castle Ottawa Quality Assessment Scale (NOS)	http://www.ohri.ca/programs/clinical_epidemiology/nosgen.doc	Used to assess the quality of non-randomized studies with its design, content and ease of use directed to the task of incorporating the quality assessments in the interpretation of meta-analytic results. Has been recommended by Cochrane nonrandomized studies methods working group

Epidemiology Outcomes: Case Control Studies	SIGN 50	http://www.sign.ac.uk/guidelines/fulltext/50/checklist4.html	Checklist used by chiropractic best practices guidelines committee for assessing the quality of case control studies.
	STROBE	http://www.strobe-statement.org/Checklist.html	provides guidance on how to report observational research well
	New Castle Ottawa Quality Assessment Scale (NOS)	http://www.ohri.ca/programs/clinical_epidemiology/nosgen.doc	Used to assess the quality of non-randomized studies with its design, content and ease of use directed to the task of incorporating the quality assessments in the interpretation of meta-analytic results. Has been recommended by Cochrane nonrandomized studies methods working group
Epidemiology Outcomes: Observational Studies	MOOSE	http://jama.ama-assn.org/cgi/content/full/283/15/2008	Proposal of items for reporting meta-analysis of observational studies in epidemiology
	Sanderson S et al.	Sanderson S, Tatt ID, Higgins JPT. Tools for assessing quality and susceptibility to bias in observational studies in epidemiology: a systematic review and annotated bibliography. *Intl J Epidemiol* 2007; 36: 666–676.	Assessment of many tools identified for the quality of observational studies in epidemiology. The authors chose specific domains and criteria for evaluating each tool's content on methods for selecting study participants, methods for measuring exposure and outcome variables, sources of bias, methods to control confounding, statistical methods and conflict of interest.
	AHRQ	http://www.ahrq.gov/clinic/epcsums/strengthsum.htm	Considers five key domains: comparability of subjects, exposure or intervention, outcome measurement, statistical analysis, and funding or sponsorship. systems that cover these domains represent acceptable approaches for assessing the quality of observational studies

(Continued)

Table 1.1 ***Published Quality Reporting Criteria of Evidence*—Cont'd**

Type of research	Quality scoring system	Where to go to	Description
Epidemiology Outcomes: N of 1	NCI Best Case Series Criteria	http://www.cancer.gov/cam/bestcase_criteria.html	Process that evaluates data about patients who have been treated with alternative approaches and is designed to evaluate data from cancer patients who have received alternative treatments
	Guyatt Guidelines	Guyatt G, Sackett D et al. A clinician's guide for conducting randomized trials in individual patients CMAJ 1988; 139: 497–503.	Guyatt lays some guidelines for conducting and assessing N of 1 randomized controlled trials
Qualitative Case Reports	McMaster University Occupational Therapy evidence based practice research group	http://www-fhs.mcmaster.ca/rehab/ebp//pdf/qualguidelines.pdf	Guidelines for critical review of qualitative studies developed by the McMaster University Occupational Therapy evidence based practice research group
	Qualitative Evaluation Framework by National Centre for Social Research RAND Research	http://www.pm.gov.uk/files/pdf/Quality_framework.pdf	A framework for assessing research evidence developed by the Government chief social researcher's office
	Malterud K. assessment scale	Malterud K Qualitative Research: Standards, challenges and guidelines Lancet 2001; 358: 485.	Guidelines for authors and reviewers of qualitative research

to date for research within each of the domains discussed in this book. Various checklists exist for helping investigators think about these quality criteria when reviewing or constructing research. One such checklist (the Likelihood of Validity Evaluation or LOVE) is described below, but many others are available, as listed in Table 1.1. A unique aspect of the LOVE is the inclusion of criteria for 'model validity' combined with internal and external validity.

MODEL VALIDITY

In addition to internal and external validity, previously described, CAM research also requires evaluation of 'model validity', which assesses the likelihood that the research has adequately addressed the unique theory and therapeutic context of the CAM system being evaluated (Jonas & Linde 2002). Many CAM systems arise outside developed countries or western theories so cross-tradition and cross-disciplinary research, involving experts in both conventional medicine and CAM, is often required (Jonas 1997). Some standardized treatments can produce marked variations that may be culture-specific; consequently results from one cultural environment may not always translate to another, particularly with respect to differences in informed consent (Bergmann et al. 1994; Kirsch 1999; Moerman 2000). Model validity refers to the fact that the research must be a fair exemplar of the practice in use and the method chosen to test it must reflect the goals and context of the audience that will use the consequent information.

THE LIKELIHOOD OF VALIDITY EVALUATION

Table 1.2 shows a checklist of the main quality criteria for evaluating internal, external and model validity. For convenience, these criteria have been drawn from a variety of quality rating scales (including Scottish Intercollegiate Guidelines Network (SIGN) 50, CONSORT, Cochrane and others) and are collated and summarized in an approach called the Likelihood of Validity Evaluation (LOVE) system, which has been applied to the evaluation of several areas of CAM research (Jonas & Linde 2002). Section 1 addresses internal validity and includes criteria such as randomization, baseline comparability, change of intervention, blinding, outcomes, statistical analysis and sample issues. Section 2 addresses external validity and includes criteria such as generalizability, reproducibility, clinical significance, therapeutic interference and outcomes. Section 3 addresses model validity and includes criteria especially important to whole-systems research. This includes representativeness, informed consent, methods matching, model congruity and context. Finally, Section 4 addresses reporting clarity that includes how well an article or report accurately describes the study.

Model validity criteria highlight a number of conceptual and contextual issues of which the investigator should be aware of when conducting research on CAM (Levin et al. 1997; Vickers et al. 1997; Eskinasi 1998; Egger & Davey 2000). CAM interventions are complex and in general do not consist of a single isolated entity; this is very similar to many of the interventions in primary

Table 1.2 *The Likelihood of Validity Evaluation (LOVE) guidelines – an adaptation of the various scoring systems for the main types of validity needed in complementary and alternative medicine research*	
Dimension	**Main criteria**
Internal validity	**Randomization**
How likely is it that the effects reported are due to the independent variable (the treatment)?	Was subject assignment to treatment groups done randomly and in a concealed manner?
-	**Baseline comparability**
	Were gender, age and prognostic factors balanced?
	Change of intervention
	Was there loss to follow-up, contamination, poor compliance?
	Blinding
	Did the patients, practitioners, evaluators, analysts know who got the treatment?
	Outcomes
	Were the objectivity, reliability and sensitivity of the outcome assessed?
	Analysis
	Was the number treated large? Were *P*-values significant? Were multiple outcomes measured and analysed?
External validity	**Generalizability**
How likely is it that the observed effects would occur outside the study and in different settings?	Was there a range of patients as would be seen in practice or were there multiple or narrow inclusions and exclusions? Was the study done at several sites with similar results?
	Reproducibility
	Was what was done clear? Were confidence intervals reported? Was the treatment transferable to other practitioners?
	Clinical significance
	Was the effect size big enough to make a difference? Is the condition in need of this type of treatment? Were any preferences determined? Was adherence good?
	Therapeutic interference
	Was there flexibility in varying the treatment? Was feedback on the outcomes available? Is the treatment feasible in most (or your) practice settings?
	Outcomes
	Were the outcomes clinically relevant? Were the outcomes checked for importance with the patients? Were any important outcomes missing?
Model validity	**Representativeness/accuracy**
How likely is it that the study accurately reflects the system under investigation?	Were the therapists well trained and experienced? Was the treatment strategy adequate? Was the treatment clearly described?
	Informed consent
	Was the informed consent comprehensive? Was it effective – did patients understand it? Did it generate expectations different from practice?

Table 1.2 *The Likelihood of Validity Evaluation (LOVE) guidelines – an adaptation of the various scoring systems for the main types of validity needed in complementary and alternative medicine research—Cont'd*	
Dimension	**Main criteria**
	Methodology matching
	Were the goals of the study clear and limited? Did the investigators select the correct research method to achieve the goals? See the citation categories
	Model congruity
	Were the patients classified, was the treatment determined and were the outcomes assessed according to the system of the practice being assessed?
	Context/meaning
	Did the patients/practitioners believe in the therapy? How well was the intervention adapted to the culture, family, meaning of the patient?
Reporting quality	**Comprehensive**
How likely is it that the report accurately reflects what was found in the study?	Can you address the above criteria?
	Clarity
	Could you reproduce this study? How clear and accurate is the information presented?
	Conclusions
	Were the conclusions and reporting format (e.g. relative versus absolute improvement rates, strength of wording) appropriate to the data collected?

Reproduced from LOVE version 4, copyright 2000 WB Jonas, used with permission.

care (general practice) or surgery (Gabbay & le May 2004). For example, acupuncture is a treatment within TCM and is itself highly variable. Acupuncture has often been considered a single intervention, but evidence suggests that the treatment of addictions such as smoking withdrawal may be employing entirely different neurophysiological mechanisms to those involved in the treatment of chemotherapy-related nausea and vomiting (Lewith & Vincent 1995). As a consequence, trial design may need to be entirely different for acupuncture when applying this intervention in differing clinical contexts with different underlying mechanisms. It may be appropriate to use sham acupuncture when the underlying mechanism is point-specific (as in the treatment of nausea) but entirely inappropriate to depend on point specificity for the design of the placebo when the underlying mechanisms are themselves not point-specific, as in the treatment of addiction.

Modern clinical trial methodology tends to make specific assumptions which may not apply to all aspects of CAM research. Therefore our methodology needs to be applied with an understanding of the science and the CAM intervention involved, and underpinned by theoretical ideas about the underlying mechanisms involved in the intervention. This will allow us to consider how to design research properly with appropriate controls that fit the CAM 'model' under study; in other words, with a high degree of 'model validity'.

While research that maximizes internal, external and model validity is the ideal, the realities of the CAM research environment often make the ideal difficult to achieve. First, funding levels for CAM are quite small compared to research in conventional medicine. Thus, large, multicentred pragmatic or three-armed studies (in which both placebo and standard care comparison groups exist) are few and far between. Research on mechanisms with adequate product quality are unlikely to be supported, such as those required for multi-component herbal products. The sceptical attitudes to CAM in many conventional circles, the competitive nature of new products and practices and the low profit potential of many CAM products and practices keep CAM research off the priority list for many governments and private funders. Rarely is there a critical mass of experienced researchers for conducting complex studies or mentors and a clear career path for training CAM investigators. Thus, CAM research continues to produce a continual stream of pilot and small studies or larger studies that address rather focused questions providing incremental information. In the context of so many questions about CAM practices, it is not surprising that the public often has no evidence for making decisions about CAM practices.

THE ABSENCE OF EVIDENCE

CAM has been very much the poor relation of research in the context of the EU, UK and US environments. The current UK CAM research budget is 0.0085% of medical research spending (Lewith 2007). When placed against the context of CAM use in the UK (15% per annum and 50% lifetime use), this is hardly an adequate distribution of research funding as far as the population's use of CAM is concerned. While the total expenditure in the US is substantially larger, it is still miniscule in proportion to CAM use. Consequently there is very limited research evidence within the whole field. Oxman (1994), one of the fathers of EBM, makes it very clear that the absence of evidence of effectiveness should not be interpreted as being synonymous with the absence of clinical effect. A pervasive problem in CAM is the inappropriate interpretation of limited and inadequate data, an approach which substantially misrepresents the underlying priniciples of rigorous EBM.

APPLYING RESEARCH STRATEGIES IN CAM

So far we have discussed different research methodologies, the types of evidence they provide and the preferences and goals various audiences have when applying evidence. There is much that we don't know about this area of medicine and we are curently struggling to apply rigorous scientific approaches to a very 'underinvestigated' clinical area. Our intention is to use the principles outlined in this chapter as a 'staging post' for future strategic development while recognizing that, as our evidence base grows, our approaches to obtaining and translating evidence into clincial practice will change. Within this cultural reality how does one use these principles when choosing research methods in CAM? Figure 1.5 provides a stepwise decision tree for mapping out an appropriate research sequence for the type of evidence needed in any given circumstance. As discussed, the decision to use evidence begins by first defining the research question (Vickers et al. 1997; Linde & Jonas 1999) and then by clarifying who will primarily use the resulting information and for what purpose. We hope that this will allow researchers to define their questions better and subsequently their chosen methodology; however, the final decision to pursue a particular method depends on a number of factors, including:

- the complexity of the condition and therapy being investigated
- the type of evidence sought (causal, descriptive, associative)
- the purpose for which the information will be used
- the methods that are available, ethical and affordable.

In Figure 1.5 we outline a CAM research decision tree map that illustrates the relationship between study goals, the type of information being sought on a practice and the type of methodology that will be most appropriate for providing that evidence. This is at the core of establishing model validity.

MATCHING GOALS AND METHODS IN CLINICAL RESEARCH

The first step in selecting an appropriate research method is clearly defining what evidence is needed, particularly in relationship to how it will be used (Feinstein 1989). Each research method has its own purpose, value and limitations. To summarize, when defining concepts, constructs and terms and when assessing the relevance of an outcome measurement, qualitative methods, with their indepth interviews and content analysis, are the most appropriate approach. When seeking associations of variables, surveys, cross-sectional or longitudinal studies with methods that allow for factor analysis, regression analysis or a combination of both, such as structural equation modelling, are the most useful. When trying to measure the overall impact of a complex intervention delivered in a clinical context, pragmatic trials and outcomes methods should be applied. When attempting to isolate and prove specific theoretical effects of treatment on selected outcomes, or determine the relative merit of whole-practice systems, placebo-controlled or pragmatic RCTs are the method of choice, respectively.

CHOOSING RESEARCH METHODS IN CAM

The research question, main audience and the utility of a research project will anchor the methodology (Figure 1.5). For example, in multimodality practices that are often not well described (e.g. spiritual healing, lifestyle therapies) and where the interest is on impact on chronic disease, outcomes research or pilot trials are the best initial approach (domain 3A in Figure 1.5). In well-described modalities that are safe and not expensive where effectiveness (not efficacy) may be the main interest (e.g. acupuncture, homeopathy), outcomes data coupled with decision analysis may provide the best strategic approach (domain 3B in Figure 1.5) (Dowie 1996). For many natural products, where the active or standard constituents are variable, basic science (e.g. laboratory characterization and safety

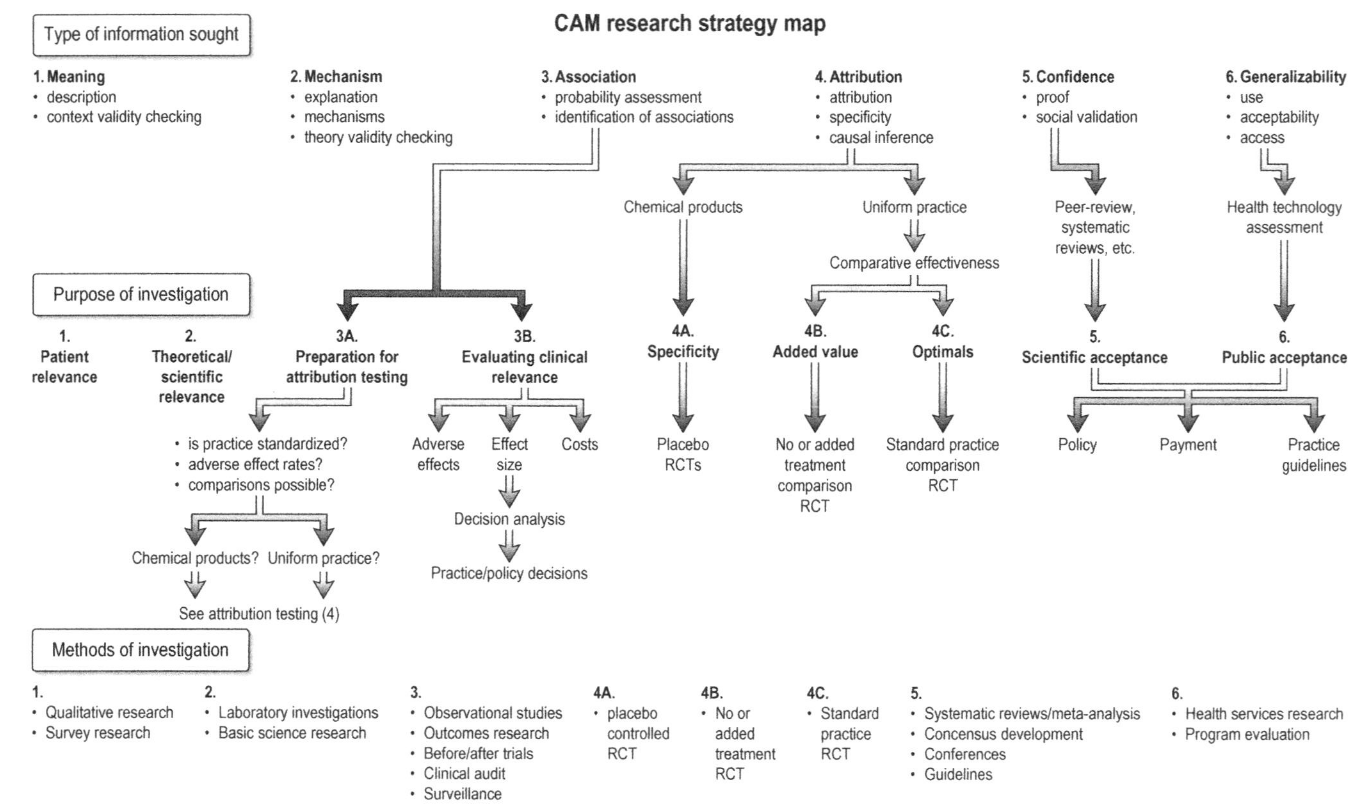

FIGURE 1.5 Complementary and alternative medicine (CAM) research strategy map. RCT, randomized controlled trial. *Adapted with permission from Jonas & Linde (2002).*

data) is needed prior to clinical research (domain 2 in Figure 1.5). Products that are well characterized but have potential direct adverse effects need placebo-controlled or standard comparison RCTs provided their public health implications warrant such an investment. Placebo studies of natural products are more useful for making regulatory decisions (e.g. product marketing and claims) than for individual clinical decisions (domain 4A in Figure 1.5). The US National Institutes of Health's study of the efficacy of St John's wort for depression, using a large, three-armed, multicentred, placebo-controlled trial, is an example of this latter approach (Shelton et al. 2001; Hypericum Depression Trial Study Group 2002). It is a widely used treatment, has significant potential drug–herb interactions (through the P450 system) and is treating an important, common clinical condition (domain 2 in Figure 1.5).

A physician considering referral of a patient with back pain for acupuncture will want to know what kind of patients local acupuncturists see, how they are treated, whether these patients are satisfied with treatment and their outcomes. This type of data comes from practice audit (observational research), surveys and qualitative research (domains 3B and 1 in Figure 1.5) (Cassidy 1998a, b). For these situations, information from local practice audits may be more valuable than relying on the results of small (or large) placebo-controlled trials done in settings where the practitioners and populations may be quite different. Data collection, monitoring and interpretation of observational studies must be as carefully performed as experimental studies. Finally, when exploring theories and data that do not fit into current assumptions about causality (e.g. energy healing or homeopathy), a carefully thought-out basic science strategy is needed. Given the public interest and the implications for science of these areas, it is irresponsible for the scientific community to ignore them completely (Jonas 1997).

Within RCTs (domain 4 in Figure 1.5) there are several goals that determine which design and sequence of studies are most appropriate. If the goal is obtaining information on the specificity of molecular or procedural effects (e.g. drug effects), placebo controls are required (domain 4A in Figure 1.5). Placebo controls cannot provide information about added value from a therapy (domain 4B in Figure 1.5), which requires a no treatment or standard treatment control (e.g. hypericum versus antidepressant control). Research summaries (domain 5 in Figure 1.5) and generalizability (domain 6 in Figure 1.5) require systematic reviews and health technology assessment, respectively. Examples of these two are the National Institutes of Health Consensus Conference statement on acupuncture (1997), which influenced public decisions on reimbursement for acupuncture. A similar approach used by the former Agency for Health Care Policy and Research's practice guideline on low-back pain and manipulation and the subsequent establishment of chiropractic services in the USA (Bigos & Bowyer 1994).

Use of this decision tree, along with quality standards for each of the research methods listed, provides a rational strategy for selecting the most appropriate type of evidence, assures quality for each method and so combines rigour and relevance for creating EBP in a pluralistic health care environment.

SPECIAL CAM RESEARCH ISSUES

We have now reviewed different research methods, strategies for selecting appropriate methods for obtaining evidence and criteria available for assessing research quality when using those methods. There are additional issues of which all investigators should be aware when designing and conducting research. Issues that often become of particular importance to CAM research include:

- sample and population selection
- differing diagnostic classification
- ensuring adequate treatment
- the interaction of placebo and non-placebo factors
- selection of theory-relevant or patient-relevant outcomes
- the risk of premature hypotheses without pilot data
- assumptions about randomization
- blinding and unconscious expectancy
- learning and therapeutic growth
- the nature of 'equipoise' in CAM
- risk stratification for determining 'adequate' levels of proof

SAMPLE AND POPULATION SELECTION

Recruitment for clinical trials underpins their generalizability. We have previously discussed the tension between internal and external validity and their relevance to recruitment in any study. CONSORT flow charts identify the number of individuals approached for a study and consequently give a percentage of the number recruited. A good example of this problem in conventional medicine is the evaluation of Antabuse, a pharmacological treatment that makes alcoholics vomit if they continue to take the medication daily. Trials evaluating Antabuse suggested that it was very effective; however, only 9% of the alcoholics approached agreed to be recruited, making it difficult to generalize about the effect of Antabuse in the broad population (Howard et al. 1990). All studies should explicitly consider population selection and breath of application.

DIAGNOSTIC CLASSIFICATION

When groups are defind as 'homogeneous' conventionally and recruited to a clinical trial they may not be homogeneous when evaluated from the perspective of another medical tradition. The differing diagnostic taxonomies of CAM systems may need to be addressed within a research context. The diagnosis of osteoarthritis may represent over a dozen classifications when evaluated by TCM. A 'standardized' treatment may approximate the 'average' syndrome and this simplifies the treatment strategy. However, this standardized treatment may be suboptimal and so risk producing 'false-negative' results within the trial – a sign of poor model validity. Subjects with irritable-bowel syndrome treated with individualized TCM herbs improved for longer than those given a standardized approach and both groups did better than the placebo group (Bensoussan & Menzies 1998). A three-arm study design allows for the evaluation of this aspect of model validity.

In addition to a three-armed trial, a double selection design can be used, in which group selection is done according to both conventional medicine and the alternative whole system. Shipley & Berry (1983) tested the homeopathic remedy *Rhus toxicum* on a conventinally homogeneous group of osteoarthritis patients without individual homeopathic classification and reported no effect over placebo. Fisher et al. (1989), in a follow-up study, used a double selection approach that provided both good internal validity and model validity. Patients met criteria for fibromyalgia and *Rhus tox*, producing a group 'homogeneous' for both medical systems. In this study those treated with homeopathic *Rhus tox* did better than those given placebo.

ADEQUATE TREATMENT

Pilot data should always be obtained to ensure adequate treatment is being tested in a clinical trial. This is frequently omitted. For example, a study of acupuncture for human immunodeficiency virus (HIV)-associated peripheral neuropathy published in the *Journal of the American Medical Association* reported negative results. Many acupuncturists report good results in this condition (Shlay et al. 1998), but use considerably more treatments than in the *Journal of the American Medical Association* study. The treatment being tested must be optimal or at least representative for a defined group of providers and piloted for that condition. This is certainly not the case for asthma treated with acupuncture, as only two trials used the same points (Linde et al. 1996).

We would suggest the combination of a detailed literature review and an expert panel approach, designed to build consensus around best practices (Ezzo et al. 2000; Flower & Lewith 2007).

THE INTERACTION OF PLACEBO AND NON-PLACEBO FACTORS

It is typical to see 70–80% effectiveness reported from open practices in both conventional and alternative medicine (Roberts et al. 1993; Jonas 1994; Guthlin et al. 2004; Witt et al. 2005b). Traditional medicine systems, various mind–body approaches and psychological and spiritual systems often attempt to induce self-healing by manipulating the MAC effects on illness; MAC is often confused with placebo, which itself interacts with non-placebo elements of therapy in complex ways (Bergmann et al. 1994; de Craen et al. 1999; Moerman 2002). Arthur Kleinman's classic study on why healers heal illustrates the importance of these contextual issues (Kleinman et al. 1978; Moerman & Jonas 2002).

OUTCOMES SELECTION

Outcomes that are objective and easy to measure, or well known, are often selected instead of more difficult patient-oriented, subjective outcomes, though the latter may be more relevant. Eric Cassell (1982) has pointed out that, because of an overemphasis on finding a 'cure', researchers may seek more objective, disease-oriented outcomes that move away from gaining knowledge that may help in the more subjective, healing process of the illness, a core goal of medicine. The investigator, in the name of 'rigour', may try to maximize internal validity by using objective measures instead of measures that are meaningful to patients. For example, many physicians deem 'pain relief' a fuzzy, non-objective outcome. However, for patients suffering from pain, its relief is the only really relevant outcome.

While non-patient-centred outcomes selection is not a unique issue for CAM it may be one of the main reasons for CAM's popularity. Cassidy (1998a, b) conducted interviews with over 400 patients visiting acupuncturists. Most patients did not experience a 'cure' but they continued acupuncture treatment because of other factors such as an improved ability to 'manage' their illness and a sense of well-being. Measuring these outcomes may require including qualitative research methods, or developing and validating new measurement instruments. Researchers may settle for popular outcome measures, such as the SF-36 (Guthlin & Walach 2007), while forgoing more individualized outcome measures, such as the Measure Your own Medical Outcome Profile (MYMOP) (Paterson 1996; Paterson & Britten 2003). Recently, a database of CAM-relevant outcome measures has been developed and posted online: IN-CAM Outcomes Database (www.outcomesdatabase.org).

HYPOTHESIS TESTING

Hypothesis-focused research allows investigators to identify cause-and-effect relationships. This is a powerful method for confirming or refuting theories about treatment–outcome associations. But by focusing on a particular theory-driven causal link we risk 'fixing' our conclusions about the value of a therapy, which in turn may restrict the investigation of other, possibly better approaches (Heron 1986). Given the small resources invested in CAM research, potentially superior CAM practices may never see the light of evidence, compared to better-funded and profitable treatments.

Once treatments are established they become the 'standard of care'. After this, alternative treatments are ethically more difficult to investigate. Lifestyle therapy for coronary artery disease (CAD) is an example. Current standard-of-care treatments for CAD are oriented around an anatomically based hypothesis of CAD. Coronary artery bypass grafting (CABG), balloon angiography and stents are all established treatments of CAD. An extensive industry has developed around these procedures and with it the economic and political interests to sustain these treatments. Lifestyle therapy can also successfully treat CAD but is based on a non-anatomical hypothesis of CAD aetiology not tied to a reimbursement and other industry drivers. It may be that lifestyle therapy is better than CABG for treatment of CAD in certain populations given its low cost, preventive potential, reduction in fatigue and improvement in well-being (Blumenthal & Levenson 1987; Haskell et al. 1994; McDougall 1995; Ornish et al. 1998), but this is difficult to investigate as it is unethical to mount placebo-controlled trials in this life-threatening situation. Revealing partial causes runs the risk of preventing the discovery of potentially more beneficial therapies based on other hypotheses. Research strategies for chronic disease need to have the flexibility to test multiple hypotheses (Horwitz 1987; Coffey 1998; Gallagher & Appenzeller 1999).

ASSUMPTIONS ABOUT RANDOMIZATION

When the results of observational and randomized studies are different it is usually assumed the randomized study is more rigorous and valid. This assumption has been challenged by an increasing number of studies showing that, properly done, observational studies may not differ in outcome from those that are randomized (Benson & Hartz 2000; Concato et al. 2000; Linde et al. 2007b). This does not in any way invalidate RCTs but rather suggests that much useful and important data may be collected utilizing a variety of different methods. Some practitioners of complex traditional or alternative medical systems believe that randomization can interfere with a therapy (by eliminating choice), obscure our awareness and so bias outcome. For example, TCM is based not on direct cause-and-effect assumptions but on an assumption that 'correspondences' occur between system levels (biological, social, psychological, environmental) (Porkert 1974). An assumption in TCM theory is that if a practice influences one level it can affect all others. Thus, finding direct cause-and-effect links may be less important for a TCM practitioner than to establish accurate correspondences between the body and season (Unshuld 1985). From this perspective extensive efforts to establish isolated causal links between intervention components and outcome (as done in non-pragmatic RCTs) are of less interest than in western medicine (Lao 1999).

BLINDING AND UNCONSCIOUS EXPECTANCY

Blinding or masking is primarily used to control for expectation effects in clinical studies and to reduce assessment bias. Although there is no foolproof method to ensure successful blinding, it is still an important part of quality research (Begg et al. 1996). Some alternative treatments, such as certain herbal preparations and superficial acupuncture techniques, can be at least partially blinded. Special attention is needed to match smell and taste in herbal products. When giving acupuncture, the practitioner cannot be completely blinded, except with special types of acupoint stimulation, such as with ultrasound or laser. Homeopathy or healing is more easily double-blinded than most conventional drugs but complex behavioural or lifestyle programmes cannot be delivered blind. Controlling for time and attention can often be achieved and it is possible to code groups and so do blind measurement of outcomes and analysis. For example, equal time and the presence of a sham therapist can be incorporated into studies of therapeutic touch (Gordon et al. 1998). In most traditional medical systems such as Ayurvedic or Native American medicine, a deep connectivity to all information about a therapy is assumed to coexist and complete blinding is not believed ever to be achievable. These systems assume that expectation effects are largely unconscious (Rigby 1988). In fact, a therapy in a traditional system often tries to enhance these unconscious expectation effects by manipulation of 'spirits' or 'energy' and the patient's belief system associated with them (Jonas 1999). From this perspective masking and sham interventions simply eliminate our awareness of the therapeutic agent, but not the agent itself, however implausible we may think this to be. There is evidence that autonomic and physiological effects occur unconsciously (such as reactions to music when under anaesthesia), something that many traditional medical systems would predict (Bennett 1986; Blankfeild 1991; Radin 1997). Unconscious expectancies may influence outcomes in clinical trials. For example, the physiological effects of 'active' placebos (drugs that produce 'side-effects' but not the therapeutic effect) in studies of antidepressants can influence outcomes even within double-blind studies (Greenberg et al. 1992; Kirsch & Sapirstein 1998). These assumptions should not be used as an excuse for conducting or accepting poor-quality research but they do make a case for non-experimental (observational) studies and non-blind studies.

LEARNING AND THERAPEUTIC GROWTH

Many CAM therapies involve teaching and learning, such as biofeedback, meditation, imagery and hypnosis. The skill and ability of the teacher (therapist) and the student (patient) may affect outcome (Kim et al. 2006). Blinding in such clinical trials is not usually possible and if it were, it would reduce the very processes upon which the effects of the intervention are thought to be based. Some physiological reactions may change, even during a single therapeutic episode, and so the degree of blindness may also change, altering equipoise, expectation effects and the relative efficacy of the 'active' treatment. The goal of many of these therapies is to increase the patient's awareness of unconscious processes and enhance self-efficacy.

THE NATURE OF EQUIPOISE IN CAM

Preferences have important consequences for clinical research, especially in CAM where patient preferences and belief may be high. Randomization is ethical only when equipoise exists between treatment groups (Black 1996). This can occur only when efficacy is truly ambiguous and there are no strong preferences for any therapy. Equipoise is present by definition when new drugs are tested, especially if no established therapy exists, and placebo controls are then ethically acceptable. This situation often does not exist in CAM. If patients are using or avoiding CAM therapies, it is often because of strong preferences and beliefs which may influence outcomes (Furnham & Kirkcaldy 1996; Fonnebo et al. 2007).

Recruitment to RCTs is problematic in these cases and good clinical studies have either been abandoned or the process of randomization dropped because of the refusal of patients to enter such studies (von Rohr et al. 2000; Katz et al. 2005). Randomization processes in conventional studies have been subverted by well-meaning health care practitioners, a problem that may also happen in CAM research (Schulz et al. 1995). In addition, research may be contaminated when subjects use alternative therapies that interact with the treatments being tested. For example, over 16% of patients in clinical trials at the US National Institutes of Health Clinical Center were using herbal therapies and not reporting this to the investigators (Sparber et al. 2000). The opposite trend might also be a problem: if patients on a trial for a CAM intervention take conventional drugs in addition to the CAM treatment, and do so differently in the control or treatment group, the outcome may be biased.

RISK STRATIFICATION AND 'ADEQUATE' EVIDENCE

Most therapies become used and often accepted before good evidence on their efficacy is available (Eddy 1990). Acupuncture provides a current CAM example: there is a growing acceptance of acupuncture in general, even in the absence of proof for its effectiveness for most conditions. The clear safety of acupuncture (Melchart et al. 2004) makes many clinicians and researchers willing to recommend it with less evidence than other higher-risk interventions. This type of risk stratification is a useful step in deciding what type of evidence is needed for balancing rigour, relevance and cost in EBP. For many therapies and conditions observational research may be initially sufficient for clinical decisions about best practices. For example, few patients or physicians would recommend against the use of a low-cost and inexpensive therapy (e.g. mind–body or homeopathic treatment) for a non-life-threatening disease (e.g. seasonal allergies) if outcomes data indicated that it was safe and benefited patients (Linde & Jonas 1999).

IMPROVING STANDARDS OF EVIDENCE-BASED MEDICINE FOR CAM

CAM needs to keep pace with developments in EBM. Recycled debates about the value and exclusivity of RCT data for making binary decisions about the use of CAM in health care are of little value. This has often led to critiques of the relevance of EBM to CAM which frequently lack any acknowledgement of the complexity within EBM. A clear example relates to observational data; the question is no longer should it be included, but how, and can we distinguish good from bad observational data?

Improved approaches to EBM, such as those being developed in mainstream medicine, need to be applied to CAM. Frameworks for such advances have been produced such as the 'evidence house' and the circular model (Jonas 2002; Jonas & Linde 2002). It is time for the CAM field to go beyond simplistic approaches to EBM and develop improved standards that rationally use all types of scientific information in a thoughtful, targeted and systematic way and are sufficiently robust and relevant for use in clinical settings (Christianson et al. 2007).

CONCLUSION: CAM AND EVOLUTION OF THE SCIENTIFIC METHOD

We hope that this chapter will act as a guide to the complex and sometimes confusing landscape of CAM research. The first essential process in any research project is to define the question you wish to answer and then subsequently the best method available to provide that answer. Within this medical arena CAM has a part to play in the development of medical research. Over 100 years ago William James pointed out the important role of the unconventional in the advancement of science. He said: 'Round about the accredited and orderly facts of every science there ever floats a sort of dust-cloud of exceptional observations, of occurrences minute and irregular and seldom met with, which it always proves more easy to ignore than to attend to. Anyone will renovate his science who will steadily look after the irregular phenomena, and when science is renewed, its new formulas often have more the voice of the exceptions in them than of what were supposed to be the rules (http://www.quotegeek.com/index.php?action=viewcategory&categoryid=152).'

The rigour of conventional science has undoubtedly improved clincial decision-making and CAM has much to learn from these approaches. However, unconventional practices are often used as a testing ground for new research ideas and scientific methods. Pioneers of modern clinical trial methods include Franklin, who began the idea of blinding (Rapport des Commissionaires Chargés par le Roi de l'Examen du Magnétisme Animal 1784), Haygarth (1801), who added sham treatments to the mix, and Fisher, who showed how randomization improved 'likelihood' estimation (Green 2002). Blinding and randomization became essential parts of medical research often after they were first applied to unorthodox practices such as mesmerism, psychic healing and homeopathy (Kaptchuk 1998a, b). The continuing march toward global medicinal excellence challenges us to define explicitly the terms 'rigorous research' or 'scientifically established' and demonstrate the evidence upon which quality criteria are based (Moher 1998). Good-quality research in CAM helps us develop the decision-making process for a strategic approach to medical research in general. A creative tension between established science and its frontiers can advance knowledge and help us understand both the benefits and limitations of the scientific process for health care. The ongoing interaction between orthodox and unorthodox medicine is the opportunity for developing new research strategies and clarifying the appropriate role of science in the service of healing.

In the same way we would expect that a thoughtful analysis and debate about the problems surrounding CAM research would benefit the whole medical research community and agenda. It is likely that many therapies will never be fully 'scientifically established', in the sense that they will fill in all the evidence domains described in this chapter. Decisions about what is 'sufficient' for particular audiences and uses (individual, practice, regulatory, public health) requires careful examination of both the value and limits of science in guiding the contextual management of disease as well as in the investigation of alternative strategies for gaining evidence. Science answers incremental and isolated questions and research can never answer all the questions of interest to every audience. Scepticism about unorthodox practices is great and so rigorous evidence is often required before such practices are accepted. Such rigour is important and it should be applied in a balanced and contextualized manner to all of medicine; for instance we may need different types and quality of evidence for the treatment of cancer compared to tension headache. While medicine is served by science, the practice of medicine is still an art that should use scientific evidence when and where it is needed and helpful. Yet, even with the best of evidence, we will usually have to be content with only partial knowledge when trying to judge if our actions truly help the patients we seek to serve.

REFERENCES

Astin, J.A., Stone, J., Abrams, D.I., et al., 2006. The efficacy of distant healing for human immunodeficiency virus – Results of a randomized trial. Altern. Ther. Health Med. 12, 36–41.

Barnes, P., Powell-Griner, E., McFann, K., et al., 2002. Complementary and alternative medicine use among adults: United States. Advance Data from Vital and Health Statistics. Available online at: http://www.cdc.gov/nchs/data/ad/ad343.pdf.

Barnes, P.M., Bloom B., and Nahin R.L., 2007. Complementary and Alternative Medicine Use Among Adults and Children: United States. National Health Statistics Report 12, 1–24. http://nccam.nih.gov/news/2008/nhsr12.pdf

Bausell, R.B., Lao, L., Bergman, S., et al., 2005. Is acupuncture analgesia an expectancy effect? Preliminary evidence based on participants perceived assignments in two placebo-controlled trials. Eval. Health Prof. 28 (1), 9–26.

Begg, C., Cho, M., Eastwood, S., 1996. Improving the Quality of Reporting of randomized controlled trials. JAMA 276 (8), 637–639 649.

Bennett, H., 1986. Pre-operative instructions for decreased bleeding during spine surgery. Anesthesiology 65 (3A), 245.

Benson, K., Hartz, A.J., 2000. A comparison of observational studies and randomized controlled trials. N. Engl. J. Med. 342, 1878–1886.

Bensoussan, A., Menzies, R., 1998. Treatment of irritable bowel syndrome with Chinese herbal medicine. JAMA 280, 1585–1589.

Bergmann, J., Chassany, O., Gandiol, J., et al., 1994. A randomised clinical trial of the effect of informed consent on the analgesic activity of placebo and naproxen in cancer pain. Clin. Trials Metaanal. 29, 41–47.

Bigos, S., Bowyer, O., 1994. Acute low back problems in adults: Clinical practice guidelines. US Department of Health and Human Services, Public Health Services, Rockville, Maryland December.

Bishop, F.L., Yardley, L., Lewith, G.T., 2008. Treat or Treatment: A qualitative study conceptualising patients use of complementary and alternative medicine. Am. J. Public Health 98, 1700–1705.

Bivins, R., 2007. Alternative Medicine? A History. Oxford University Press, Oxford.

Black, N., 1996. Why we need observational studies to evaluate the effectiveness of health care. Br. Med. J. 312, 1215–1218.

Blankfeild, R., 1991. Suggestion, relaxation, and hypnosis as adjuncts in the care of surgery patients: a review of the literature. Am. J. Clin. Hypn. 33 (3), 172–186.

Blumenthal, J.A., Levenson, R.M., 1987. Behavioral approaches to secondary prevention of coronary heart disease. Circulation 76 (1 Pt 2), I130–I137.

Brinkhaus, B., Witt, C.M., Jena, S., et al., 2006. Acupuncture in patients with chronic low back pain: a randomized controlled trial. Arch. Intern. Med. 166, 450–457.

Callahan, D., 2002. Introduction. In: Callahan, D. (Ed.), The Role of Complementary and Alternative Medicine: Accommodating Pluralism. Georgetown University Press, Washington, DC, pp. vii.

Campbell, N.C., Murray, E., Darbyshire, J., et al., 2007. Designing and evaluating complex interventions to improve health care. BMJ 334 (7591), 455–459.

Cassell, E., 1982. The Nature of suffering and the goals of medicine. N. Engl. J. Med. 306 (11), 639–645.

Cassell, E., 1991. The Nature of Suffering and the Goals of Medicine. Oxford University Press, Oxford.

Cassidy, C.M., 1998a. Chinese medicine users in the United States Part I: utilization, satisfaction, medical plurality. J. Altern. Complement. Med. 4 (1), 17–27.

Cassidy, C.M., 1998b. Chinese medicine users in the United States Part II: preferred aspects of care. J. Altern. Complement. Med. 4 (2), 189–202.

Christianson, J., Finch, M., Findlay, B., et al., 2007. Reinventing the Hospital Experience. Health Administration Press, Chicago, IL.

Clancy, C.M., Cronin, K., 2005. Evidence-based decision-making: global evidence, local decisions. Health Aff. (Millwood) 24 (1), 151–162.

Clouser, K.D., Hufford, D.J., O'Connor, B.B., 1996. Medical ethics and patient belief systems. Altern. Ther. Health. Med. 2 (1), 92–93.

Coffey, D.S., 1998. Self-organization, complexity and chaos: the new biology for medicine. Nat. Med. 4 (8), 882–885.

Concato, J., Shah, N., Horwitz, R.I., 2000. Randomized, controlled trials, observational studies, and the hierarchy of research designs. N. Engl. J. Med. 342, 1887–1892.

Cook, T.D., Campbell, D.T., 1979. Quasi-Experimentation Design and Analysis Issues for Field Settings. Rand McNally, Chicago.

Coulter, I.D., Khorsan, R., 2008. Is health services research the Holy Grail of complementary and alternative medicine research? Altern. Ther. Health Med. 14 (4), 40–45.

Coulter, I., Shekelle, P., Mootz, R., et al., 1995. The use of expert panel results: The RAND Panel for appropriateness of manipulation and mobilization of the cervical spine. J. Topics in Clinical Chiropractic 2 (3), 54–62.

Crabtree, B.F., Miller, W.L., 1999. Doing Qualitative Research (Research Methods for Primary Care). Sage, Thousand Oaks, CA.

Dean, M.E., Coulter, M.K., Fisher, P., et al., 2006. Reporting data on homeopathic treatments (RedHot): a supplement to CONSORT*. Forsch Komplement. Med. 13 (6), 368–371.

de Craen, A.J.M., Moerman, D.E., Heisterkamp, S.H., et al., 1999. Placebo effect in the treatment of duodenal ulcer. Br. J. Clin. Pharmacol. 48, 853–860.

Dowie, J., 1996. Evidence based medicine. Needs to be within framework of decision-making based on decision analysis [letter; comment]. BMJ 313 (7050), 170 discussion 170–171.

Eddy, D.M., 1990. Should we change the rules for evaluating medical technologies? In: Gelijns, A.C. (Ed.), Modern Methods of Clinical Investigation, vol. 1. National Academy Press, Washington D.C., pp. 117–134.

Egger, M., Davey, S., 2000. Systematic reviews in health care: meta-analysis in context. British Medical Journal Books, London.

Eisenberg, D.M., Davis, R.B., Ettner, S.L., 1998. Trends in alternative medicine use in the United States. JAMA 280, 246–252.

Ernst, E., 2000. Prevalence of use of complementary/alternative medicine: A systematic review. Bull. World Health Organ. 78 (2), 252–257.

Eskinaski, D.P., 1998. Factors that shape alternative medicine. JAMA 280, 1621–1623.

Ezzo, J., Berman, B., Hadhazy, V.A., et al., 2000. Is acupuncture effective for the treatment of chronic pain? A systematic review. Pain 86 (3), 217–225.

Feinstein, A.R., 1989. Epidemiologic analyses of causation: The unlearned scientific lessons of randomized trials. J. Epidemiol. 42, 481–489.

Fisher, P., Ward, A., 1994. Complementary medicine in Europe. BMJ 309 (6947), 107–111.

Fisher, P., Greenwood, A., Huskisson, E.C., et al., 1989. Effect of homoeopathic treatment of fibrositis (primary fibromyalgia). BMJ 299, 365–366.

Flower, A., Lewith, G.T., 2007. Seeking an oracle: using the Delphi process to develop practice guidelines for the treatment of endometriosis with Chinese herbal medicine. J. Complement. Altern. Med. 13, 969–976.

Fonnebo, V., Grimsgaard, S., Walach, H., et al., 2007. Researching complementary and alternative treatments – the gatekeepers are not at home. BMC Med. Res. Methodol. 7 (7).

Friedson, E., 1998. A Study of the Scoiology of Applied Knowledge. University of Chicago Press, Chicago.

Furnham, A., Kirkcaldy, B., 1996. The health beliefs and behaviours of orthodox and complementary medicine clients. Br. J. Clin. Psychol. 35, 49–61.

Gabbay, J., le May, A., 2004. Evidence based guidelines or collectively constructed "mindlines?" Ethnographic study of knowledge management in primary care. BMJ 329, 1013–1017.

Gallagher, R., Appenzeller, T., 1999. Beyond Reductionism. Science 284, 79.

Gordon, A., Merenstein, J.H., D'Amico, F., et al., 1998. The effects of therapeutic touch on patients with osteoarthritis of the knee. J. Fam. Pract. 47 (4), 271–277.

Graham, R.E., Ahn, A.C., Davis, R.B., et al., 2005. Use of complementary and alternative medical therapies among racial and ethnic minority adults: results from the 2002 National Health Interview Survey. J. Natl. Med. Assoc. 97 (4), 535–545.

Green, S., 2002. The origins of modern clinical research. Clin. Orthopaed. Res. 405, 311–319 325.

Greenberg, R.P., Bornstein, R.F., Greenberg, M.D., et al., 1992. A meta-analysis of antidepressant outcome under "blinder" conditions. J. Consult. Clin. Psychol. 60, 664–669.

Guthlin, C., Lange, O., Walach, H., 2004. Measuring the effects of acupuncture and homoeopathy in general practice: An uncontrolled prospective documentation approach. BMC Public Health 4, (6).

Guthlin, C., Walach, H., 2007. MOS-SF 36 – Structural equation modeling to test the construct validity of the second-order factor structure. European Journal of Assessment 23, 15–23.

Haskell, W.L., Alderman, E.L., Fair, J.M., et al., 1994. Effects of intensive multiple risk factor reduction on coronary atherosclerosis and clinical cardiac events in men and women with coronary artery disease. The Stanford Coronary Risk Intervention Project (SCRIP). Circulation 89 (3), 975–990.

Haygarth, J., 1801. Of the Imagination, as a Cause and as a Cure of Disorders of the Body: exemplified by Fictitious Tractors and Epidemical Convulsions. R Cruttwell, Bath, UK.

Haynes, R.B., 2006. Of studies, syntheses, synopses, summaries, and systems: the "5S" evolution of information services for evidence-based health care decisions. ACP J. Club 145 (3), A8.

Heron, J., 1986. Critique of conventional research methodology. Complementary Medicine Research 1 (1), 10–22.

Hill, A., 1971. Chapter 20: Clincial trials. In: Hill, A. (Ed.), Principle of Medical Statistics. The Lancet, London, pp. 245–254.

Horwitz, R.I., 1987. Complexity and contradiction in clinical trial research. Am. J. Med. 82 (3), 498–510.

House of Lords Select Committee on Science and Technology, 2000. 6th Report, Session 1999–2000. Complementary and Alternative Medicine 6.

Howard, K.I., Cox, W.M., Saunders, S.M., et al., 1990. Attrition in substance abuse comparative treatment research: The illusion of randomization. In: Psychotherapy and Counseling in the Treatment of Drug Abuse. National Institute of Drug Abuse, Rockville, pp. 66–79.

Hyland, M.E., Whalley, B., Geraghty, A.W.A., 2007. Dispositional predictors of placebo responding: A motivational interpretation of flower essence and gratitude therapy. J. Psychosom. Res. 62, 331–340.

Hypericum Depression Trial Study Group, 2002. Effect of *Hypericum perforatum* (St. John's wort) in major depressive disorder. A randomized controlled trial. JAMA 287, 1807–1814.

Jadad, A., 1998. Randomized Controlled Trials: A User's Guide. BMJ Books, London.

Jonas, W., 1994. Therapeutic labeling and the 80% rule. Bridges 5 (2), 1, 4–6.

Jonas, W.B., 1997. Researching alternative medicine. Nat. Med. 3 (8), 824–827.

Jonas, W., 1999. Models of medicine and models of healing. In: Jonas, W., Levin, J. (Eds.), Essentials of Complementary and Alternative Medicine. Lippincott Williams and Wilkins, Philadelphia.

Jonas, W., 2001. The evidence house. West. J. Med. 175, 79–80.

Jonas, W., 2002a. Evidence, ethics and evaluation of global medicine. In: Callahan, D. (Ed.), The Role of Complementary and Alternative Medicine: Accommodating Pluralism. Georgetown University Press, Washington, DC, pp. 122–147.

Jonas, W., 2002b. Policy, the public and priorities in alternative medicine research. Ann. Am. Acad. Political Soc. Sci. 583, 29–43.

Jonas, W.B., 2005. Building an evidence house: challenges and solutions to research in complementary and alternative medicine. Forsch. Komplementarmed. Klass. Naturheilkd. 12 (3), 159–167.

Jonas, W., Callahan, D., 2002. Evidence, ethics and evaluation of global medicine. In: Callahan, D. (Ed.), The Role of Complementary and Alternative Medicine: Accommodating Pluralism. Georgetown University Press, Washington, DC, pp. 122–147.

Jonas, W., Linde, K., 2002. Chapter 24. Conducting and evaluating clinical research on complementary and alternative medicine. In: Gallin, J. (Ed.), Principles and Practice of Clinical Research. Academic Press, San Diego, pp. 401–426.

Kalauokalani, D., Cherkin, C.D., Sherman, K.J., et al., 2001. Lessons from a trial of acupuncture and massage for low back pain. Spine 26 (13), 1418–1424.

Kaptchuk, T.J., 1998a. Intentional ignorance: A history of blind assessment and placebo controls in medicine. Bull Hist. Med. 72, 389–433.

Kaptchuk, T.J., 1998b. Powerful placebo: the dark side of the randomised controlled trial. Lancet 351, 1722–1725.
Katz, T., Fisher, P., Katz, A., et al., 2005. The feasibility of a randomised, placebo-controlled clinical trial of homeopathic treatment of depression in general practice. Homeopathy 94, 145–152.
Kim, D.M., Wampold, B.E., Bolt, D.M., 2006. Therapist effects in psychotherapy: A random-effects modeling of the National Institute of Mental Health Treatment of Depression Collaborative Research Program data. Psychotherapy Research 16, 161–172.
Kirsch, I., 1999. How Expectancies Shape Experience. American Psychological Association, Washington, DC.
Kirsch, I., Sapirstein, G., 1998. Listening to Prozac but hearing placebo: A meta-analysis of antidepressant medication. Prevention & Treatment 1, 2a. http://journals.apa.org/prevention.
Kleinman, A., Eisenberg, L., Good, B., 1978. Culture, illness, and care: clinical lessons from anthropologic and cross-cultural research. Ann. Intern. Med. 88 (2), 251–258.
Lao, L., 1999. Traditional Chinese medicine. In: Jonas, W., Levin, J. (Eds.), Essentials of Complementary and Alternative Medicine. Lippincott Williams and Wilkins, Philadelphia.
Levin, J.S., Glass, T.A., Kushi, L.H., et al., 1997. Quantitative methods in research on complementary and alternative medicine. A methodological manifesto. NIH Office of Alternative Medicine. Med. Care 35 (11), 1079–1094.
Lewith, G., 2007. Funding for CAM. BMJ 335, 951.
Lewith, G.T., Vincent, C., 1995. The evaluation of the clinical effects of acupuncture. A problem reassessed and a framework for future research. Pain Forum 4 (1), 39.
Linde, K., Jonas, W.B., 1999. Evaluating complementary and alternative medicine: The balance of rigor and relevance. In: Jonas, W.B., Levin, J.S. (Eds.), Essentials of Complementary and Alternative Medicine. Lipincott Williams & Wilkins, Philadelphia, PA, pp. 57–71.
Linde, K., Worku, F., Stor, W., et al., 1996. Randomised clinical trials of acupuncture for asthma – a systematic review. Forsch. Komplementarmed. 1, 148–155.
Linde, K., Streng, A., Jurgens, S., et al., 2005. Acupuncture for patients with migraine: a randomized controlled trial. JAMA 293, 2118–2125.
Linde, K., Witt, C.M., Streng, A., et al., 2007a. The impact of patient expectations on outcomes in four randomized controlled trials of acupuncture in patients with chronic pain. Pain 128, 264–271.
Linde, K., Streng, A., Hoppe, A., et al., 2007b. Randomized trial vs. observational study of acupuncture for migraine found that patient characteristics differed but outcomes were similar. J. Clin. Epidemiol. 60 (3), 280–287.
MacPherson, H., White, A., Cummings, M., et al., 2001. Standards for reporting interventions in controlled trials of acupuncture: the STRICTA recommendations. Complement. Ther. Med. 9 (4), 246–249.
Malterud, K., 2001. Qualitative research: standards, challenges, and guidelines. Lancet 358 (9280), 483–488.
Marwick, C., 1998. Alterations are ahead at the OAM. JAMA 280, 1553–1554.
McDougall, J., 1995. Rapid reduction of serum cholesterol and blood pressure by a twelve-day, very low fat, strictly vegetarian diet. J. Am. Nutr. 14 (5), 491–496.
Melchart, D., Weidenhammer, W., Reitmayr, S., et al., 2004. Prospective investigation of adverse effects of acupuncture in 97 733 patients. Arch. Intern. Med. 164, 104–105.
Melchart, D., Streng, A., Hoppe, A., et al., 2005. Acupuncture in patients with tension-type headache: randomised controlled trial. Br. Med. J. 331, 376–382.
Miller, W.L., Crabtree, B.F., 1994. Qualitative analysis: how to begin making sense. Fam. Pract. Res. J. 14 (3), 289–297.
Moerman, D.E., 2000. Cultural variations in the placebo effect: ulcers, anxiety, and blood pressure. Med. Anthropol. Q. 14 (1), 51–72.
Moerman, D.E., 2002. Meaning, Medicine, and the "Placebo Effect". Cambridge University Press, Cambridge.
Moerman, D.E., Jonas, W.B., 2002. Deconstructing the placebo effect and finding the meaning response. Ann. Intern. Med. 136, 471–476.
Moher, D., 1998. CONSORT: an evolving tool to help improve the quality of reports of randomized controlled trials. Consolidated Standards of Reporting Trials. JAMA 279 (18), 1489–1491.
Mykhalovskiy, E., Weir, L., 2004. The problem of evidence-based medicine: directions for social science. Soc. Sci. Med. 59 (5), 1059–1069.
NIH Consensus Statement Online, 1997. November 3–5. http://www.healthy.net/scr/article.asp?Id=2492.

Nilsen, E.S., Myrhaug, H.T., Johansen, M., et al., 2006. Methods of consumer involvement in developing healthcare policy and research, clinical practice guidelines and patient information material. Cochrane Database Syst. Rev. 3, CD004563.

O'Connor, B., 2002. Personal experience, popular epistemology and complementary and alternative medicine research. In: Callahan, D. (Ed.), The Role of Complementary and Alternative Medicine: Accommodating Pluralism. Georgetown University Press, Washington, DC, pp. 54–73.

Ornish, D., Scherwitz, L.W., Billings, J.H., et al., 1998. Intensive lifestyle changes for reversal of coronary heart disease. JAMA 280, 2001–2007.

Oxman, A.D., 1994. Checklists for review articles. BMJ 309, 648–651.

Paterson, C., 1996. Measuring outcomes in primary care: a patient generated measure, MYMOP, compared with the SF-36 health survey. BMJ 312, 1016–1020.

Paterson, C., Britten, N., 2003. Acupuncture for people with chronic illness: Combining qualitative and quantitative outcome assessment. J. Altern. Complement. Med. 9, 671–681.

Pelletier, K.R., Marie, A., Krasner, M., et al., 1997. Current trends in the integration and reimbursement of complementary and alternative medicine by managed care, insurance carriers, and hospital providers. Am. J. Health Promot. 12 (2), 112–123.

Porkert, M., 1974. The theoretical foundations of chinese medicine – systems of correspondence. MIT Press, Cambridge.

Radin, D., 1997. Unconscious perception of future emotions: An experiment in presentiment. Journal of Scientific Exploration 11, 163–180.

Rampes, H., Sharples, F., Maragh, S., et al., 1997. Introducing complementary medicine into the medical curriculum. J. R. Soc. Med. 90, 19–22.

Rapport des Commissionaires Chargés par le Roi de l'Examen du Magnétisme Animal, 1784. Imprimerie Royale, Paris, pp. 19–37.

Rees, R., 2002. Improving patient care in complementary medicine: using clinical audit. In: Lewith, G., Jonas, W., Walach, H. (Eds.), Clinical Research in Complementary Therapies: Principles, Problems and Solutions. Churchill Livingstone, London, pp. 109–128.

Rigby, B., 1988. New perspectives in medical practice: the psychophysiological approach of Maharishi Ayurveda. Modern Science and Vedic Science 2 (1), 77–87.

Roberts, A.H., Kewman, D.G., Mercier, L., et al., 1993. The power of nonspecific effects in healing: implications for psychosocial and biological treatments. Clin. Psychol. Rev. 13, 375–391.

Sackett, D.L., Rennie, D., 1992. The science of the art of the clinical examination. JAMA 267 (19), 2650–2652.

Sackett, D.L., Haynes, R.B., Guyatt, G.H., et al., 1991. Clinical Epidemiology: A Basic Science for Clinical Medicine. Little, Brown, Boston.

Schaffner, K., 2002. Assessments of efficacy in biomedicine: The turn toward methodological pluralism. In: Callahan, D. (Ed.), The Role of Complementary and Alternative Medicine: Accommodating Pluralism. Georgetown University Press, Washington, DC, pp. 1–14.

Scharf, H.P., Mansmann, U., Streitberger, K., et al., 2006. Acupuncture and knee osteoarthritis – a three-armed randomized trial. Ann. Intern. Med. 145, 12–20.

Schulz, K.F., Chalmers, I., Hayes, R.J., et al., 1995. Empirical evidence of bias. Dimensions of methodological quality associated with estimates of treatment effects in controlled trials. JAMA 273, 408–412.

Shelton, R.C., Keller, M.B., Gelenberg, A., et al., 2001. Effectiveness of St. John's wort in major depression. A randomized controlled trial. JAMA 285, 1978–1986.

Shipley, M., Berry, H.G.B., 1983. Controlled trial of homoeopathic treatment of osteoarthritis. Lancet 8316, 97–98.

Shlay, J.C., Chaloner, K., Max, M.B., et al., 1998. Acupuncture and amitriptyline for pain due to HIV-related peripheral neuropathy: a randomized controlled trial. Terry Beirn Community Programs for Clinical Research on AIDS. JAMA 280 (18), 1590–1595.

Sirois, F., Purc-Stephenson, R., 2008. Consumer decision factors for initial and long-term use of complementary and alternative medicine. Complementary Health Practice Review 13, 3–19.

Smith, G.C.S., Pell, J.P., 2003. Parachute use to prevent death and major trauma related to gravitational challenge: systematic review of randomised controlled trials. Br. Med. J. 327, 1459–1561.

Sox, H.C., Greenfield S., 2009. Comparative Effectiveness Research: A Report from the Institute of Medicine. Annals of Internal Medicine. 151, 203–205.

Sparber, A., Wootton, J.C., Bauer, L., et al., 2000. Use of complementary medicine by adult patients participating in HIV/AIDS

clinical trials. J. Altern. Complement. Med. 5, 415–422.
Stolberg, M., 1996. Die Homeopathie auf dem Prüfstein. Der erste Doppelblindversuch der Medizingeschichte im Jahr 1835. Münchner Medizinische Wochenschrift 138, 364–366.
Stroup, D.F., Berlin, J.A., Morton, S.C., et al., 2000. Meta-analysis of observational studies in epidemiology: a proposal for reporting. Meta-analysis Of Observational Studies in Epidemiology (MOOSE) group. JAMA 283 (15), 2008–2012.
Thomas, K.J., MacPherson, M., Thorpe, L., et al., 2006. Randomised controlled trial of a short course of traditional acupuncture compared with usual care for persistent non-specific low back pain. BMJ 333, 623.
Tindle, H.A., Davis, R.B., Phillips, R.S., et al., 2005. Trends in use of complementary and alternative medicine by US adults: 1997–2002. Altern. Ther. Health. Med. 11 (1), 42–49.
Travers, J., Marsh, S., Williams, M., et al., 2007. External validity of randomised controlled trials in asthma: to whom do the results of the trials apply? Thorax 62 (3), 219–223.
Unshuld, P.U., 1985. Medicine in China. A History of Ideas. University of California Press, Berkeley.
Verhoef, M.J., Lewith, G., Ritenbaugh, C., et al., 2004. Whole systems research: moving forward. Focus on Alternative and Complementary Therapies 9, 87–90.
Verhoef, M.J., Vanderheyden, L.C., Fonnebo, V., 2006. A whole systems research approach to cancer care: why do we need it and how do we get started? Integr. Cancer Ther. 5 (4), 287–292.
Vickers, A., Cassileth, B., Ernst, E., et al., 1997. How should we research unconventional therapies? A panel report from the conference on Complementary and Alternative Medicine Research Methodology, National Institutes of Health. Int. J. Techno. Assess. Health Care 13 (1), 111–121.
Vickers, A., Cassileth, B., Ernst, E., et al., 1997. How should we research unconventional therapies? A panel report from the Conference on Complementary and Alternative Medicine Research Methodology, National Institutes of Health. Int. J. Technol. Assess. Health Care 13 (1), 111–121 Winter.
Vickers, A.J., Rees, R.W., Zollman, C.E., et al., 2004. Acupuncture for chronic headache in primary care: large, pragmatic, randomised trial. BMJ 328, 744.
von Rohr, E., Pampallona, S., van Wegberg, B., et al., 2000. Experiences in the realisation of a research project on anthroposophical medicine in patients with advanced cancer. Schweizer medizinische Wochenschrift 130, 1173–1184.
Walach, H., Falkenberg, T., Fonnebo, V., et al., 2006. Circular instead of hierarchical: methodological principles for the evaluation of complex interventions. BMC Med. Res. Methodol. 6, 29.
Warkentin, R., 2000. Creative response to alternative medicine: Clients of a modern Finnish healer in a northwestern Ontario city. Qual. Health Res. 10, 214–224.
Wetzel, M.S., Eisenberg, D.M., Kaptchuk, T.J., 1998. A survey of courses involving complementary and alternative medicine at United States medical schools. JAMA 280, 784–787.
White, P., Lewith, G., Prescott, P., et al., 2004. Acupuncture versus placebo for the treatment of chronic mechanical neck pain. Ann. Intern. Med. 141, 911–919.
Witt, C., Keil, T., Selim, D., et al., 2005a. Outcome and costs of homoeopathic and conventional treatment strategies: A comparative cohort study in patients with chronic disorders. Complement. Ther. Med. 13, 79–86.
Witt, C.M., Lüdtke, R., Baur, R., et al., 2005b. Homeopathic medical practice: Long term results of a cohort study with 3981 patients. BMC Public Health 5, 115.
Witt, C., Brinkhaus, B., Jena, S., et al., 2005c. Acupuncture in patients with osteoarthritis of the knee: a randomised trial. Lancet 366, 136–143.
Witt, C., Jena, S., Brinkhaus, B., et al., 2006. Acupuncture for patients with chronic neck pain. Pain 125, 98–106.
Wonderling, D., Vickers, A.J., Grieve, R., et al., 2004. Cost effectiveness analysis of a randomised trial of acupuncture for chronic headache in primary care. BMJ 328, 747.
World Health Organization, 2003. Traditional medicine: Report by the secretariat. World Health Organization, Geneva 31 March.

Qualitative research methods: a focus on understanding experiences and meaning

Marja J. Verhoef • Heather S. Boon

2

CHAPTER CONTENTS

INTRODUCTION

A wealth of information about complementary and alternative medicine (CAM) use is currently available. Although estimates vary, it is clear that many people are using CAM, often in conjunction with conventional health

DOI: 10.1016/B978-0-443-06956-7.00002-1

care treatments. Surveys tell us that reasons for CAM use include everything from 'because it is natural and safe' to 'because no conventional treatments have helped' or 'because it allows me to play a more active role in my care' (Boon et al. 2000, 2003). Usually survey respondents are asked to select 'all that apply' from a list of general predetermined statements. However, in order to understand why people use CAM, we need to know more than percentages and measures of association. Making a decision to use CAM or assessing whether CAM works is dependent on a wide range of factors, such as individual patient and provider characteristics and beliefs, the patient–provider relationship and the patient's social networks.

Further, many randomized controlled trials (RCTs) have looked at whether certain CAM therapies are efficacious, which usually means assessing if they change some predetermined biomedical parameter such as blood pressure or tumour size (Morreale et al. 1996; Goertz et al. 2002; Streitberger et al. 2003). These trials, however, do not tell whether and how patient-related factors contribute to evidence of efficacy.

Qualitative research methods are the most appropriate approach to understanding phenomena such as why and how people decide to use CAM, or why and how complex CAM interventions work. Qualitative research is based on the assumptions underlying a naturalistic research paradigm. These assumptions are related to the nature of reality, the relationship between the researcher and the research participant and the notion that phenomena are time-, context- and value-bound (Lincoln & Guba 1985). These assumptions make qualitative research eminently suitable to examine complex phenomena related to CAM and set the context for understanding what kind of questions are best answered using qualitative methods and what data collection methods or analysis techniques are best suited to find these answers.

This chapter is divided into two parts. In the first part we review the theoretical underpinnings of qualitative research and identify the different qualitative approaches including their associated data collection techniques and analyses. In the second part of the chapter we focus on how qualitative methods can be used in CAM research.

OVERVIEW OF QUALITATIVE RESEARCH METHODS

QUALITATIVE THEORY

Research paradigms define the world view and thus the context in which research takes place (Lincoln & Guba 2000). Three primary concepts are encompassed in paradigms: ontology (beliefs about the nature of reality); epistemology (what is knowable or what can be studied); and methodology (the best way of gaining knowledge about the world). Table 2.1 summarizes some of the fundamental differences between qualitative and quantitative paradigms of inquiry.

Quantitative research is generally approached from a positivist or realist ontological perspective. Generally speaking, this perspective embraces the idea that there is a 'real' world that can be observed and understood (Lincoln & Guba 2000). In contrast, qualitative research is based on a constructionist

Table 2.1 *Qualitative versus quantitative research*

Research approach	Qualitative	Quantitative
Ontology (beliefs about the nature of reality)	Constructionist/relativist	Positivist/realist
Epistemology (theory of knowledge)	Interpretivist/transactional	Objectivist/duallist
Research purpose	To explore little-known areas, describe complex processes or everyday experiences, develop theories or explanatory models, or to generate new ideas	To describe attitudes, opinions, practices; predict or assess associations; measure change; establish cause and effect; add to knowledge base; test ideas or hypotheses
Research question	What? Why? How? (classification/meaning)	How many? Strength of association? (enumeration/causation)
Design	Maximizes flexibility: natural setting, process-oriented	Maximize scientific rigour: highly controlled (outcome-oriented), often experimental design
Reasoning	Inductive	Deductive
Sampling	Purposive (evolving)	Statistical (predetermined)
Data collection	Indepth interviews, focus groups, observation	Structured interviews, questionnaires, administrative records, clinical tests
Measurement	Researcher as instrument ('insider view'/subjective)	Psychosocial/physiological instruments ('outsider view'/objective)
Data reduction	Phrases/categories/themes	Means/categories/codes
Data analysis	Coding/categorizing/comparing	Statistical inference/statistical estimation

Based on Verhoef & Vanderheyden (2007).

(also known as a social constructivist) paradigm which is closely aligned with the ontological assumption of relativism (Schwandt 2000). Those who adopt this paradigm generally reject the idea that there is an intrinsic reality that one can 'find' or 'know'. This perspective emphasizes that 'truth' is both socially constructed and historically situated. A key underlying assumption is that all human knowledge is developed, transmitted and maintained through social processes (Berger & Luckmann 1967). Research guided by this paradigm generally strives to uncover ways in which individuals and groups perceive reality and participate in its creation. This approach is particularly well suited to research that attempts to understand individuals' perceptions of the world and their relationships within the world.

Quantitative and qualitative researchers also differ in terms of their epistemological approaches. While quantitative researchers approach questions from a dualist or objectivist standpoint (the assumption that it is possible to find an objective truth that is perspective-free), qualitative researchers take an interpretivist or transactional approach. This perspective suggests that the qualitative researcher and the research participants are inseparably linked, mutually creating knowledge in an interdependent manner to facilitate understanding of the phenomena under study (Lincoln & Guba 2000). This perspective is particularly suited to understanding personal experiences, how individuals make sense of experiences and the meanings they attach to their experiences. Thus, qualitative research assists in understanding individuals' actions and interactions. A key approach in this tradition is called symbolic interactionism (Schwandt 1994). A fundamental assumption of this approach is that to understand the world, one must analyse individuals' actions and interactions. This involves actively engaging those who are being studied (Blumer 1969; Schwandt 1994).

The theoretical context briefly described above sets the context for how and when qualitative methods are best chosen. Qualitative research answers questions that include the words 'why' and 'how'. Why do people choose to use CAM? How is acupuncture experienced? Why do some people do better in clinical trials than others? How does a homeopathic consultation have an impact on an individual's life? Qualitative research is particularly useful to describe areas in which currently not much is known; explore social processes (e.g. decision-making); develop instruments (e.g. quantitative surveys); and create theoretical models.

APPROACHES TO QUALITATIVE INQUIRY

Multiple approaches exist to qualitative research, each of which is rooted in different philosophical traditions resulting in different ways of framing the problem and, thus, the inquiry. We briefly discuss five common approaches (Creswell 1998; DePoy & Gitlin 1998).

Ethnography

This approach is rooted in anthropology and is concerned with the description and interpretation of cultural patterns of groups and the understanding of the cultural meanings people use to organize and interpret their experiences. In such studies the researcher studies the meaning of behaviour, language and interactions of the 'culture-sharing' group, for example a hospital, a health unit, or the different ways in which pain is expressed by men and women.

Phenomenology

The purpose of phenomenology is to uncover the meaning of how humans experience phenomena through the description of those experiences as they are lived by individuals. For example, what is the meaning of healing to women with cancer, or, what is the meaning of fear of dementia in ageing people? This approach is different from ethnography because it focuses on experiences from the perspective of the individual rather than understanding a group or cultural pattern.

Grounded theory

Grounded theory is a method that is primarily used to develop a theory or conceptual model. Usually the researcher begins with a broad query in a particular topic area and then collects relevant information about the topic. As data collection continues, each new piece of information is reviewed, compared and contrasted with earlier collected information. From this constant comparison process commonalities and dissimilarities among categories of information become clear and ultimately a theory that explains the observations is inductively developed. For example, this approach could be used to develop a theory of how people diagnosed with cancer decide whether or not to use CAM or to explain why some people refuse conventional treatment options.

Case study

Case studies include either indepth analyses of single cases or comparison across multiple cases (Yin 2003). Usually data collection spans a variety of sources including documents, interviews and observation. Data from different sources are triangulated (i.e. information collected using different strategies is used to examine the same phenomenon from different perspectives) to provide an indepth view of each case. When multiple cases are available, analysis is first completed on a case-by-case basis and then cross-case comparisons are made (Miles & Huberman 1994; Stake 2006). For example, this approach may facilitate identification of success factors for integrative clinics where each clinic is analysed as a separate case.

Biography

A biographical study is the investigation of an individual and his or her experiences as told to the researcher or found in documents and archival material (Creswell 1998). Life history inquiry is a form of a biographical study, and this focuses on the individual life course. This type of research is concerned with eliciting life experiences and with how individuals interpret and attribute meanings to these experiences (DePoy & Gitlin 1998).

DATA COLLECTION STRATEGIES

Rather than an etic perspective, as used in quantitative research, in which understanding is developed by those who are external to the group or population under study, qualitative researchers explore reality from an emic perspective – 'understanding life from the perspective of the participants in the setting under study' (Morse & Field 1995). This means that data collection examines everyday life in an uncontrolled naturalistic setting. Since qualitative research has been embraced by a number of different social science disciplines (e.g. anthropology, sociology and philosophy), each with different epistemological underpinnings, a number of different methods for data collection have been developed.

Qualitative data can be gathered from interviews, focus groups, recordings of conversations, direct (or recorded) observations and documents of all kinds. Choice of a data collection strategy is driven primarily by the research question. Other factors that are likely to influence the data collection strategy include constraints of the setting, the potential participants and resources available to the researcher (Creswell 1998). Each of these strategies is further outlined below.

Personal interviews

Interviews are the main data collection method employed by qualitative researchers. Interviewing techniques vary from semistructured interview schedules that ensure all participants are asked to discuss the same topics to completely unstructured interviews or narratives where the participant primarily determines what is discussed (Berg 1995; Morse & Field 1995). Unstructured interviews are generally used when the researcher knows very little about the topic and is unable to prepare a series of questions because s/he doesn't know what to ask. In this case it is best simply to let the participants tell their stories. Semistructured interviews are used for more focused inquiries where the researcher knows many of the key topics of interest. Questions are worded so that they are open-ended and the interviewer should allow the participant to guide the order in which the topics are discussed. For example, if the participant begins talking about question 5 when answering question 2, the interviewer should follow the participant's lead by probing about question 5. The questions that have been skipped can be addressed later in the interview. To enhance semistructured interviews it is important to maintain a conversational flow with the participants. Interviews are usually audio-recorded. Face-to-face interviews are best to establish rapport with the participant; however, telephone interviews can facilitate data collection across greater physical distances. An advantage of individual interviews is the ability to elicit information about a specific process or changes over time. Interviews allow the investigation of indepth personal experiences of phenomena and can be particularly useful when discussing sensitive (personal) topics. The two main disadvantages of individual interviews are the fact that they can be time-consuming and expensive. For example, usually no more than two interviews can be scheduled in a single day and analysis of individual interview transcripts is often very time-intensive. Costs related to travel, interviewer time and transcription can make individual interviews too expensive for large studies.

Focus groups

One way to minimize costs and decrease data collection time is to interview participants in groups, usually called focus groups. Typically, focus groups consist of six to eight individuals who share some characteristics (e.g. disease diagnoses; experience of a therapy) and a trained moderator leads the group through a discussion of predetermined topics (Morgan 1998). Focus groups are very useful for gathering a wide range of opinions quickly or to develop consensus guidelines in a group process. Another advantage of focus groups is the ability to capture and analyse interactions between individuals attending the group, for example, one participant trying to explain his/her point of view to another participant, or disagreements that arise between group members. This also emphasizes the need for a skilled moderator who can ensure everyone has an opportunity to express his/her views and that one participant does not unduly influence the opinions of others. Since it is necessary to schedule multiple individuals to attend each group, focus groups do not work well with individuals who are difficult to schedule, such as busy physicians.

Observation

Observation is another way to explore the interaction of participants with each other (Lincoln & Guba 1985). The main purpose of observation is to collect data about participants in a natural setting. Observation is often used to provide breadth and context that cannot be achieved by interviews alone. However, it can be time-consuming and expensive, so it needs to be justified based on the research question and the value it can add needs to be clearly specified (Morse & Field 1995; Creswell 1998). Consent is an important issue to consider when designing a study that includes an observational component. Generally ethics boards permit observational data collection in public spaces without obtaining the informed consent of those being observed. However, observation of patients in health care settings, or clinicians interacting with each other in integrated clinics, requires the consent of those being observed. Observational strategies are generally categorized by the degree of researcher involvement in the setting and range from complete participation of the researcher (e.g. a naturopathic doctor who is also a PhD student observing how fellow practitioners interact with patients and other clinicians in an integrative clinic) to complete observer (e.g. a sociologist observing patients receiving acupuncture treatments). The former is challenging due to issues related to informed consent (ensuring consent of those being observed or justifying why the intent to observe cannot be disclosed to those being observed) and the difficulty the participant observer is likely to have with objectivity (it is difficult to maintain the work role while taking a researcher perspective). The latter has the disadvantage of not permitting the researcher to ask questions or clarify what is happening, which can lead to misinterpretation of what is being observed. In practice, normally some compromise between these two extremes is found to be the best way to collect data using observation techniques (Lincoln & Guba 1985; Morse & Field 1995).

Existing documents

Finally, any written document can be used for qualitative inquiries. Diaries, letters, personal notes and official documents can all inform the investigation. Although qualitative analysis is most easily performed on written texts, increasingly photographs, works of art, videos and performance art are also considered as sources of data for qualitative inquiry. Ultimately, the source of data and the data collection technique should be driven by the research question.

SAMPLING

One issue relevant to all types of data collection is the choice of the sample. There are two principles that guide sample selection: appropriateness and adequacy (Kuzel 1992; Morse & Field 1995). Appropriateness refers to a focus on choosing participants who will best be able to help answer the question. As qualitative research is intensive and time-consuming, it is important to focus on those individuals who can provide the richest insight into the phenomenon of interest. If one selected a random sample, it is inevitable that many participants would know little about the topic under investigation. Thus 'random selection is not only useless to the aims of qualitative research, but may be a source of invalidity' (Morse & Field 1995). Therefore, qualitative researchers are encouraged to undertake theoretical sampling (also sometimes called purposeful or purposive sampling) to use theoretical insights or knowledge to choose participants best able to inform the investigation (Berg 1995; Boyatzis 1998; Creswell 1998). Adequacy refers to ensuring enough data is collected to answer the question in a full and rich way (Morse & Field 1995). Qualitative researchers attempt to continue data collection to the point of saturation – the point at which no new information is emerging with respect to the key themes emerging from the investigation and all negative cases have been investigated (Morse & Field 1995; Creswell 1998). There is some debate about how one knows that saturation has been achieved. A general rule of thumb is that one continues data collection until no new information has emerged from the last two to three interviews or equivalent. Guest et al. (2006) argue that the time to reach saturation is approximately 12 interviews. However, it is likely that this will vary depending on the focus of the question, the homogeneity versus heterogeneity of the participants (or their views on the topic of interest) and on the amount of detail required to answer the research question fully.

DATA ANALYSIS

Qualitative inquiry is an iterative process in which data collection and analysis occur simultaneously and continually inform each other (Boyatzis 1998). As soon as data collection begins, the researcher should be preparing for data analysis. Interviews and focus groups should be transcribed so they can be coded as soon as possible. As with data collection, there are a number of different ways in which qualitative data can be analysed. For example, data analysis can be theory-driven, driven by prior knowledge or data or inductive (Boyatzis 1998). However most approaches involve the following basic steps: comprehending, synthesizing (or decontextualizing), theorizing and recontextualizing (Morse & Field 1995). Although these steps generally occur sequentially (e.g. you cannot synthesize something until you understand it fully), the entire process is very much circular with much looping back to earlier steps and data collection itself (i.e. data analysis might identify the need to change the interview guide).

A special type of analysis is narrative analysis, which is distinct from the analysis of narratives (Hurwitz et al. 2004; Finlay & Ballinger 2006). This approach holds that the narrative, or the story line, constitutes the social reality of the narrator. It assumes that life and narrative are inseparable and that the narrative not only shapes a person's experiences, but also becomes experience. A person's account is organized in particular ways that facilitate understanding or meaning ascribed by the participant to his or her experience. Through their stories people make sense of their experiences. Discourse and conversational analyses are forms of narrative analysis. These types of analysis share a focus on talk and conversation as constructing social truths and also as being indicative of the wider systems of meaning that inform how the social world is understood (Hurwitz et al. 2004; Finlay & Ballinger 2006).

One of the underlying key premises in qualitative data collection and analysis is the importance of staying 'grounded' in the data. That is, staying true to what participants are saying. The first step in data analysis is simply 'making sense of' the data. Most qualitative researchers do this by some kind of content analysis: careful reading of the verbatim transcripts or textual material to identify topics or themes (Berg 1995; Morse & Field 1995; Boyatzis 1998). These topics or themes are given names and detailed descriptions of what the theme concerns, when it occurs and any qualifications or exclusions, to facilitate coding (Boyatzis 1998). Segments of transcripts (pieces of text) pertaining to a specific topic receive a similar code and will be grouped in the same category. New categories emerge from the data as new topics arise. A variety of computer programs facilitate data management, but only the researcher can create the coding scheme from the raw data. Comprehension is achieved when the researcher is able to identify all the key topics or themes relevant to the research question and can 'richly' describe 'what is going on'. Saturation is reached and comprehension completed when the interviewer grows 'bored' because s/he has already 'heard' everything being said (Krefting 1991; Morse & Field 1995).

Synthesizing is the process of identifying and describing regularities or patterns in the data. This occurs when the researcher can describe aggregate-level stories (e.g. these types of patients use acupuncture due to their specific beliefs and experiences). This process helps the researcher identify critical factors that are necessary to explain variation in the data by comparing themes across subsamples. It is important to note that these factors arise from the data during analysis and are not identified a priori (Morse & Field 1995; Boyatzis 1998). Theorizing (or hypothesis testing) 'is the process of constructing alternative explanations and holding these against the data until the best fit that explains the data most simply is obtained' (Morse & Field 1995). This is a process of active trial and error, falsification and verification, seeking negative cases and testing theories against ongoing data collection (Berg 1995). This process is often the key to appropriate sampling (called theoretical sampling) because the developing theory dictates what other viewpoints need to be sampled. Finally, recontextualizing is the process of placing the emergent theory of the specific dataset into the context of the wider literature and exploring its applicability in other settings (Morse & Field 1995). The researchers' findings need to be linked to previously published works and other theories to demonstrate how the new findings broaden understanding and advance disciplines of inquiry.

ASSESSING THE QUALITY OF QUALITATIVE RESEARCH

As in quantitative research, evaluation of the quality of the research findings is important; however, the traditional forms of evaluating reliability and validity in quantitative research do not apply in qualitative research as these concepts are rooted in a quantitative positivist paradigm. The purpose of qualitative research is understanding of phenomena rather than prediction and control (Stake 2006). In qualitative research, the term 'trustworthiness', the degree to which the research findings can be believed, has gained most acceptance as a criterion for evaluating qualitative research. For instance, Lincoln & Guba (1985) proposed four criteria for judging the soundness of qualitative research and explicitly offered these as an alternative to more traditional quantitatively oriented criteria. Their proposed criteria and the 'analogous' quantitative criteria are listed in Table 2.2. Several strategies have been identified to assess each of the four criteria (Lincoln & Guba 1985; Krefting 1991). A common strategy to establish credibility is member checking, which is a technique that consists of continually testing the researcher's interpretations and conclusions with study participants. Transferability can be assessed by thoroughly describing participants' characteristics, the research context as well as the assumptions that were central to the research. Audit trails that carefully describe the decisions (such as coding or interpretation) made by the investigator help to assess dependability. Code–recode procedures and peer examination are other strategies. Confirmability can also be assessed by audit trails. Another common strategy is triangulation, which consists of the use of multiple methods or perspectives to collect and interpret data about a phenomenon and assess whether there is convergence.

QUALITATIVE RESEARCH METHODS APPLIED TO CAM

As we described before, qualitative research is important when we want to explore and understand complex processes, to understand the meaning people give to their experiences or to assess how they make sense of these experiences. Qualitative research is also helpful when we need to develop conceptual models or theories that help us understand complex phenomena.

Table 2.2 ***Criteria to assess trustworthiness in qualitative research as compared to standards in quantitative research***

Criteria for evaluating quantitative research	Criteria for evaluating qualitative research
Internal validity	Credibility: the extent to which the results and interpretations of qualitative research are believable from the perspective of the study participants
External validity	Transferability: the extent to which a study's findings can be transferred (generalized) to other contexts or settings
Reliability	Dependability: the extent to which others can logically follow the processes and procedures used in the study and find the same or similar concepts, themes or pattern, given the same data, context and perspective
Objectivity	Confirmability: the extent to which research findings, conclusions and recommendations are supported by the data

Based on Krefting (1991) and Guba (1981).

Qualitative research is often considered to be compatible with a holistic perspective that views human experience as complex and cannot be understood by using reductionistic methods (Janesick 1994; Boyatzis 1998). A holistic paradigm assumes that meaning in human experience is derived from an understanding of individuals in their social environments, that multiple realities exist and that our view of reality is determined by events viewed through individual lenses or biases (Boyatzis 1998). It is therefore not surprising that qualitative research has such an important role to play in CAM research, as many CAM healing systems are holistic in nature.

Qualitative research can be conducted as a stand alone approach to explore and understand issues related to CAM, or to develop conceptual models or theories. However, qualitative research can also be used in combination with quantitative research methods to add understanding to quantitative methods and facilitate data triangulation. Examples of each of these applications are presented and discussed below in order to demonstrate the practical relevance of qualitative research.

EXAMPLES OF QUALITATIVE RESEARCH

Understanding meaning shifts

Many CAM interventions emphasize patients' developing understanding of health and illness. Stibich & Wissow (2006) examined how perceptions of health and illness changed in the context of wellness acupuncture. To this end they asked graduating acupuncture students to select three patients and ask them to write a letter about the benefits of acupuncture. A total of 367 letters were received. The letters were analysed using a grounded-theory approach to identify meaning shifts. Five shifts were identified: (1) from a goal of fixing the problem to a goal of increasing health; (2) from symptoms as problems to symptoms as teachers; (3) from healing as passive to healing as active; (4) from being dominated by illness to moving beyond illness; and (5) from regarding the practitioner as a technician to regarding the practitioner as a healer/friend. Numerous quotes are used in the paper to support these changes. In an attempt to assess the transferability of these themes we conducted a secondary analysis of transcripts from qualitative interviews with cancer patients receiving integrative care and found that these shifts could also be identified in this population (Verhoef & Leis 2008). The suggested link between meaning and health led Stibich & Wissow (2006) to look for models that explain how meaning shifts can be created. As such this work has great potential for informing and enhancing clinical practice.

Assessing outcomes of CAM interventions

A common concern in CAM efficacy/effectiveness research is that the current arsenal of outcome measures may not be sufficient to assess outcomes experienced by people receiving CAM interventions or integrated care. Bell et al. (2003) identified that changes homeopathic practitioners witnessed in their patients extend beyond health-related domains to a much broader view of the individual's entire scope and flow of life experience, such as personal perception, creativity, sense of freedom and 'feeling less stuck'. Qualitative analysis of interviews that explored patients' experiences of homeopathy (Bell et al. 2004) and of integrative care (reported in Berg 1989) confirmed that several of these outcomes, including 'unsticking' and transformation, occur in patients who receive CAM or integrative health care interventions (Koithan et al. 2007). This information is currently being used by a research team headed by Dr Ritenbaugh (University of Arizona, USA) to develop a quantitative instrument to measure where patients are in their transformation process. As long as CAM interventions are being evaluated using conventional physical, psychological and quality of life measures, we will not be able to identify benefits that are specific to whole-system CAM interventions. In fact, using outcome measures that do not target individualized and holistic outcomes may result in bias and compromise clinical relevance. Qualitative analysis is a useful tool to identify and assess the outcomes patients describe as being most relevant.

Developing a conceptual model of CAM decision-making

Given the rise of CAM use it is important to know how patients make the decision to use CAM. Balneaves et al. (2007) have developed a model that explains how women with breast cancer make the decision to use CAM. Participants were recruited from clinical oncology settings, an integrative care clinic and community support groups in Vancouver, Canada. Investigators used grounded-theory methodology and conducted semistructured interviews. The resulting conceptual model is called 'bridging the gap'. All participants aimed at making treatment decisions that would help them survive cancer and improve their well-being. In the context of their knowledge and beliefs about conventional medicine and CAM as well as their social networks, women contemplated which therapies would help them maximize the benefits and minimize the chances of harm. Once they identified CAM therapies they often moved into a complex and confusing process of gathering and filtering information about these therapies and trying to figure out which ones were credible and which ones were not. They were often confronted by contradictory information and recommendations about the safety and the value of these therapies and started to feel there was a gap between the two worlds of conventional medicine and CAM. Faced with these paradigmatic differences, but wanting to make a treatment choice that would be best for their health and be congruent with their knowledge and beliefs, women engaged in three different decision-making processes of 'bridging the gap'. These included:

1. Taking one step at the time in choosing CAM therapies: women in this group tended to live alone and received little guidance from their health care professionals regarding CAM. They expressed high levels of anxiety and conflict in making decisions about CAM, therefore they tended to slow down or step back and not use CAM during active treatment, or only CAM treatments that were non-invasive and non-controversial.
2. Playing it safe with regard to CAM decisions: women in this group had limited experience with CAM use and engaged in more conservative

treatment decision-making processes. They preferred CAM therapies that were science-based and could be used alongside conventional treatment.

3. Bringing it all together: women in this group tended to focus not only on their cancer but also on their overall well-being. All had previously used CAM. They chose conventional practitioners who were open to CAM and used their intuition to select therapies and practitioners. In general they were confident decision-makers.

Again the results of this study provide direction for health care practitioners regarding the need for education and decision support strategies to ensure the safety and well-being of women with breast cancer.

RELEVANCE OF QUALITATIVE STUDIES

While these studies provide information that informs and potentially improves patient care, they also have limitations. They are particularly limited because they each include only a small, and very specific, select group of people who were able and willing to talk indepth about their feelings and experiences. For example, in the first study, no letters were received from patients who had not benefited from acupuncture. This limits the generalizability of the results. However, the results are very useful to develop hypotheses that can be tested by additional research or to explore potential practical implications of the results. This is why it is important to combine qualitative research with quantitative methods. Qualitative research can develop ideas, hypotheses or models that can then be tested in qualitative research, or on the other hand, qualitative research could follow quantitative research and be used to explain the meaning of quantitative associations, for example between receiving integrative care and patient outcomes.

Somewhat along the same line it has become clear that, while there has been an accumulation of qualitative studies in recent years, little cumulative understanding is gained from them. If the findings are to have an impact and to inform clinical practice and policy-making, they must be situated in a larger context, be accessible and be presented in a usable format (Sandelowski et al. 1997). Over the past years, conducting a metasynthesis (also referred to as qualitative meta data analysis, qualitative meta-analysis and meta-ethnography) has been raised as a strategy to generalize the results from a range of qualitative studies (Noblit & Hare 1988; Sandelowski & Barroso 2003; Thorne et al. 2004). Sandelowski & Barroso (2003) have defined qualitative metasynthesis as 'a form of systematic review or integration of qualitative research findings that are themselves interpretive syntheses of data, including phenomenologies, ethnographies, grounded theories and other integrated and coherent descriptions of phenomena, events or cases'. No metasyntheses have been published yet in the field of CAM; however, several projects are under way.

COMBINED METHODS RESEARCH

Combining qualitative and quantitative methods is helpful to understand many aspects of CAM practice and CAM use. It is particularly relevant with respect to the evaluation of CAM interventions. CAM interventions or CAM systems, such as naturopathic medicine, homeopathy or traditional Chinese medicine, are often complex, as: (1) many are based on philosophies that differ from the philosophy underlying biomedical interventions; (2) their outcomes often cover a wide range of domains and are holistic in nature; (3) the context of the interventions, such as patients' expectations, the patient–provider (healing) relationship, patient and provider characteristics and physical surroundings, often plays an important and complex role in bringing about changes; and (4) the processes of the interventions need to be considered, as healing is often not linear. Process is sometimes also seen as part of the context (see Chapter 1). While many may argue that it is impossible to combine two opposing forms of inquiry, positivist and naturalist, a more pragmatic perspective suggests that using both will enhance understanding of the phenomenon under study, and, thus, the usability of the results. The Institute of Medicine (2005) has argued in its chapter on the need for innovative research designs that qualitative research can provide extremely valuable information to help interpret the results of effectiveness studies or to design these studies in the best possible way. The authors argue that the richest information will come from the combined results of studies with different designs. Two examples of combining both types of research follow.

Adding qualitative inquiry to randomized controlled trials

Evaluating complex CAM interventions is challenging for an RCT design as it means standardizing individualized treatment; controlling for non-specific and placebo effects, such as the impact of patient preferences, hopes and expectations; the impossibility of blinding; and a focus on group rather than individual results. As qualitative inquiry is an approach that is very suitable to address the impact of several of these issues, it is sometimes added to an RCT design. For example, Brazier et al. (2006) added qualitative interviews to an RCT assessing the effect of a 2-week residential yogic breathing, movement and meditation programme aimed at improving mental health, health status and stress reduction among people living with human immunodeficiency virus (HIV)/acquired immunodeficiency syndrome (AIDS). They found only minor differences between the experimental and control groups; however, qualitative results showed that participants experienced personal growth processes following the intervention. They described how 'living' began to feel more meaningful and conscious, and they began to feel everything, pleasant and unpleasant, with greater intensity – but this greater self-awareness also included greater awareness of changes, stress, pain and discomfort. These results illuminate the trial results and aid the development of more sensitive evaluation approaches for future research.

In another study Stalpers et al. (2005) conducted an RCT to determine whether hypnotherapy reduced anxiety and improved quality of life in cancer patients. No statistical differences in anxiety and quality of life were found; however, qualitative interviews, including an open-ended questionnaire, showed that the majority of patients felt their mental and overall well-being had improved and all patients in the hypnotherapy group would recommend such therapy to other patients. The authors suggest that the increased attention of doing the interviews might have been responsible for the changes. However, the qualitative inquiry reveals a number of potential explanations that could be further explored and tested. Studies such as the above identify how qualitative research can explain issues related to the meaning of the intervention, outcomes, process and context of the intervention.

Early-phase research

While early-phase research or phase I trials are not uncommon designs, Aickin (2007) and Fønnebø (2007) have pointed out the importance of this type of study with respect to CAM trials. Many CAM approaches are un- or underresearched and it is not feasible to investigate them all using large studies that will present definitive results. Early-phase studies are intended to get answers to many design questions, such as: What patients should be targeted for the intervention? Who is willing to accept the intervention? Is placebo really placebo or part of the intervention? Can CAM and conventional practitioners deliver the treatment under circumstances that differ from their normal practice? What are appropriate outcome measures? Are there different versions of the intervention? Do practitioners agree on the nature of the intervention? In order to address such questions, Aickin suggests that the sample size should be small, as in this phase, in which much is unknown, we will find that some research approaches will not work. He also suggests that measurement should be intensive to learn as much as possible about those data that are relevant and those that are not. Most importantly, such studies will only be successful if both quantitative and qualitative inquiry is used. In fact, qualitative research will serve as a 'corrective check on researcher bias' via the use of techniques that solicit unstructured responses from participants.

RELEVANCE OF COMBINED METHODS RESEARCH

Given the relevant and useful findings resulting from combining qualitative research with RCTs, it is time to reconsider the use of RCTs only with respect to CAM interventions. Qualitative methods are able to explain trial results as they get at the heart of what CAM interventions mean to patients by examining the meaning of choosing CAM, the meaning of healing, the healing experience and issues related to the patient–provider relationship. Second, early-phase research followed by a carefully developed RCT is a more sensible approach than moving quickly to expensive large-scale RCTs, which often show limited effects and leave one to wonder what exactly made (or did not make) the difference. Early-phase research also assists in identifying whether an RCT is possible, and if it is not, whether a modified RCT design is a feasible option. Such designs include, for example, pragmatic trials, preference trials and factorial designs, which may be a better option than a classical RCT. Such designs are discussed in the publication by the Institute of Medicine (2005).

CONCLUSION

Qualitative research has much to offer to CAM research. However, in and of itself it is limited, as is quantitative research. Combining qualitative and quantitative methods is the preferred direction for many CAM-related issues. This fits very well with the increasing call for well-coordinated programmes of research that allow proper development of the best methodological approach. Programmes of research might be best facilitated by collaboration across countries and disciplines. In addition, by combining both qualitative and quantitative approaches, model, internal and external validity of the results will be increased.

REFERENCES

Aickin, M., 2007. The importance of early phase research. J. Altern. Complement. Med. 13 (4), 447–450.

Balneaves, L.G., Truant, T.L.O., Kelly, M., et al., 2007. Bridging the gap: decision-making processes of women with breast cancer using complementary and alternative medicine (CAM). Support. Care Cancer 15 (8), 973–983.

Bell, I.R., Koithan, M., Gorman, M.M., et al., 2003. Homeopathic practitioner views of changes in patients undergoing constitutional treatment for chronic disease. J. Altern. Complement. Med. 9 (1), 39–50.

Bell, I.R., Koithan, M., DeToro, D., 2004. Outcomes of homeopathic treatment: patient perceptions and experiences. FACT 9, 21.

Berg, B., 1989. Qualitative research methods for the social sciences. Allyn and Bacon, Toronto.

Berg, B.L., 1995. Qualitative research methods for the social sciences. second ed. Allyn and Bacon, Needham Heights, MA.

Berger, P., Luckmann, T., 1967. The social construction of reality: a treatise in the sociology of knowledge. Penquin, London.

Blumer, H., 1969. Symbolic interaction. University of California Press, Berkeley, CA.

Boon, H., Stewart, M., Kennard, M.A., et al., 2000. Use of complementary/alternative medicine by breast cancer survivors in Ontario: prevalence and perceptions. J. Clin. Oncol. 18 (13), 2515–2521.

Boon, H., Westlake, K., Stewart, M., et al., 2003. Use of complementary/alternative medicine by men diagnosed with prostate cancer: prevalence and characteristics. Urology 62 (5), 849–853.

Boyatzis, R., 1998. Transforming qualitative information: thematic analysis and code development. Sage Publications, Thousand Oaks, CA.

Brazier, A., Mulkins, A., Verhoef, M., 2006. Evaluating a yogic breathing and meditation intervention for individuals living with HIV/AIDS. Am. J. Health Promot. 20 (3), 192–195.

Creswell, J.W., 1998. Qualitative inquiry and research design: choosing among five traditions. Sage Publications, Thousand Oaks, CA.

DePoy, E., Gitlin, L.N., 1998. Introduction to research: understanding and applying multiple strategies. Mosby, London.

Finlay, L., Ballinger, C., 2006. Qualitative Research for Allied Health Professionals. Challenging Choices. John Wiley, West Sussex, UK.

Fønnebø, V., 2007. Early phase methodology is needed in CAM and conventional research endeavors. J. Altern. Complement. Med. 13 (4), 397–398.

Goertz, C.H., Grimm, R.H., Svendsen, K., et al., 2002. Treatment of Hypertension with Alternative Therapies (THAT) study: a randomized clinical trial. J. Hypertens. 20 (10), 2063–2068.

Guba, E., 1981. Criteria for assessing the trustworthiness of naturalistic inquiries. Educational Resources Information Center Annual Review Paper 29, 75–91.

Guest, G., Bunce, A., Johnson, L., 2006. How many interviews are enough? An experiment with data saturation and variability. Field Methods 18 (1), 59–82.

Hurwitz, B., Greenhalgh, T., Skultans, V. (Eds.), 2004. Narrative Research in Health and Illness. Blackwell Publishing, Oxford, UK.

Institute of Medicine of the National Academies, 2005. Need for innovative designs in research on CAM and conventional medicine. Complementary and alternative medicine in the United States. National Academies Press, Washington, DC, pp. 108–128.

Janesick, V., 1994. The dance of qualitative research design: metaphor, methodolatry and meaning. In: Denzin, N., Lincoln, Y. (Eds.), Handbook of qualitative research. Sage Publications, Thousand Oaks, CA, pp. 209–219.

Koithan, M., Verhoef, M., Bell, I.R., et al., 2007. The process of whole person healing: 'unstuckness' and beyond. J. Altern. Complement. Med. 13 (6), 659–668.

Krefting, L., 1991. Rigor in qualitative research – the assessment of trustworthiness. Am. J. Occup. Ther. 45 (3), 214–222.
Kuzel, A.J., 1992. Sampling in qualitative inquiry. In: Crabtree, B., Miller, W.L. (Eds.), Doing qualitative research. Sage Publications, Newbury Park, CA, pp. 31–44.
Lincoln, Y., Guba, E., 1985. Naturalist inquiry. Sage Publications, Newbury Park, CA.
Lincoln, Y., Guba, E., 2000. Paradigmatic controversies, contradictions, and emerging concluences. In: Denzin, N., Lincoln, Y. (Eds.), Handbook of qualitative research. Sage Publications, Thousand Oaks, CA, pp. 163–188.
Miles, M., Huberman, A., 1994. Qualitative data analysis: an expanded sourcebook, second ed. Sage Publications, London.
Morgan, D.L., 1998. The focus group guidebook. Sage Publications, Thousand Oaks, CA.
Morreale, P., Manopulo, R., Galati, M., et al., 1996. Comparison of the antiinflammatory efficacy of chondroitin sulfate and diclofenac sodium in patients with knee osteoarthritis. J. Rheumatol. 23 (8), 1385–1391.
Morse, J., Field, P., 1995. Qualitative research methods for health professionals, second ed. Sage Publications, Thousand Oaks, CA, pp. 21, 80, 128.
Noblit, G.W., Hare, R., 1988. Meta-ethnography: synthesizing qualitative studies. Sage Publications, Newbury Park, CA.
Sandelowski, M., Barroso, J., 2003. Creating metasummaries of qualitative findings. Nurs. Res. 52 (4), 226–233.
Sandelowski, M., Docherty, S., Emden, C., 1997. Focus on qualitative methods – qualitative metasynthesis: issues and techniques. Res. Nurs. Health 20, 365–371.
Schwandt, T., 1994. Constructivist, interpretivist approaches to human inquiry. In: Denzin, N., Lincoln, Y. (Eds.), Handbook of qualitative research. Sage Publications, Thousand Oaks, CA, pp. 118–137.
Schwandt, T., 2000. Three epistemological stances for qualtitative inquiry: interpretivism, hermeneutics, and social constructionism. In: Denzin, N., Lincoln, Y. (Eds.), Handbook of qualitative research. Sage Publications, Thousand Oaks, CA, pp. 379–399.
Stake, R., 2006. Mutliple case study analysis. Guilford Press, New York.
Stalpers, L.J.A., da Costa, H.C., Merbis, M.A.E., et al., 2005. Hypnotherapy in radiotherapy patients: A randomized trial. Int. J. Radiat. Oncol. Biol. Phys. 61 (2), 499–506.
Stibich, M., Wissow, L., 2006. Meaning shift: findings from wellness acupuncture. Altern. Ther. Health Med. 12 (2), 42–48.
Streitberger, K., Friedrich-Rust, M., Bardenheuer, H., et al., 2003. Effect of acupuncture compared with placebo-acupuncture at P6 as additional antiemetic prophylaxis in high-dose chemotherapy and autologous peripheral blood stem cell transplantation: a randomized controlled single-blind trial. Clin. Cancer Res. 9 (7), 2538–2544.
Thorne, S., Jensen, L., Kearney, M.H., et al., 2004. Qualitative metasynthesis: reflections on methodological orientation and ideological agenda. Qual. Health Res. 14 (10), 1342–1365.
Verhoef, M.J., Leis, A., 2008. From studying patient treatment to studying patient care: arriving at methodologic crossroads. Hematol. Oncol. Clin. North Am. 22 (4), 671–682.
Verhoef, M.J., Vanderheyden, L.C., 2007. Combining qualitative methods and RCTs in CAM intervention research. In: Adams, J. (Ed.), Researching complementary and alternative medicine. Routledge, London, pp. 72–86.
Yin, R., 2003. Case study research, third ed. Sage Publications, Thousand Oaks, CA.

FURTHER READING

Cresswell, J.W., 2006. Qualitative Inquiry and Research Design: Choosing Among Five Approaches, second ed. Sage Publications, Thousand Oaks, CA.
DiCicco-Bloom, B., Crabtree, B.F., 2006. Qualitative Interviews. Med. Education 40 (9), 314–321.
Morgan, D.L., Krueger, R.A., 1998. The Focus Group Kit. Sage Publications, Thousand Oaks, CA.
Patton, M.Q., 2002. Qualitative Research and Evaluation Methods, third ed. Sage Publications, Thousand Oaks, CA.
Wolcott, H.F., 2001. Writing Up Qualitative Research, second ed. Sage Publications, Thousand Oaks, CA.

The role of outcomes and observational research in evaluating integrative medicine

3

William 'Mac' Beckner • William Harlan

CHAPTER CONTENTS

INTRODUCTION

Methods that are used in conventional medical research are designed to produce a successive hierarchy of scientific inquiry that, in turn, produces improved and therefore more rigorous evidence upon which to make clinical decisions. Typically described in a structured hierarchy are clinical observations, case studies, retrospective and prospective case series, followed by cohort studies with historical and concomitant non-randomized controls. Open-label randomized controlled trials (RCTs), and blinded, placebo-controlled RCTs are listed at the top of the hierarchy. They offer the most internal validity and minimization of bias and are considered by many to be the most reliable evidence for evaluation of modern medical interventions. This hierarchical structure (Figure 3.1) is based on a pharmacological model designed to produce the most definitive evidence of efficacy and harms and lead to regulatory approval. This hierarchy tends to undervalue the important evidence developed from observational studies and the contributions such studies make to generalizablity, long-term evaluation of efficacy and harms and to hypothesis generation as well as explanation of mechanisms underlying response to interventions.The hierarchal approach reaches its limitations when one considers the complexities

DOI: 10.1016/B978-0-443-06956-7.00003-3.

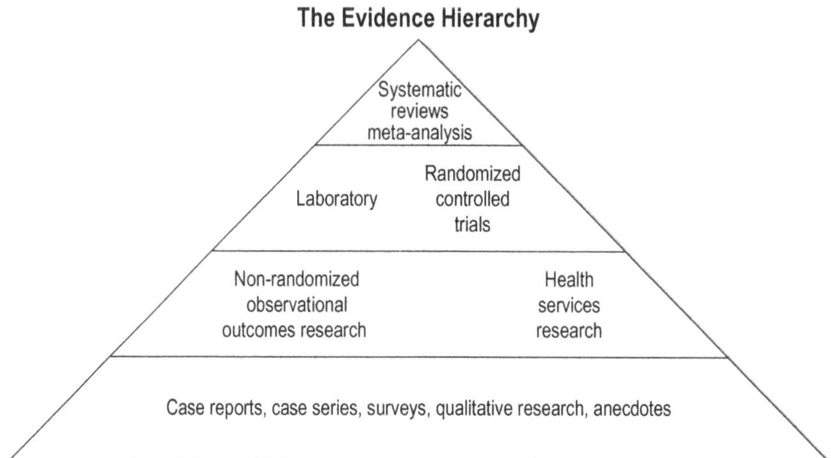

FIGURE 3.1 The evidence hierarchy. *Adapted with permission from Jonas (2001).*

of clinical decision-making and the various types of evidence needed for an evidence-based approach that is relevant within the context of clincial practice.

HISTORY AND VALUE OF RCTS IN THE EVALUATION OF MEDICAL INTERVENTIONS

One can argue that the first clinical trial dates back to approximately 600 BC when Daniel of Judah conducted what is probably the earliest recorded clinical trial (Book of Daniel). He compared the health effects of the vegetarian diet with those of a royal Babylonian diet over a 10-day period. It was a short and simple comparison of the health effects of the vegetarian diet with the royal Babylonian diet. The trial had obvious deficiencies by contemporary medical standards (10-day duration, allocation bias, ascertainment bias and confounding by divine intervention), but the report has remained influential for more than two millennia (Jadad 1998).

Credit for the modern randomized trial is usually given to Sir Austin Bradford Hill (1952). The Medical Research Council trials on streptomycin for pulmonary tuberculosis are rightly regarded as a landmark that ushered in a new era of medicine. Since Hill's pioneering achievement, the methodology of the RCT has been increasingly accepted and the number of reported RCTs has grown exponentially. The Cochrane Library now lists approximately 550 000 such trials, and they provide the basis for meta-analysis and contribute to what is currently called 'evidence-based medicine' (Cochrane Collaboration 2008).

GENERAL PRINCIPLES OF RCTS

The RCT is one of the most powerful tools of research, simple in concept but complex in execution. In essence, the RCT is a study in which treatments are allocated at random so participants receive one of several clinical interventions (Jadad 1998). Usually, the term 'intervention' refers to medical treatment, but it should be used in a much wider sense to include any clinical intervention that may have an effect on health status. Such clinical interventions include prevention strategies, screening programmes, diagnostic tests, behavioural and educational approaches, complementary and alternative medicine approaches, surgical and manipulative procedures, and devices, as well as the type or setting for provision of health services (Jadad 1998).

RCTs are powerful tools for conducting research, mainly because randomizing patients to receive or not receive the intervention balances the comparison groups with respect to factors influencing the outcomes. Thus, any significant differences between groups in the outcome event can be attributed to the intervention and not to some other identified or unidentified factor.

ISSUES AND LIMITATIONS RELATED TO RCTS

Randomized trials are designed to provide unbiased answers to specific hypotheses and theories regarding efficacy and harms of interventions on a well-defined and measured clinical outcome. Despite the strong internal validity that is designed into the trial there are important limitations. Trials are expensive to conduct and the results are very specific to the questions addressed and the populations in which they are conducted and their generalizability is often limited, particularly in pharmaceutical trials. Further, the populations selected for RCTs are based on the minimum number estimated to provide a statistically reliable result and the study groups are relatively homogeneous and limited in severity of disease and comorbidities. Duration of follow-up is usually constrained, as is populational diversity. These limit the ability to extrapolate the findings to the 'real' groups found in the usual practice setting. Further, limited comparisons are made between competing therapeutic approaches, thus leaving larger questions of comparative effectiveness unanswered. The result can be a limited application to the therapeutics of both traditional and integrated practices.

An excellent example of the issues that can arise with RCTs can be seen in the publications on mammography screening. The most important references concern the article by Miettinen et al. (2002; Larsson et al. 1997) linking screening for breast cancer with mammography and an apparently substantial reduction in fatalities and the responses that it elicited (Silverman & Altman 1996; Tabar et al. 2001). While the strongest conclusions and inferences can be reached when there is concordance between research using different methods (e.g. RCT and prospective cohort methods), such agreement is not always found, such as the different conclusions reached by cohort versus RCT studies of hormone replacement therapy in postmenopausal women (Chlebowski et al. 2003; Wassertheil-Smoller et al. 2003), antioxidant supplements to prevent cancer (Bardia et al. 2008) or decreased risk of dementia/cancer in patients using statins (Shepherd et al. 2002).

Additionally, RCTs may not be the most appropriate tool for the assessment of interventions that have rare outcomes or outcomes that take a long time to develop. In such instances, other study designs, such as case-control studies or cohort studies, may be more appropriate. In other cases, RCTs may not be feasible because of financial constraints or because of the expectation of low compliance or high drop-out rates.

Integrative medicine (IM) poses additional challenges to the RCT model. It may involve complex models of disease causation that are often treated with complex interventions that involve both specific and non-specific treatment effects (Jonas et al. 2006). Further, many of these interventions are non-pharmacologic in nature and do not lend themselves to testing of a single treatment element. There are challenges in finding credible control interventions and blinding procedures for a multifactorial 'systems' approach rather than a simple treatment regimen. Further, there is increasing pressure that research in IM provides results that are meaningful in real-life clinical practice (Boon et al. 2007). In such cases, the use of large prospective cohort studies can often afford a broader and longer-term assessment of several treatment exposures and clinical outcomes. However, the findings may be biased by selection of therapies for patients which are made based on physician or patient preferences. When treatment effects are quantitatively small or moderate the biased selection of therapies may blur or distort the true differences.

RESEARCH IN COMPLEMENTARY AND INTEGRATIVE MEDICINE

The research base for IM interventions has increased dramatically in recent years (Vickers 2000), yet there is not a critical mass of research evidence about IM and the effect of these approaches on health care to inform policy-makers and consumers adequately and uniformly on the effectiveness of these interventions. One challenge for research is how to determine the therapeutic effectiveness of interventions and thus this concerns the definition of 'effectiveness'. Another challenge is that interventions in IM are often multifaceted with complex unknown interactions among the components. Therapies delivered as a multifactorial 'system' rather than simple treatment regimen present challenges to design studies that are rigorous yet provide results that are meaningful in real-life clinical practice.

Challenges are further compounded by clinician–patient interactions; patient goals and priorities; the effects of meaning and context; patient self-care; environmental factors and social policies affecting health quality; and system factors affecting availability of resources that promote health, health behaviours or health care. Research should also focus on patient-centred care in the context of family, culture and community. Many clinical trials in the field of IM have used RCT methodologies, evaluating single components from a wider system of care in treating a specific medical condition (e.g. St John's wort for depression, a specific set of acupuncture points for headaches, a protocol of chiropractic adjustments for low-back pain or melatonin for insomnia).

It is beyond the scope of this chapter to provide a summary of all the clinical trials conducted in the field, but a recent search of PubMed found nearly 6500 RCTs under the medical subject heading of complementary therapies. In some cases, there have been enough studies on a particular treatment and condition to result in a systematic review or meta-analysis. Nearly 3000 systematic reviews and 400 meta-analyses are found in Medline when using the complementary therapies subject heading. The Cochrane Database of

Systematic Reviews had published 384 systematic reviews related to complementary therapies as of December 2009. Summaries of those reviews have been published (He et al. 2007; Bausewein et al. 2008; Bjelakovic et al. 2008; Dickinson et al. 2008; Hornerber et al. 2008; Maratos et al. 2008; Priebe et al. 2008; Zhu et al. 2008).

THE ROLE OF OUTCOMES RESEARCH AND OBSERVATIONAL STUDIES IN INTEGRATIVE MEDICINE

In conventional medicine, observational studies have provided important insights regarding the role of exposures to clinical outcomes: smoking, radiation, hormone levels and high-meat diets in the development of different kinds of cancer, lipids and coronary disease, hypertension and stroke, and sleeping position and sudden infant death syndrome (Rothwell & Bhatia 2007). Traditional biomedical research focuses on one particular disease outcome, but integrative care often addresses multiple health concerns within a single individual. These issues call for innovative research models to address the challenges inherent in testing simultaneous treatments for multiple health concerns. For example, in the case of many chronic conditions such as rheumatological diseases, chronic pain and chronic bowel diseases, IM interventions are often sought as a last resort. In such cases, an argument can be made that the study of outcomes of an effective treatment collected in large enough numbers and with methodologic rigour can be of more value than an RCT, regardless of whether the effects are due to specific or non-specific treatment effects.

An example of the value of observational research combined with an RCT in complementary and integrative medicine can be seen in recent German studies involving acupuncture and pain. A systematic review of randomized trials in patients suffering from osteoarthritis of the knee considered the available evidence as promising, but further, rigorous trials were considered necessary. In the study the Program for the Evaluation of Patient Care with Acupuncture (PEP-Ac) used a combined approach of both randomized trials and a large-scale observational study (Melchart et al. 2004). The large-scale observational study of osteoarthritis, which included 736 patients, showed that patients experience clinically relevant improvement after a treatment cycle with acupuncture. Side-effects were infrequent and minor, and the amount of pain medication consumed by patients decreased considerably (Linde et al. 2005).

In parallel with this study, the authors conducted an RCT comparing acupuncture with minimal acupuncture (superficial needling of non-acupuncture points) and a wait list control in patients with osteoarthritis of the knee (Witt et al. 2005). In this trial, therapeutically adequate acupuncture was significantly superior to both minimal acupuncture and waiting list control after 8 weeks. After 6 and 12 months, differences between acupuncture and minimal acupuncture were no longer significant. Absolute improvement in the Western Ontario and McMaster universities (WOMAC) index was slightly higher than that observed in the observational study and changes for the pain disability index and physical health were very similar in the two studies. Additionally, results were in accordance with the promising results from a review of randomized trials on acupuncture for osteoarthritis of the knee (Ezzo et al. 2000) as well the large randomized trial by Berman et al. (2004). Overall, the available evidence from both observational studies and RCTs suggests that acupuncture is effective in the treatment of osteoarthritis of the knee. However, a relevant part of the effect might be due to unspecific needling effects or placebo effects which favour continued investigations of complementary and integrative medicine with large multisite observational studies.

MEASURING NON-SPECIFIC EFFECTS

In a clinical trial, patients improve for multiple reasons. These include regression to the mean of repeated measurements, spontaneous remission, natural course, biased reporting, non-specific therapeutic effects and specific therapeutic effects. These effects are often generally referred to as the 'placebo effect' and they can account for improvements in up to 60% of patients for some conditions (Kaptchuk et al. 2008). Historically, placebo effects have been considered more a nuisance than a useful therapeutic effect because of the need to control such effects within the context of placebo-controlled trials for pharmacologic treatments. Further, the efficacy observed in the placebo arm may sometimes be significantly superior to no treatment or standard medical care (Linde et al. 2005; Melchart et al. 2005; Brinkhaus et al. 2007; Haake et al. 2007). The interaction and context of an integrative encounter are likely to increase this non-specific effect. Instead of considering the placebo effect as of secondary importance, it might be more apt to consider the placebo effect as 'contextual healing', an aspect of healing that has been produced, activated or enhanced by the context of the clinical encounter(35) that maximizes contextual healing, including the environment of the clinical setting, cognitive and affective communication of practitioners and the ritual of administering the treatment (Kaptchuk et al. 2002).

A core aspect of IM is the importance of the relationship between practitioner and patient (Chang et al. 1983; Quinn et al. 2003) that has been incorporated into the evolving concept of 'relationship-centred care' (Deng 2008). Relationship-centred care focuses on the importance of human relationships, with experience of the patient being at the centre of care. Additionally, a more integrative approach towards patient care entails incorporating biopsychosocial interdisciplinary content emphasizing compassion, communication, mindfulness, respect and social responsibility. Studies measuring the clinical impact of the relationship between practitioner and patient and outcomes of the training of clinician healers (Novack et al. 1999; Miller et al. 2003) are ripe areas for future outcomes research in IM. Enhancing research efforts towards harnessing the non-specific therapeutic effect rather than controlling for it is likely to offer expanded tools and additional insight into patient care. In situations where it is important to separate the specific effect from 'contextual healing', optimal effort needs to be placed towards validating a placebo control before pursuing large multicentre RCTs.

With the complexities involved in conducting research in IM, Jonas (2001) argues that perhaps the best model of evidence is one that balances both reality and relevance in the evaluation of complex interventions such as physiotherapy, surgery and integrative practices (Figure 3.2). There is an essential tension between internal validity (rigour and the removal of bias) and external

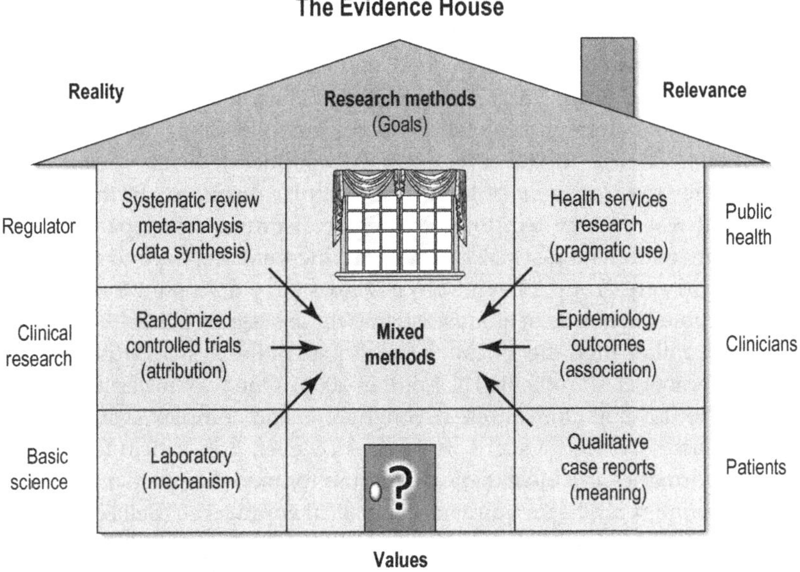

FIGURE 3.2 The evidence house. *Adapted with permission from Jonas (2001).*

validity (generalizability) in the hierarchical model and this weakness, Jonas argues, warrants a multiplicity of methods, using different designs, counterbalancing their individual strengths and weaknesses to arrive at pragmatic but equally rigorous evidence. The 'evidence house' (Jonas 2001) (Figure 3.2) seeks to lateralize the main knowledge domains in science in order to highlight their purposes by aligning methodologies that isolate specific effects (those with high internal validity potential) and those that seek to explore utility of practices in real clinical settings (those with high external validity potential).

INCORPORATING OUTCOMES INTEGRATIVE MEDICINE AND WHOLE-SYSTEMS RESEARCH

Researchers can make use of outcome measurement tools developed in conventional disciplines of medicine, especially those emphasizing functional performance in addition to structural integrity and those taking into consideration the psychological and societal impact of disease (Coons et al. 2000). Such outcomes have been collected in rheumatology (Ward 2004), neurology (von Steinbuechel et al. 2005; Miller & Kinkel 2008), geriatric (Burns et al. 2000; Demers & McKelvie 2000), rehabilitation (Andresen & Meyers 2000; Donnelly & Carswell 2002) and pain and palliative care (Turk et al. 2002). They form a foundation from which IM researchers can build a truly global outcome measurement system. Another consideration in IM research is how to evaluate multimodality health care approaches.

There is an impetus for 'whole-systems' research, which strives to examine the effect of a multimodality health care approach to provide individualized treatment. The belief is that this will more accurately evaluate the health care currently being provided to patients and is an increasingly frequent trend in IM research. There are several articles in the literature urging IM researchers to consider research methods beyond the RCT (Cardini et al. 2006; Boon et al. 2007; Fonnebo et al. 2007). One example of whole-systems research is the study by Ritenbaugh et al. (2008), who examined the effect of whole-system traditional Chinese medicine versus naturopathic medicine versus standard of care for the treatment of tempromandibular disorders. In this study, improvement was seen in temporomandibular disorders when participants were randomized to whole-systems treatment interventions beyond that seen in the standard care group. Several investigators have discussed the need to use more complex methods of analysis so that these systems of health care can be examined, rather than the efficacy of each part of the system (Ritenbaugh et al. 2003; Verhoef et al, 2005; Bell & Koithan 2006). One way to capture these outcomes is to develop clinical research networks and complex system analysis tools to assess whole-systems research. However, it is critical to engage skilled bioinformatics and biostatistical expertise for modelling and analysis as these more complex studies require new statistical approaches (Bell & Koithan 2006). Researchers should be encouraged to add qualitative measures to studies because they can provide a source of data for unexpected outcomes and a way to measure the broader effects of a whole system, such as IM (Verhoef et al. 2005). As these new study designs mature it will be important for IM researchers to consider the range of effects IM treatments may have for patients, and thus to measure a broad area of outcomes in order to detect these effects.

CAPTURING THE IMPACT OF PERSONALIZED INTEGRATIVE CARE IN THE ERA OF GENOMIC MEDICINE

Personalized medicine is just beginning on a long journey of discovery that will include genomics and genetic influences on conditions and their development (and response to environmental exposures) and the individual response to treatments. Genomics refers to the study of all the genes of a cell, or tissue, at the DNA (genome), mRNA (transcriptome) or protein (proteome) levels. It is well known that individuals respond differently to risk exposure and interventions. Proposing a research agenda for incorporating genomic medicine into IM is described in Chapter 4. As new and innovative tools and technologies for genomic discovery become available they can be utilized to advance current knowledge of processes of healing and repair that fit into observational research approaches. A discovery model for genomic associations in IM could mirror what Weston & Hood (2004) call P4 medicine – predictive, preventive, personalized and participatory. In such a model health care interventions, both conventional and integrative care, would no longer be conceptualized in terms of disease, but rather in terms of mediating health and wellness.

CLEAR AND RIGOROUS REPORTING OF OBSERVATIONAL STUDIES

For outcomes research to be of value to health care decision-making it should be reported transparently so that readers can follow what was planned, what was done, what was found and what conclusions were drawn. The credibility of research depends on a critical assessment by peers of the strengths and weaknesses in study design, conduct and analysis. An analysis of epidemiological studies published in general medical and specialist journals found that the rationale behind the choice of potential confounding variables was often not reported (Pocock et al. 2004). Only a few reports of case-control studies in psychiatry explained the methods used to identify cases and controls (Lee et al. 2007). In a survey of longitudinal studies in stroke research, 17 of 49 articles (35%) did not specify the eligibility criteria (Tooth et al. 2005). Others have argued that without sufficient clarity of reporting, the benefits of research might be achieved more slowly (Bogardus et al. 1999) and that there is a need for guidance in reporting observational studies. Transparent reporting is also needed to judge whether and how results can be included in systematic reviews (Juni et al. 2001). However, in published observational research important information is often missing or unclear. Recommendations on the reporting of research can improve reporting quality. The Consolidated Standards of Reporting Trials (CONSORT) statement was developed in 1996 and revised 5 years later (Moher et al. 2001). Many medical journals support this initiative and require the reporting format of CONSORT, which has helped to improve the quality of reports of randomized trials (Egger et al. 2001; Plint et al. 2006). Similar initiatives have followed for the reporting of meta-analyses of randomized trials (Moher et al. 1999) and diagnostic studies (Bossuyt et al. 2003).

Recently, researchers have established a network of methodologists, researchers and journal editors to develop recommendations for the reporting of observational research: the Strengthening the Reporting of Observational Studies in Epidemiology (STROBE) statement. The STROBE statement was designed to help researchers when writing up analytical observational studies, support editors and reviewers who are considering such articles for publication and help readers when critically appraising published articles. Adopting the STROBE checklist for research in IM observational studies can serve a wide range of purposes, on a continuum from the discovery of new findings to the confirmation or refutation of previous findings (Vandenbroucke 2004). While some studies may be essentially exploratory and raise interesting hypotheses, others may pursue clearly defined hypotheses in available data.

The ultimate goal of outcomes research is to guide clinical practice and its efficient utilization to maximize benefits and to minimize patient harms. When formulating clinical guidelines, two factors are in play: strength of evidence and burden/risk to the patient. Because it is not always possible to have definitive evidence on safety and effectiveness and clinical decisions have to be made with limited information (Deng 2008), burden and risk to the patient need to be taken into account. Although the highest level of evidence is desirable for every health intervention, it is simply not possible to achieve this goal. Limited research resources have to be allocated according to priorities. Therefore, interventions or therapies having high risk or burden (economic/time/effort) to patients and society should meet a higher standard in strength of evidence, often in the form of multiple RCTs, to be utilized for regulatory or reimbursement approval and in clinical practice. Those with low or little risk/burden can be incorporated into practice even when the highest level of evidence is not available (McCrory et al. 2007). Implicit in this understanding is the notion that both the clinician and patient understand and agree with respect to: the problem; the goal of therapy; the evidence regarding safety and effectiveness of the therapy being considered; the extent to which it is accessible, affordable and of high and consistent quality; and availability of similar information about integrative treatments (or a combination of treatments) under consideration.

Using a combined strategy that utilizes both observational and outcomes research and RCTs enables methods to be modified so that the concerns of all stakeholders are taken into account. This ensures that as far as possible what is being assessed under experimental conditions is consistent with everyday IM practice. Unless evidence is generated in a way that satisfies such criteria, it is unlikely to have an impact.

REFERENCES

Andresen, E.M., Meyers, A.R., 2000. Health-related quality of life outcomes measures. Arch. Phys. Med. Rehabil. 81 (12 Suppl. 2), S30–S45.

Bardia, A., Tleyjeh, I.M., Cerhan, J.R., et al., 2008. Efficacy of antioxidant supplementation in reducing primary cancer incidence and mortality: systematic review and meta-analysis. Mayo Clin. Proc. 83 (1), 23–34.

Bausewein, C., Booth, S., Gysels, M., et al., 2008. Non-pharmacological interventions for breathlessness in advanced stages of malignant and non-malignant diseases. Cochrane Database Syst. Rev. (2): CD005623.

Bell, I.R., Koithan, M., 2006. Models for the study of whole systems. Integr. Cancer Ther. 5 (4), 293–307.

Berman, B.M., Lao, L., Langenberg, P., et al., 2004. Effectiveness of acupuncture as adjunctive therapy in osteoarthritis of the knee: a randomized, controlled trial. Ann. Intern. Med. 141 (12), 901–910.

Bjelakovic, G., Nikolova, D., Gluud, L.L., et al., 2008. Antioxidant supplements for prevention of mortality in healthy participants and patients with various diseases. Cochrane Database Syst. Rev. (2): CD007176.

Bogardus Jr., S.T., Concato, J., Feinstein, A.R., 1999. Clinical epidemiological quality in molecular genetic research: the need for methodological standards. JAMA 281 (20), 1919–1926.

Boon, H., Macpherson, H., Fleishman, S., et al., 2007. Evaluating complex healthcare systems: a critique of four approaches. Evid. Based Complement. Alternat. Med. 4 (3), 279–285.

Bossuyt, P.M., Reitsma, J.B., Bruns, D.E., et al., 2003. Towards complete and accurate reporting of studies of diagnostic accuracy: The STARD Initiative. Ann. Intern. Med. 138 (1), 40–44.

Brinkhaus, B., Witt, C.M., Jena, S., et al., 2007. Physician and treatment characteristics in a randomised multicentre trial of acupuncture in patients with osteoarthritis of the knee. Complement. Ther. Med. 15 (3), 180–189.

Burns, R., Nichols, L.O., Martindale-Adams, J., et al., 2000. Interdisciplinary geriatric primary care evaluation and management: two-year outcomes. J. Am. Geriatr. Soc. 48 (1), 8–13.

Cardini, F., Wade, C., Regalia, A.L., et al., 2006. Clinical research in traditional medicine: priorities and methods. Complement. Ther. Med. 14 (4), 282–287.

Chang, J.D., Eidson, C.S., Dykstra, M.J., et al., 1983. Vaccination against Marek's disease and infectious bursal disease. I. Development of a bivalent live vaccine by co-cultivating turkey herpesvirus and infectious bursal disease vaccine viruses in chicken embryo fibroblast monolayers. Poult. Sci. 62 (12), 2326–2335.

Chlebowski, R.T., Hendrix, S.L., Langer, R.D., et al., 2003. Influence of estrogen plus progestin on breast cancer and mammography in healthy postmenopausal women: the Women's Health Initiative Randomized Trial. JAMA 289 (24), 3243–3253.

Collaboration, C., 2009. The Cochrane Library. Update Software [cited 2009 December 10]; Available from: www.update-software.com/cochrane.

Coons, S.J., Rao, S., Keininger, D.L., et al., 2000. A comparative review of generic quality-of-life instruments. Pharmacoeconomics 17 (1), 13–35.

Daniel, Book of Daniel 1, 1–21. The Bible.

Demers, C., McKelvie, R.S., 2000. Exercise training for patients with chronic heart failure reduced mortality and cardiac events and improved quality of life. West. J. Med. 172 (1), 28.

Deng, G., 2008. Integrative Cancer Care in a US Academic Cancer Centre: The Memorial Sloan-Kettering Experience. Curr. Oncol. 15 (Suppl. 2), s108 es68–71.

Dickinson, H.O., Campbell, F., Beyer, F.R., et al., 2008. Relaxation therapies for the management of primary hypertension in adults. Cochrane Database Syst. Rev. (1), CD004935.

Donnelly, C., Carswell, A., 2002. Individualized outcome measures: a review of the literature. Can. J. Occup. Ther. 69 (2), 84–94.

Egger, M., Juni, P., Bartlett, C., 2001. Value of flow diagrams in reports of randomized controlled trials. JAMA 285 (15), 1996–1999.

Ezzo, J., Berman, B., Hadhazy, V.A., et al., 2000. Is acupuncture effective for the treatment of chronic pain? A systematic review. Pain 86 (3), 217–225.

Fonnebo, V., Grimsgaard, S., Walach, H., et al., 2007. Researching complementary and alternative treatments – the gatekeepers are not at home. BMC Med. Res. Methodol. 7, 7.

Haake, M., Muller, H.H., Schade-Brittinger, C., et al., 2007. German Acupuncture Trials (GERAC) for chronic low back pain: randomized, multicenter, blinded, parallel-group trial with 3 groups. Arch. Intern. Med. 167 (17), 1892–1898.

He, J.L., Xiang, Y.T., Li, W.B., et al., 2007. Hemoperfusion in the treatment of acute clozapine intoxication in China. J. Clin. Psychopharmacol. 27 (6), 667–671.

Hill, A., 1952. The clinical trial. N. Engl. J. Med. (247):113–119.

Horneber, M.A., Bueschel, G., Huber, R., et al., 2008. Mistletoe therapy in oncology. Cochrane Database Syst. Rev. (2), CD003297.

Jadad, A. (Ed.), 1998. Randomised controlled trials: a user's guide: London. BMJ Books, England.

Jonas, W.B., 2001. The evidence house: how to build an inclusive base for complementary medicine. West. J. Med. 175 (2), 79–80.

Jonas, W.B., Beckner, W., Coulter, I., 2006. Proposal for an integrated evaluation model for the study of whole systems health care in cancer. Integr. Cancer. Ther. 5 (4), 315–319.

Juni, P., Altman, D.G., Egger, M., 2001. Systematic reviews in health care: Assessing the quality of controlled clinical trials. BMJ 323 (7303), 42–46.

Kaptchuk, T., Eisenberg, D., Komaroff, A., 2002. Pondering the placebo effect. Newsweek 140 (23), 71 3.

Kaptchuk, T.J., Kelley, J.M., Deykin, A., et al., 2008. Do 'placebo responders' exist? Contemp. Clin. Trials 29 (4), 587–595.

Larsson, L.G., Andersson, I., Bjurstam, N., et al., 1997. Updated overview of the Swedish Randomized Trials on Breast Cancer Screening with Mammography: age group 40–49 at randomization. J. Natl. Cancer Inst. Monogr. (22)57–61.

Lee, W., Bindman, J., Ford, T., et al., 2007. Bias in psychiatric case-control studies: literature survey. Br. J. Psychiatry 190, 204–209.

Linde, K., Streng, A., Jurgens, S., et al., 2005. Acupuncture for patients with migraine: a randomized controlled trial. JAMA 293 (17), 2118–2125.

Maratos, A.S., Gold, C., Wang, X., et al., 2008. Music therapy for depression. Cochrane Database Syst. Rev. (1), CD004517.

McCrory, D.C., Lewis, S.Z., Heitzer, J., et al., 2007. Methodology for lung cancer evidence review and guideline development: ACCP evidence-based clinical practice guidelines, 2nd edition. Chest 132 (Suppl. 3), 23S–28S.

Melchart, D., Hager, S., Hager, U., et al., 2004. Treatment of patients with chronic headaches in a hospital for traditional Chinese medicine in Germany. A randomised, waiting list controlled trial. Complement. Ther. Med. 12 (2–3), 71–78.

Melchart, D., Streng, A., Hoppe, A., et al., 2005. The acupuncture randomised trial (ART) for tension-type headache – details of the treatment. Acupunct. Med. 23 (4), 157–165.

Miettinen, O.S., Henschke, C.I., Pasmantier, M.W., et al., 2002. Mammographic screening: no reliable supporting evidence? Lancet 359 (9304), 404–405.

Miller, W.L., Crabtree, B.F., Duffy, M.B., et al., 2003. Research guidelines for assessing the impact of healing relationships in clinical medicine. Altern. Ther. Health Med. 9 (Suppl. 3), A80–A95.

Miller, D.M., Kinkel, R.P., 2008. Health-related quality of life assessment in multiple sclerosis. Rev. Neurol. Dis. Spring; 5 (2), 56–64.

Moher, D., Cook, D.J., Eastwood, S., et al., 1999. Improving the quality of reports of meta-analyses of randomised controlled trials: the QUOROM statement. Quality of Reporting of Meta-analyses. Lancet 354 (9193), 1896–1900.

Moher, D., Schulz, K.F., Altman, D.G., 2001. The CONSORT statement: revised recommendations for improving the quality of reports of parallel-group randomised trials. Lancet 357 (9263), 1191–1194.

Novack, D.H., Epstein, R.M., Paulsen, R.H., 1999. Toward creating physician-healers: fostering medical students' self-awareness, personal growth, and well-being. Acad. Med. 74 (5), 516–520.

Plint, A.C., Moher, D., Morrison, A., et al., 2006. Does the CONSORT checklist improve the quality of reports of randomised controlled trials? A systematic review. Med. J. Aust. 185 (5), 263–267.

Pocock, S.J., Collier, T.J., Dandreo, K.J., et al., 2004. Issues in the reporting of epidemiological studies: a survey of recent practice. BMJ 329 (7471), 883.

Priebe, M.G., van Binsbergen, J.J., de Vos, R., et al., 2008. Whole grain foods for the prevention of type 2 diabetes mellitus. Cochrane Database Syst. Rev. (1), CD006061.

Quinn, J.F., Smith, M., Ritenbaugh, C., et al., 2003. Research guidelines for assessing the impact of the healing relationship in clinical nursing. Altern. Ther. Health Med. 9 (Suppl. 3), A65–A79.

Ritenbaugh, C., Hammerschlag, R., Calabrese, C., et al., 2008. A pilot whole systems clinical trial of traditional Chinese medicine and naturopathic medicine for the treatment of temporomandibular disorders. J. Altern. Complement. Med. 14 (5), 475–487.

Ritenbaugh, C., Verhoef, M., Fleishman, S., et al., 2003. Whole systems research: a discipline for studying complementary and alternative medicine. Altern. Ther. Health. Med. 9 (4), 32–36.

Rothwell, P.M., Bhatia, M., 2007. Reporting of observational studies. BMJ 335 (7624), 783–784.

Shepherd, C.E., McCann, H., Thiel, E., et al., 2002. Neurofilament-immunoreactive neurons in Alzheimer's disease and dementia with Lewy bodies. Neurobiol. Dis. 9 (2), 249–257.

Silverman, W.A., Altman, D.G., 1996. Patients' preferences and randomised trials. Lancet 347 (8995), 171–174.

Tabar, L., Vitak, B., Chen, H.H., et al., 2001. Beyond randomized controlled trials: organized mammographic screening substantially reduces breast carcinoma mortality. Cancer 91 (9), 1724–1731.

Tooth, L., Ware, R., Bain, C., et al., 2005. Quality of reporting of observational longitudinal research. Am. J. Epidemiol. 161 (3), 280–288.

Turk, D.C., Monarch, E.S., Williams, A.D., 2002. Cancer patients in pain: considerations for assessing the whole person. Hematol. Oncol. Clin. North Am. 16 (3), 511–525.

Vandenbroucke, J.P., 2004. When are observational studies as credible as randomised trials? Lancet 363 (9422), 1728–1731.

Verhoef, M.J., Lewith, G., Ritenbaugh, C., et al., 2005. Complementary and alternative medicine whole systems research: beyond identification of inadequacies of the RCT. Complement. Ther. Med. 13 (3), 206–212.

Vickers, A., 2000. Recent advances: complementary medicine. BMJ 321 (7262), 683–686.

von Steinbuechel, N., Richter, S., Morawetz, C., et al., 2005. Assessment of subjective health and health-related quality of life in persons with acquired or degenerative brain injury. Curr. Opin. Neurol. 18 (6), 681–691.

Ward, M.M., 2004. Rheumatology care, patient expectations, and the limits of time. Arthritis Rheum. 51 (3), 307–308.

Wassertheil-Smoller, S., Hendrix, S.L., Limacher, M., et al., 2003. Effect of estrogen plus progestin on stroke in postmenopausal women: the Women's Health Initiative: a randomized trial. JAMA 289 (20), 2673–2684.

Weston, A.D., Hood, L., 2004. Systems biology, proteomics, and the future of health care: toward predictive, preventative, and personalized medicine. J. Proteome Res. 3 (2), 179–196.

Witt, C., Brinkhaus, B., Jena, S., et al., 2005. Acupuncture in patients with osteoarthritis of the knee: a randomised trial. Lancet 366 (9480), 136–143.

Zhu, X., Proctor, M., Bensoussan, A., et al., 2008. Chinese herbal medicine for primary dysmenorrhoea. Cochrane Database Syst. Rev. (2), CD005288.

Laboratory research and biomarkers

Hakima Amri • Mones Abu-Asab • Wayne B. Jonas • John A. Ives

4

CHAPTER CONTENTS

INTRODUCTION

Laboratory research in complementary and alternative medicine (CAM) is a challenging topic due to the complexity of biological systems, the heterogeneity of CAM modalities and the diversity in their application. Scientists are well aware of the complexity of biological systems. To compensate for this complexity biological scientists attempt to isolate single components and study them outside their milieu. This has led to simplifying the research hypothesis for determining the effect of a single chemical enzymatic reaction, the impact of loss or gain of a substrate on a cellular pathway or the effect of a receptor/ligand on molecular signals. Extrapolations and correlations of the findings to a disease state or a specific pathophysiological pathway are then drawn. The experiments are performed in a test tube using a cocktail of ingredients, on cell or tissue extracts or on laboratory animals. Laboratory research like this is often

DOI: 10.1016/B978-0-443-06956-7.00004-5

translated to clinical research where trials are performed on human subjects. Thus, laboratory research encompasses both basic science and the clinical aspects of investigative science. Answering scientific questions by extrapolating from less to more complex systems has been the approach in conventional basic science research. This approach has led to the deciphering of important action mechanisms at cellular, molecular and genetic levels.

However, are these mechanisms reported to the scientific community in a comprehensive framework? In most cases the answer is no. Each new discovery is reported in the respective research field, to the respective experts in the field, to answer one specific question. Science has gradually become so compartmentalized and scientists so specialized that if you want to know more about a specific oncogene, for example, there is only one expert for you to contact. Clearly this is not an optimal approach as there are about 24 500 protein-coding genes and around 3400 cell lines from over 80 different species, including 950 cancer cell lines held at the ATCC Global Bioresource Center (Clamp et al. 2007) (http://www.atcc.org). The problem is exacerbated with highly specialized journals, which scientists from other fields often do not even read. Furthermore, standards and validation of procedures are still at the centre of scientific debates, especially at a time when leading-edge technology is advancing faster than their laboratory application. All these factors lead one to conclude that laboratory research has become so scattered that it is a challenge to paint a big picture that could be translated to the clinic.

In these times of 'compartmentalized' science there is a crying need for a comprehensive framework. It is within this context that CAM finds itself and through its renaissance putting pressure on decades of this unchallenged conventional scientific construct. To achieve a successful CAM renaissance, however, we must strive for the quality of evidence reached in conventional biomedical research over the decades (Jonas 2005). To establish a laboratory science, like any other biomedical endeavour, CAM must successfully pass the main domains of evidence checkpoints: hypothesis-driven experimental design, model validity, specificity, reproducibility and action mechanism or conceptual framework defining dependent and independent variables. This is especially difficult because CAM in general and CAM laboratory research in particular are adding layers of complexity, heterogeneity and diversity to the already fragmented conventional scientific paradigm. The validation of CAM modalities requires the most rigorous scientific testing and clinical proof involving product standardization, innovative biological assays, animal models, novel approach to clinical trials, as well as bioinformatics and statistical analyses (Yuan & Lin 2000).

Is there a process that could reconcile both sides of CAM and conventional science, bringing together a scientific community that values open-mindedness and constructive criticism and take advantage of the state-of-the art technological advances science has successfully accomplished? We believe so. Recent advances in bioinformatics, biotechnology and biomedical research tools encourage us to predict that CAM laboratory research is positioned to move from cataloguing phenomenology to developing novel and innovative paradigms that could benefit both houses of 21st-century medicine.

This chapter addresses the laboratory design and methodology used to measure changes in an organ or whole organism in response to a CAM modality. These methods cover tissue culture and animal models, integrative approaches of data generation from proteomics, mass spectrometry, genomic microarray, metabolomics, nuclear magnetic resonance and imaging, as well as analytical methods for the identification of novel effects of CAM modalities and that may qualify as biomarkers. We also provide the CAM researcher with an overview of the challenges faced when designing bench experiments and a general idea about the cutting-edge technology currently available to carry out evidence-based laboratory science in CAM.

CAM RESEARCH: REVERSE-COURSE HYPOTHESIS

Reports on the efficacy of CAM modalities to treat disorders and chronic diseases vary considerably in terms of their quality and scientific rigour (Giordano et al. 2003; Jonas 2005). This can be attributed to the lack of systematic and scientific basis for most of these modalities, as well as the wide variability of responses and outcomes often seen in CAM practices. Anecdotal data of a modality's success alone do not meet the standards of evidence-based science and it is unlikely that experimental laboratory research alone will provide adequate substantiation for some CAM modalities (Moffett et al. 2006).

Some hold the assumption that CAM research should not necessarily be hypothesis-driven. This feeling is associated with the fact that many modalities of CAM have been practised for hundreds of years and thus the feeling that is there is no need for research because the clinical practice already exists. However, this runs counter to evidence-based medicine and the scientific process itself. Scientific research is hypothesis-driven. A properly designed experiment will attempt to falsify a null hypothesis and support an alternative hypothesis – the study hypothesis. The latter is an educated guess based on observation or preliminary data. Formulating hypotheses in CAM research is, in many cases, perceived as unnecessary because there already exist hundreds of years of CAM practice and experience.

The goal of many active research programmes in CAM today is to attempt to develop mechanistic understandings of CAM modalities through systematic scientific research that goes beyond anecdotal reports. With this in mind, CAM laboratory research is emulating the already-established conventional science paradigm, i.e. relating the effect of a particular active ingredient in a plant extract to its action on a specific biochemical pathway in vivo and thus elucidate its potential mechanism of action. The effects of *Ginkgo biloba* and St John's wort on humans have been relatively well described. Specifically, *Ginkgo biloba* has been shown to have an impact on blood circulation (McKenna et al. 2001; Wu et al. 2008) while St John's wort appears to improve mild depression (Kasper et al. 2006, 2008). In addition, these two plants have often been studied in rat models where various mechanisms are being investigated but, in most cases, with a weak or no link to the original health conditions for which these plants are prescribed (Amri et al. 1996; Pretner et al. 2006; Hammer et al. 2008; Higuchi et al. 2008; Ivetic et al. 2008; Lee et al. 2008). As of January 2010, a PubMed search using the key words 'Ginkgo biloba and rats' and 'St John's wort and rats' yielded 533 and 233 entries, respectively, covering a variety of mechanisms of action.

The usual progression in biomedical research is to start with a cell-free or tissue culture model, progress to intact or genetically engineered animal models, advance to pilot studies in humans and, finally, run tests in more elaborate clinical trials. In much of CAM research taking place today we are seeing this paradigm run in reverse. Often, in a CAM research laboratory, the starting assumption is that the CAM modality under study has worked for hundreds of years in humans and now there is an attempt to understand the mechanism of action. To do so, the researchers first organize human pilot studies, followed by the use of animal models and then conclude with research to define action mechanisms at the cellular and molecular levels using test tubes – the reverse of the usual order (Figure 4.1) (Fonnebo et al. 2007).

This viewpoint is illustrated in the studies performed by Jacobs and colleagues (2000, 2006). They performed two separate clinical studies of homeopathy and homeopathic principles. In one, the homeopathic treatment of children with diarrhoea was tailored to their symptom constellations. In the other, the subjects were given the same homeopathic regimen ignoring symptomatic variability. Although these studies tested assumptions within homeopathy they were designed without clearly elucidated mechanisms to construct hypotheses around. As another example, *Ginkgo biloba* is already used by thousands of patients in the hope that it will improve memory and counter some of the other effects of ageing, though a recent clinical trial demonstrated no effect on Alzheimer's disease (DeKosky et al. 2008). The mechanisms by which effects might occur are not understood. Because of this gap Amri and colleagues (1997, 2003) studied the action mechanisms of *Ginkgo biloba*.

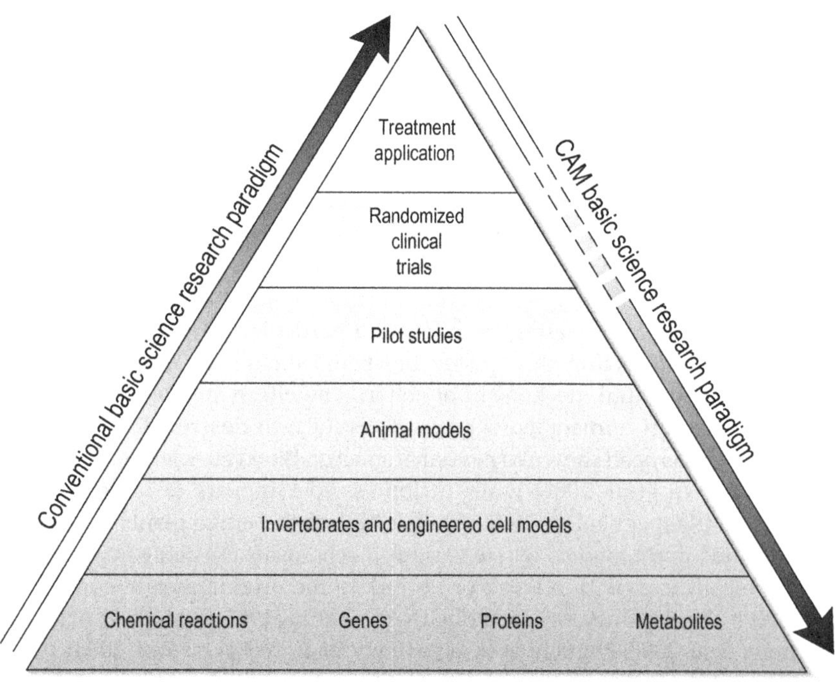

FIGURE 4.1 The course of research development in both conventional and complementary and alternative medicine basic science.

They demonstrated the beneficial effects of *Ginkgo biloba* in controlling the corticosterone synthesis by the adrenal gland (cortisol equivalent in humans) in rats in vivo, ex vivo and in vitro at the molecular and gene regulation levels. The authors also showed that the whole extract had better effects than its isolated components by reducing corticosterone levels while keeping adrenocorticotrophic hormone levels low, which indicates that *Ginkgo biloba* whole extract affected the adrenal–pituitary negative-feedback loop (Figure 4.2).

In both examples the standard experimental design has been altered in order to respect the CAM treatment efficacy premise and the laboratory research rigour. In the case of the homeopathic clinical trials, the investigators administered individualized remedies, which is a deviation from the conventional trials where one pharmaceutical drug is given to all subjects. The effect of *Ginkgo biloba* extract, on the other hand, while clinically tested in humans, has almost all of its mechanistic research done in the animal and cellular models, as well as the molecular aspect to elucidate its mechanism of action.

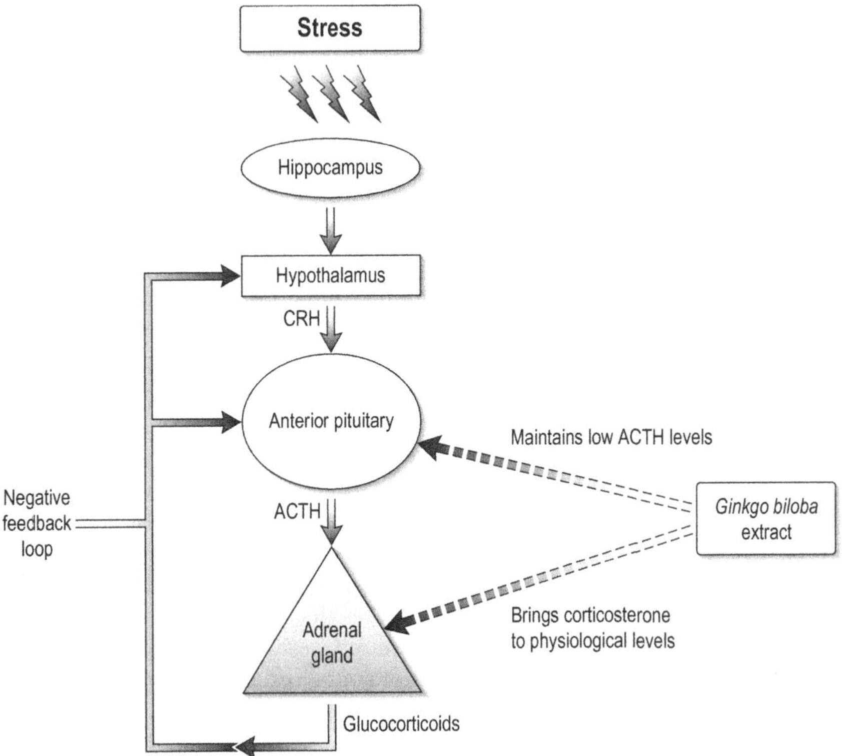

FIGURE 4.2 Summary of the effect of *Ginkgo biloba* extract on the hypothalamus–pituitary–adrenal (HPA) axis in the rat model. Stress stimulates the HPA axis to overproduce corticosterone; treatment with *Ginkgo biloba* extract decreases corticosterone levels while maintaining physiological adrenocorticotrophic hormone (ACTH) levels. The downward arrows represent stimulation, the arrows on the far left represent inhibition and dashed arrows represent normalizing effects. CRH, corticotrophin-releasing hormone.

One of the big problems within CAM research is combining what are often old traditions within CAM practices, such as the assignment of treatment based upon traditional – often not scientifically validated – diagnostic techniques such as taking of pulses in traditional Chinese medicine (TCM), or the symptom constellation used in homeopathy, with modern reductionist scientific approaches. Because of this, the field of CAM research is in great need of established standards without compromising the CAM practice itself but performing the research within a rigorous scientific framework. We also believe that in this era of postgenome and systems biology, laboratory testing of CAM modalities has not yet fully employed integrative high-throughput methods, such as microarray gene expression and protein mass spectrometry. These techniques enable the screening of large numbers of specimens at significantly improved rates and can provide the blueprint for finding potential biomarkers (Cho 2007; Abu-Asab et al. 2008).

EXPERIMENTAL DESIGN

When setting up a study, a significant effort should be placed at the early planning stage to avoid potential biases during the conduct of the study and in order to produce meaningful data and analysis. The planning starts by clearly defining the objectives of the study, then outlining the set of experiments that the researcher will conduct to test their hypothesis. The experimental design should include all the elements, conditions and relations of the consequences; these include: (1) selecting the number of subjects – the sample, the study group or the study collection; (2) pairing or grouping of subjects; (3) identifying non-experimental factors and methods to control them (variables); (4) selecting and validating instruments to measure outcomes; (5) determining the duration of the experiment – endpoints must be suitably defined; and (6) deciding on the analytical paradigm for the analysis of the collected data.

Incorporating randomization in experiments is necessary to eliminate experimenter bias. This entails randomly assigning objects or individuals by chance to an experimental group. It is the most reliable process for generating homogeneous treatment groups free from any potential biases. However randomization alone is not sufficient to guarantee that treatment groups are as similar as possible. An experiment should include a sufficient number of subjects to have adequate 'power' to provide statistically meaningful results. That is, can we trust the results to be a good representation of the class of subjects under study, i.e. do we believe the results?

The replication of an experiment is required to show that the effectiveness of a treatment is true and not due to random occurrence. Replication increases the robustness of experimental results, their significance and confidence in their conclusions.

The question of how many replicates should be used in an experiment is an important topic that has been addressed many times and continues to be revisited periodically by statisticians whenever there is the introduction of new technologies such as microarray. The goal is to encompass the variation spectrum that may occur in a population or class; or, in the case of treatment effectiveness, to reach statistical significance. According to its website, the National Center for Complementary and Alternative Medicine (NCCAM) has concluded, based on discussions with statisticians, peer-reviewed articles, simulations and data from studies, that in microarray studies about 30 patients per class are needed to develop classifiers for biomarkers discovery (Pontzer & Johnson 2007). However, the necessary sample sizes vary for each research project depending on the conditions of the experiment (e.g. inbred (mice, rats) versus outbred populations (humans)) (Wei et al. 2004). There are published formulas and web-based programs for calculating the required study size in order to ensure that a study is properly powered (Dobbin et al. 2008).

Selection of the control group is one of the most crucial aspects of study design, especially when testing complex phenomena in the laboratory. Controls determine which part of a theoretical model is tested. For example, in acupuncture there is the ritual, needle, point and sensation to expectancy or conditioned response: which is the most important aspect of the treatment? In homeopathy or herbal therapy, is it a specific chemical, preparation, process, combination, dose or sequence of delivery? Each of the above requires different controls. Thus, selecting the control is selecting the theory. Likewise, results should state precisely what aspect of the theory is elucidated by the control treatment result differences. Additionally, the need for a control group cannot be overemphasized. This group is included to avoid experimental bias and placebo effects, focus the hypothesis and serve as a baseline for detecting differences.

This discussion outlines the standard paradigm for laboratory research in general where guidelines and standards have been established decades ago by specialized institutions such as the Clinical and Laboratory Standards Institute (CLSI) and the Clinical Laboratory Improvement Amendments (CLIA) to ensure quality standards for laboratory testing and promote accuracy, as well as for inter- and intralaboratory reproducibility. In general CAM laboratory research has not reached these levels of standardization and regulation, at least in the USA. However, applying these guidelines and standards to CAM research exposes their inadequacies and confirms the complexity of CAM modalities. Nevertheless, we believe that conducting CAM basic science research in the 21st century using newly developed as well as existing approved standards from the conventional field in conjunction with cutting-edge technology will benefit and advance CAM research.

BASIC SCIENCE RESEARCH AND CAM

STANDARDIZATION DILEMMA IN BASIC SCIENCE RESEARCH

For over a century, conventional scientific research has undergone phases of trial and error that led to establishing guidelines and standards. As a result, scientific research as conducted today is becoming high-quality, rigorous and reproducible. Tremendous effort and resources have been dedicated to developing analytical methodologies and sophisticated technologies to bring conventional scientific research to this level of standing. CAM research, however, has not received similar attention, primarily due to a confluence of historic, political and economic forces and additionally due to the complexity and heterogeneity of its constructs around mode of action. Many of these do not conform to the reductionism paradigm that dominates conventional research (Kurakin 2005, 2007).

The challenges in CAM clinical research design are covered in other sections of this book. CAM basic science research faces a number of experimental hurdles, starting with hypothesis generation based upon controversial putative cellular and molecular mechanisms and extending to choice of biological model, dosage, treatment frequency and analytical methodology, to name a few. These are not, in principle, any different from the hurdles faced in conventional research. However, as mentioned above, there is a century or more of historical experience behind the conventional approaches and models and only a few decades of serious attention to CAM modalities of healing and their possible mechanistic underpinnings. The need for standards, inherent difficulties notwithstanding, makes it essential that these issues be addressed.

Each experimental model has its strengths and weaknesses. For example, translating in vitro data to in vivo applications often does not work. This is true of all biomedical research, whether focused on CAM or not. However, it should be emphasized that the researcher must develop an awareness of the limitations of the various available models. This is important, especially, for the interpretation of the data and/or their translation to clinical research. It is crucial that CAM researchers be cognizant of these limitations and always alert to consider the extra layer of complexity that is added by the CAM modality under study.

CELLULAR MODELS

Cell lines in cultures, i.e. in vitro, are widely used in almost all fields of biomedical research. The relatively cheap cost and fast turnaround time of this technique have contributed to its ubiquity. Cell lines derived from all types of tissues and cancers are commercially available; in addition, researchers constantly introduce and characterize new cell lines. In vitro experiments, although easy to set up and carry out, are challenging in all fields of research. This is due, at least in part, to the variability among cell lines that arises from their susceptibility to genetic and phenotypic transformation and potential contamination during frequent serial passages. There have been a number of studies reporting discrepancies within cell lines with regard to their purported characteristics (Masters et al. 1988; Chen et al. 1989; Dirks et al. 1999). One solution is to use primary cell cultures (from fresh normal tissues and not transformed to become immortal). These tend to have fewer artifacts compared to transformed immortal cell lines but efforts developing strategies to use them as a cell model have been hindered by cost and time (Zhang & Pasumarthi 2008).

Despite their limitations, most of our tumour biology and gene regulation knowledge has stemmed from studying tumour cell lines. This is underscored by the over 50,000 publications reporting use of HeLa cells and over 20,000 reports describing NIH/3T3 cell line use. It is generally accepted that monolayer, three-dimensional cultures, or xenografts, cannot entirely reproduce the biological events occurring in humans. It is, thus, a challenge to create experimental cell models that capture the complex biology and diversity of human beings (Chin & Gray 2008).

In basic science, animal models remain the 'gold standard' and the crucial step before using human subjects. Certain regulatory agencies in the USA, such as the Environmental Protection Agency (EPA) and the Food and Drug Administration (FDA), are encouraging the substitution of the expensive, time-consuming and sometimes ethically problematic animal testing with the bacterial tier testing if human studies are already available (Marcus 2005). This strategy is applicable to many CAM studies where natural products have already been tested on human subjects.

ANIMAL MODELS

Animal use for food, transport, clothes and other products is as old as humanity itself. Their use in experimental research parallels the development of modern medicine, which had its roots in ancient cultures of Egypt, Greece, Rome, India and China. It is known that Aristotle and Hippocrates based their knowledge of structure and function of the human body in their respective *Historia Animalium* and *Corpus Hippocraticum* on dissections of animals. Galen carried out his experimental work on pigs, monkeys and dogs, which provided the fundamentals of medical knowledge in the centuries thereafter (Baumans 2004).

Today, animal models remain the gold standard in laboratory research for testing the efficacy and effects of treatments. In vivo animal models are used to validate in vitro data and both of these are a prerequisite for clinical trials. A wide spectrum of animals is used in basic science research. Examples include: *Caenorhabditis elegans*, zebrafish and *Drosophila* in developmental biology and genetic studies; mouse, rat, guinea pig, rabbit, cat, dog and monkey in general physiology, pharmacology and neuroscience. Each model presents its own advantages and disadvantages and should be evaluated first for cost, time effectiveness and ethical appropriateness and then for the related issues of handling and management in laboratory settings. Although many models are used today to answer fundamental scientific questions, the mouse remains the model of choice, in part because of the remarkable progress achieved in producing engineered models to mimic several pathologies.

Thirty years of cancer research and millions of dollars spent on clinical and basic science research produced the genetically engineered mouse model. There are models for almost every epithelial malignancy in humans, including transgenic, 'knockout' and 'knockdown' models. The scientific and technical ability to generate engineered animal models, where targeted conditional activation or silencing of genes and oncogenes is easily manipulated, confirms the remarkable progress achieved since Galen's era. With the discovery in the 1980s that *Myc* expression caused breast adenocarcinoma in mice mammary epithelium, the study of genes and its application in genetic engineering has exploded (Meyer & Penn 2008).

The current science and capabilities of genetic engineering are testimony to the power of reductionist thinking. This has led to further entrenchment of the reductionist approach in biomedicine and the belief that all mechanisms of biology and disease can and must be understood – understanding the action mechanisms underlying tumorigenesis in order to develop the most effective treatment. Understanding action mechanisms confers validity and credibility on biomedical research. Thus, knowing that *Myc* activation can cause breast cancer demonstrates our understanding of mechanism. On the other hand, to say that we know a homeopathic remedy that reduces prostate tumour size, or we know acupuncture reduces stress, does not address the question of mechanism. The degree to which the mechanism underlying the observed effect is understood often becomes the standard by which the quality of CAM research is judged. The conventional bias is that if the effect is confirmed, reproducible and mechanistically deciphered, then and only then will the scientific community accept it and the bench-to-bedside translation be implemented. Yet, this attitude is hypocritical.

Have we cured cancer? No. Have we deciphered cellular and molecular pathways leading to cancer development? The answer is yes. Have we developed anticancer drugs? The answer is also yes. Are they effective in curing cancer? Often, they are not. The current inability to cure cancer is one of the reasons for the observed increased use of CAM therapies among cancer patients (Miller et al. 2008; Verhoef et al. 2008). Furthermore, as the axiom 'one gene, one protein' has turned out not to be true and biological systems have proved to be far more complex than originally envisioned, the ability for pharmaceutical researchers to perform targeted drug discovery has become increasingly difficult – perhaps even impossible. More recently, a call to adopt integrative approaches to basic science research and systems biology has emerged due, at least in part, to the technological developments in the genomics and proteomics fields (see below). We feel that there is great potential for advancement of CAM basic science research employing these paradigms and new technologies. There is a philosophical synergy among integrative approaches, systems biology and CAM. CAM modalities amenable to basic science research are integrative and often affect more than one pathway, meaning that today we should be able to demonstrate the complexity of the response using the latest technologies employed by conventional researchers (van der Greef & McBurney 2005; Verpoorte et al. 2009).

IMPACT OF CUTTING-EDGE TECHNOLOGIES ON CAM RESEARCH

This section outlines novel integrative technologies measuring almost all changes in an organ or whole organism in response to a treatment. Such integrative methodologies could provide comprehensive elucidation of the effects of a CAM modality. The conventional research community is slowly moving away from simplistic and reductionism thinking and towards an inclusive mapping of all changes in the biological system. This could only benefit both basic and clinical CAM research and we encourage using it. These innovative methodologies are described below.

HIGH-THROUGHPUT SYSTEMS OF ANALYSIS: THE OMICS

New high-throughput systems of genome, proteome and metabolome analyses, such as microarray and mass spectrometry, are currently the best techniques that permit a large-scale assessment of whole-body response to treatment, while other traditional methods, such as enzyme-linked immunoassay and polymerase chain reaction, detect a limited number of gene and protein expressions at a time (Li 2007). The data produced from these newer techniques are useful for both target measurements (i.e. quantitative) and profiling (i.e. qualitative) (Abu-Asab et al. 2008). Although finding and quantifying change is achievable with the new omics, interpreting the results – establishing meaning and significance – and elucidating the pathways affected remains, as it always has been, the most difficult task a biomedical researcher faces.

We predict that, as high-throughput systems become widely used by CAM researchers, they will recast and energize CAM research because of the shared integrative characteristics of the two; they are both concerned with changes at the organismal level. CAM modalities affect systems biology of the whole organism and the high-throughput omics are the quantitative and qualitative measures of the whole systems' change.

Public databases of high-throughput data are also a great source of data that can be used to test hypotheses in preparing research proposals or before embarking on expensive laboratory experiments. The largest, publicly available and diverse data warehouse is that of the National Center for Biotechnology Information (NCBI: http://www.ncbi.nlm.nih.gov/). NCBI creates and houses public databases, conducts research in computational biology, develops software tools for analysing genome data and disseminates biomedical information in order to contribute to the better understanding of molecular processes affecting human health and disease (Barrett et al. 2009).

GENOMIC ANALYSIS

Genomic analysis here refers to the integrative study of the gene expression alterations, before and after a treatment, that could be a CAM modality. We will focus here on microarray technology because it allows a total gene expression analysis and has the ability to reveal without prejudice the shifts in whole profile. For example, microarray gene expression profiling can identify genes whose expression has changed in response to a CAM modality by comparing gene expression in cells or tissues.

Microarray chips consist of small synthetic DNA fragments (also termed probes) immobilized in a specific arrangement on a coated solid surface such as glass, plastic or silicon. Each location is termed a feature. There are tens of thousands to millions of features on an array chip. Nucleic acids are extracted from specimens, labelled and then hybridized to an array. The amount of label, which corresponds to the amount of nucleic acid adhering to the probes, can be measured at each feature. This technique enables a number of applications on a whole-genome scale, such as gene and exon expression analysis, genotyping and resequencing. Microarray analysis can also be combined with chromatin immunoprecipitation for genome-wide identification of transcription factors and their binding sites.

Because of reproducibility issues in microarray experiments (variability between runs and between different laboratories), there are a few practical considerations in the experimental design that should be followed (Churchill 2002; Yang et al. 2008). First, replicas of experimental specimens should be included in the microarray analysis (i.e. treatment groups should include multiple subjects). Second, from each subject one duplicate should also be used – two separate microarray chips for the same subject. Third, microarray chips that include multiple spots for the same gene probe should be used. This feature allows the detection of experimental or chip manufacturing problems. These guidelines need to be followed in order to obtain reliable data.

Although overall gene expression is indicative of the holistic status of a tissue, the values of a gene of interest should be independently rechecked with other methods such as quantitative real-time (QRT)-PCR to ensure the accuracy of the microarray results. It is now a routine practice to remeasure the expression values of significant genes (differentially expressed) before publishing microarray results (Clarke & Zhu 2006). Gene expression microarray studies require the extraction of messenger ribonucleic acid (mRNA) from cells or tissues; therefore, it will be an invasive procedure when applied to human and animal subjects. However, it is appropriate to use in cancer treatment animal models, tissue culture experiments and comparative plant analysis. In order to avoid experimental variability between different runs it is preferred that all specimens be hybridized to chips at the same time. Finally, microarray experiments should be designed meticulously before executing to reduce mistakes, not only to increase scientific reliability but also to reduce the cost of microarray chips, which is still substantial (Hartmann 2005).

Microarray has been used by Gao et al. (2007) to probe candidate genes involved in electroacupuncture analgesia and to understand the molecular basis of the individual differences of electroacupuncture analgesia in rats. They identified 66 differentially expressed genes and classified these into nine functional groups: (1) ion transport; (2) sensory perception; (3) synaptogenesis and synaptic transmission; (4) signal transduction; (5) inflammatory response; (6) apoptosis; (7) transcription; (8) protein amino acid phosphorylation; and (9) G-protein signalling. Another example is the exploratory study on Kososan, an antidepressant. This study suggests that gene expression profiling is possible for studying the effects of complex herbal remedies (Hayasaki et al. 2007). For more examples and a detailed description of microarray principles and practices, we recommend the excellent review of Hudson & Altamirano (2006).

PROTEOMIC ANALYSIS

In a CAM context, proteomic analysis is the study of the changes of all expressed proteins due to an application of a CAM modality. It can be applied to body tissues and fluids.

During the last decade, proteome analysis has become increasingly important. This is due to the fact that the proteomic profile is the true expression of the functionality of the biological system. Unlike genomic sequences and transcriptional profiles, proteomics is an accounting of the actual change in protein expression (Li 2007). Although protein structure, concentration and function are subjected to posttranslational modifications and degradation, protein expression provides an accurate dynamic reflection of homeostasis, as well as a dynamic measure of any reactions to stimuli and drugs.

There are two major techniques employed in the study of systems' proteomics: mass spectrometry and gel electrophoresis. Mass spectrometry is based on a machine's ability to read large sets of tandem mass spectra of laser-scattered proteins and peptides. The proteins are digested and adsorbed to a matrix chip prior to placement in the mass spectrometry machine. The most reliable mass spectrometry system in use today is the matrix-assisted laser desorption/ionization-time-of-flight (MALDI-TOF). The matrix protects the molecules from destruction by the laser beam and assists in their vaporization and ionization, while time-of-flight spectrometer determines the mass-to-charge ratio (m/z) of each protein/peptide in the specimen. There are tens of thousands of m/z values per specimen and these are the values used for quantitative and qualitative assessments as well as the identification of the protein of interest.

Two-dimensional gel electrophoresis (2-DE) is a high-resolution technique for separating proteins in acrylamide gel through two steps: first by using isoelectric focusing in the first dimension and then by mass in the second dimension. The separated proteins are then visualized by staining the gel with one of the following: Coomassie blue, silver, SYPRO Ruby and Deep Purple (Lauber et al. 2001). The 2-DE is a slow technique because it is time- and labour-intensive. Furthermore, it does not resolve proteins in low abundance and those with small molecular weight.

The various proteomic methods can be utilized to verify the identity of ingredients, or identify new bioactive agents; verify standardization; elucidate the response; decipher action mechanisms of treatment; for a priori categorizing of patients and subsequent responses; and to reveal the heterogeneity of a disease. There are numerous examples on the application of proteomics in the study of CAM. Lum 2-DE proteomics has been used to identify different species of ginseng, different parts of the same ginseng and cultured cells of ginseng and showed that the 2-DE maps of different ginseng samples contain sufficient differences to permit easy discrimination (Lum et al. 2002). The effect of the Siwu decoction on blood proteins was demonstrated through a number of proteomic techniques and shown to regulate the protein expression of bone marrow of blood deficiency in mice and thus promote the growth and differentiation of haematopoietic cells (Guo et al. 2004). Electroacupuncture treatment has been shown to induce a proteomic change in the hypothalamus (Sung et al. 2004).

METABOLOMIC ANALYSIS

For our CAM application purposes, metabolomic analysis is defined here as the detection of fingerprint changes of very large sets of small detectable metabolites in an organism due to a CAM modality treatment. Metabolites that may result from bodily responses occurring in the tissues and fluids, such as urine, saliva, serum, plasma, bile, seminal fluid, lung aspirate and spinal fluid, can be detected. Other materials that can be used are cell culture supernatant, tissue extracts and intact tissue specimens.

Metabolomics offers an additional set of data in the high-throughput data class that also includes genomics and proteomics. Because metabolites are themselves the result of the organisms, integrated biochemical machinery and pathways metabolomics may be thought of as a systems analysis of the organism. Two main methods are used in metabolomic studies: mass spectrometry and nuclear magnetic resonance (NMR). Mass spectrometry is a picogram-sensitive method that can detect thousands of metabolites in serum or urine specimens. However, it is limited by the need to carry out a separation step (by chromatography: gas chromatography, high-performance liquid chromatography, liquid chromatography) and the heterogeneous detection caused by variable ionization efficiency (Shanaiah et al. 2008). On the other hand, NMR requires little or no specimen preparation and is rapid, non-invasive and reproducible. However, it has lower sensitivity than mass spectrometry. The simplest, most reliable, accurate and reproducible NMR sequences used in metabolic study are the single-pulse or 1D nuclear Overhauser spectroscopy (NOESY).

Urine is considered an ideal biofluid for NMR analysis for diagnostic and monitoring purposes due to its low-abundant protein content, high concentration of low-molecular-weight compounds, minimum preparation and high-quality measurements (Neild et al. 1997). Furthermore, archival databases of NMR profiles allow quick comparisons of results according to NMR peaklist data, i.e. spectral search (see Human Metabolome Database at www.hmdb.ca).

NMR of serum and plasma produces sharp narrow signals from small-molecule metabolites and broad signals from proteins and lipids. The large proteins, lipoproteins and phospholipids produce a baseline distortion that is corrected by the use of NMR pulse sequence Carr–Purcell–Meiboom–Gill (CPMG). Intact tissues can be studied with NMR using the high-resolution magic angle spinning (HR-MAS) spectroscopy (van der Greef & McBurney 2005).

Additionally, metabolomics is used to establish fingerprint efficacy profiles of herbal medications and their extracts. Lu et al. (2006) established a gas chromatography-mass spectrometry fingerprint of *Houttuynia cordata* injection for quality control and were able to correlate reasonably the higher efficacy with certain fingerprints. Two-dimensional *J*-resolved NMR spectroscopy was applied to study the fingerprints of ginseng preparations and spectral data were analysed with principal component analysis (Yang et al. 2006). The authors demonstrated that the 2D NMR method can efficiently differentiate between commercial preparations and quickly assess quality control.

Due to its robustness, speed and non-invasiveness, metabolomics offers applicable profiling opportunities for diagnosis and assessment of treatments, as well as for quality and efficacy evaluation of herbal preparation.

BIOINFORMATIC ANALYSIS

Bioinformatic analysis endeavours to identify the significantly affected variables and their role in the metabolic pathways affected by treatment, classify individuals' responses to treatment and identify potential biomarkers. Raw data collected from microarray, mass spectrometry proteomics and metabolomics may require some preprocessing, such as baseline correction, alignment, binning and normalization before its analysis with a bioinformatic tool

(Kunin et al. 2008). Most datasets, especially of high-throughput omics, have a large number of variables and would not be analysed with 'pencil and paper' but rather with a bioinformatic computer program. Only through massive number crunching is it possible to perform an analysis to decipher the biologically meaningful changes that result from treatment. Analysing data from multiple datasets (acquired from different instruments for the same study group) is challenging even with current analytical paradigms. Individual variability/heterogeneity coupled with experimental noise (differences in runs within the same laboratory and between laboratories) produces a thorny bioinformatic situation. To overcome such problems we will outline two analytical paradigms, statistical and phylogenetic, highlighting their strengths and weaknesses.

STATISTICAL APPROACH

The goal of a statistical analysis is to determine whether our null hypothesis is true or false and consequently if the data support the study hypothesis. Parametric statistical methods are always applied to sampling from populations that are assumed to have a normal distribution for the variables of interest. This assumption is significant because, when comparing two samples, control versus treatment, their means are used to assess whether the treatment has influenced the variable(s) we are observing and therefore the means must accurately reflect their populations. The statistical question here becomes: How can it be inferred that the treatment mean ($\bar{x}_T$) is not equal to the control mean ($\bar{x}_C$)? All statistical tests, whether for normal distribution (*t*-distribution (for continuous numerical data), chi-square (for categorical data)) or non-normal distribution (Mann–Whitney U-test (for independent cohorts), Wilcoxon signed-rank sum test (for paired data)), aim to calculate the *P*-value, which is a measure of probability that the difference between the control and treatment groups is due to chance. The lower the *P*-value, the higher the probability the difference is caused by the treatment.

Statistical analysis permits the determination of the significantly affected variables (usually those with a *P*-value <0.05) within the specimen or a cohort of specimens. Furthermore, these significant variables can be entered into a second analysis to profile responses and for class discovery (grouping of individuals sharing similar responses, also referred to as typing). Profiling methods are either supervised or unsupervised. Supervised techniques require a training set of specimens to establish a profile for a particular class that can be later applied to identify profiles and classes (usually a combination of variables such as proteins or gene expressions), while unsupervised techniques can process the data without any prior training. Two of the most widely used unsupervised techniques are principal component analysis (PCA) and hierarchical cluster analysis (HCA) (Albanese et al. 2007; Yang et al. 2009).

Profiling with these methods is based on raw similarity from distance matrices that produces clusters of specimens (scatter plots of PCA, dendrogram of HCA, lists of mass spectrometry peaks or heat maps for microarray data). Classification (class discovery) is based on overall similarity and in some cases may have little biological relevance, i.e. low predictive power.

This point has been a source of frustration for many researchers. However, as we illustrate in the phylogenetic section below, the same data can be analysed in a phylogenetic approach to produce more biologically relevant results.

PHYLOGENETIC APPROACH

Phylogenetics is an evolutionary-based analytical approach that discriminates between ancestral and derived similarities and uses shared derived states to delimit classes and create hierarchical classification of specimens (Albert 2006; Abu-Asab et al. 2008). Biological systems are heterogeneous (or diverse) in their normal states as well as in their responses to stimuli and treatment. The many existing combinations of variables, in gene and protein expressions, are matched by an equal number of possible reactions. Therefore, a population's responses may not be homogeneous (see the section on dichotomous expressions in Abu-Asab et al. (2008a)). For a dataset that contains parameters that violate normality, we recommend phylogenetic-based analysis.

A phylogenetic approach has an added advantage: it does not use overall similarity for analysis, but rather it divides similarity between control and treatment groups into ancestral similarity (variables that are unaffected by the treatment) and derived similarity (variables affected by the treatment). This process of converting continuous quantitative data to a discontinuous qualitative format is termed polarity assessment. The variables' values for the treatment group are compared against the ranges of the control group (minimum and maximum of every variable). If a value from a treatment specimen falls within the control's range, then it is an ancestral (i.e. normal) and given the value of zero (0); otherwise it is derived and given the value of one (1). Polarity assessment produces a new matrix where the original values are replaced by 0s and 1s.

A polarity matrix can be processed with a number of algorithms. However, a parsimony phylogenetic algorithm seems to provide a multidimensional analysis that is suitable for the needs of the biomedical research community. Multidimensional analysis is defined here as one that provides a resolution of biological patterns, affected pathways and class discovery; capable of incorporating new patterns and multiple datasets (i.e. seamless and dynamic); and can be utilized in a clinical setting for early detection, diagnosis, prognosis and evaluation of treatment (Abu-Asab et al. 2008b). Furthermore, such analysis is also known to have a higher predictivity.

Parsimony phylogenetic analysis will categorize the subpopulations for variation and treatment responses on the basis of shared derived states of the variables. Shared derived states among a number of specimens represent the potential biomarkers (see the section below on biomarkers). Results of a parsimony analysis are depicted in a tree-like diagram called a cladogram. A cladogram is a concise graphical summary of data distribution, data patterns, directionality of change and general trends within the specimens. It is also the most parsimonious hypothesized hierarchical relationships for a group of specimens, because it incorporates in its analysis all of the input states (not just the statistically significant) and thus better models data heterogeneity.

ROLE OF BIOMARKERS IN CAM BASIC RESEARCH

The search for biomarkers in newly generated data is a major activity for many biomedical researchers. The goal is to find biological indicators that can be developed into non-invasive tests for early detection of disease, susceptibility, diagnosis, targeted therapy and post-treatment evaluation. Because of disease heterogeneity and human variability, no single biomarker can be expected to have a wide range of functionality and utility throughout all phases of a disease. Therefore, each disease must have a set of biomarkers to detect it at any of its phases. However, the current problems associated with biomarker discovery stem from the lack of integration among traditionally defined biomarkers (based on a pathology model) and high-throughput omics data, the provisional nature of many putative biomarkers due to the limited size of the study collection in many experiments and the failure to understand the nature of disease heterogeneity and possible existence of multiple developmental pathways.

There are a few types of biomarkers that are useful in CAM research; among these are the diagnostic, predictive, prognostic and pharmacodynamic (Sawyers 2008). A diagnostic biomarker aids in reaching or confirming a diagnosis. A predictive biomarker is useful in evaluating the possible benefits of a specific treatment. The prognostic biomarker is used in forecasting the course and outcome of the disease. While the pharmacodynamic biomarker is used in measuring the effects of a treatment on the disease, a biomarker does not necessarily have to be a unique metabolite that is specific to the disease, but rather a measure of a common parameter that is affected by the disease and can be restored by the treatment – surrogate markers (Ledford 2008).

There are several approaches to discovering biomarkers in a laboratory setting. An example of a direct approach is sorting out data from 2D gels of protein extracts taken from sick or treated subjects; it may show the disappearance of certain spots, or the appearance of new spots when compared with normal specimens. In this case, new biomarkers can be declared, but further validation should be carried out. However, in the case of omics data the situation is more difficult and has become a source of frustration and scepticism. Locating surrogate markers has been practised with success for a number of diseases; they are also fast and cheap to measure (Ledford 2008). Most researchers expected the omics data to be an easy source of many biomarkers, but this turned out to be an inflated assumption. We think that the reason behind this problem is the misunderstanding of the natures of the omics data, the disease and the definition of biomarkers in an omics context, as well as the lack of the proper bioinformatic analytical tool.

We have suggested that a quantitative statistical approach to omics data analysis is not the most suitable method of analysis and that a qualitative paradigm can better bring out informational content of the data when coupled with a phylogenetic analysis (Abu-Asab et al. 2008). For a detailed explanation of our qualitative paradigm, see the section on phylogenetic analysis, above.

STANDARDS, QUALITY AND APPLICATION IN CAM BASIC SCIENCE RESEARCH

For several years, the NCCAM at the US National Institutes of Health dedicated over 60% of its budget to clinical research and 20% to centres, but only the remaining funds to basic research, while at the same time encouraging mechanistic studies (http://nccam.nih.gov). Although it is easy to recommend that CAM be held to the same standards as conventional basic science, the complexity and intricacies of CAM, as reported in the White House Commission on CAM Policy, remain understated (Gordon 2002; White House Commission on CAM 2002).

Basic science studies are conducted in nearly all the CAM disciplines that lend themselves to the hypothesis-driven paradigm and a quick search of the literature attests to that. Essentially, CAM basic science research is following the same standards used for conventional research, i.e. use of statistically significant number of specimens or replicates, introducing internal and experimental controls, defining response specificity and reproducibility (Table 4.1). The last is perhaps the most challenging criterion. In several cases, experiments show positive results but, when repeated, sometimes in the same laboratory, do not work despite the precautions of maintaining identical experimental conditions. This is well illustrated in the work published by Yount and colleagues (2004). They investigated the effect of 30 minutes of qigong on the healthy growth of cultured human cells. A rigorous experimental design of randomization, blinding and controls was followed. While both a pilot that included eight independent experiments and a formal study that included 28 independent experiments showed positive effects, the replication study of over 60 independent experiments showed no difference between the sham and treated cells. This study represents an excellent example of CAM basic science research being held to the highest standard of experimental methodology.

This level of rigour is rarely done in CAM laboratory research. We reviewed the CAM basic and clinical research in the area of distant mental influence on

Table 4.1 ***Summary of experimental and methodological standards in complementary and alternative medicine (CAM) basic science research***

Standards	Outcomes
Experimental model	Choice of the best laboratory model to study the CAM modality
Replicates	Adequate number of replicates to achieve statistical significance
Randomization and blinding	Apply if using animal models, high-throughput screening or interventionists
Independent experiments	Replicate same experiment
Internal control	Control for intrinsic variability
Experimental control	Control for biological effect (e.g. a set not undergoing treatment)
Specificity of biologic response	Ensure that the observed effect is not an artifact (this is different from placebo)
Interlaboratory comparability	Confirm that the results are reproduced by another laboratory

living systems (DMILS) and energy medicine. The quality of research was quite mixed. While a few simple research models met all quality criteria, such as in mental influence on random number generators or electrodermal activity, much basic research in DMILS, qigong, prayer and other techniques were poor (Jonas & Crawford 2002). In setting up these evaluations, we described basic criteria needed for all such laboratory research (Jonas & Crawford 2003).

In CAM basic science research, formulating the testable hypothesis is sometimes not the major issue; it is setting up and testing the CAM practice itself. In the example of Yount et al. (2004), where they followed the most rigorous methodological and experimental designs, the practice under investigation was not a simple treatment with defined doses of a pharmaceutical compound or an antagonist of a specific receptor. Instead it was an unknown amount of energy emanating from the hands of a number of qigong practitioners.

Acupuncture is a CAM application that lends itself to use in animal models for in vivo and ex vivo evaluation of its effects. By applying electroacupuncture, researchers are in this case able to control the amount of energy delivered. However, the challenge here is the placement of the needles. Whereas in humans, needles would be placed based on meridian maps, for rats they must be placed so that the needles will not be disturbed during normal grooming while still being placed along a meridian of relevance. In addition, 20 minutes of electroacupuncture is used because this is what would be done on humans (Li et al. 2008). Should not the time and dose parameters be adjusted to the animal body size? Massage, a manipulative body-based therapy, has been tested in a rat model to show its effects on a number of physiological functions. While it is hard to envision practising Swedish massage on rats, CAM researchers have adapted this method to a massage-like stroking of the back or abdomen depending on the goal of the study. It is hard to translate the data obtained here to a clinical setting if for no other reason than the CAM application in the rat is probably not similar to massage therapy (Lund et al. 1999, 2002; Holst et al. 2005).

Mind/body-based therapies are also challenging in a laboratory setting. Although there are several studies showing the effects of meditation on cell growth (Yu et al. 2003), differentiation (Ventura 2005), water pH and temperature change, as well as on the development time of fruit fly larvae (Tiller 1997), we believe that for these studies the necessary level of methodological rigour has not been met. Independent replication has been especially problematic. On the other hand, some CAM applications, such as homeopathy, phytotherapy and dietary supplements (Ayurveda or TCM), are often translated to the laboratory setting. This is due to the fact that these practices and their products are thought of (correctly or incorrectly) as conventional interventions using pharmaceutical compounds, where dose and time course experiments can be designed (Table 4.2).

In phytotherapy, significant effort has been directed to establishing guidelines and standards to the use of herbal products in clinical research (NCCAM Interim Policy 2005). No guidelines, however, have been established for using herbal products in cell culture. Drawing from our personal experience where we used a number of herbal products on various cancer

Table 4.2 *Summary of research and analytical tools that could be applied to and are available for complementary and alternative medicine (CAM) basic science research*

	Research tools				Analytical tools		
CAM modality	**Test tube**	**Cell/ tissue**	**Animal/ preclinical**	**Genomics/ proteomics/ metabolomics**	**Biostatistics**	**Bioinformatics**	**Phylogenetics**
Whole medical systems							
Homeopathy	✓	✓	✓	✓	✓	✓	✓
Naturopathy			✓	✓	✓	✓	✓
TCM/acupuncture			✓	✓	✓	✓	✓
Ayurveda			✓	✓	✓	✓	✓
Unani			✓	✓	✓		
Mind–body medicine							
Yoga							
Meditation	✓	✓			✓		
Mind–body medicine				✓			✓
Biologically based practices							
Dietary supplements	✓	✓	✓	✓	✓	✓	✓
Botanicals	✓	✓	✓	✓	✓	✓	✓
Probiotics	✓	✓	✓	✓	✓	✓	✓
Diets			✓	✓	✓	✓	✓
Manipulative and body-based practices							
Massage			✓	✓	✓	✓	✓
Chiropractic			✓	✓	✓	✓	✓
Osteopathic			✓	✓	✓	✓	✓
Reflexology							
Energy medicine							
Veritable: electromagnetic, sound, and light therapies	✓	✓	✓	✓	✓	✓	✓
Putative: qigong, reiki, therapeutic touch		✓	✓	✓	✓	✓	✓

TCM, traditional Chinese medicine.

cell lines, plant extracts are complex mixtures that could be toxic to cells in vitro. This becomes especially critical if the outcomes of the study are cell growth and proliferation. In our studies of *Ginkgo biloba*, we performed animal studies using the whole extract (EGb761) but for the cell lines the whole extract was devoid of the proanthocyanidins that are known to bind and precipitate proteins in vitro (Hagerman & Butler 1981; Pretner et al. 2006). Precautions should be taken when analysing and interpreting experiments where whole-plant extracts are being used in cellular models.

Reproducibility is a critical issue for both conventional and CAM basic science research. An example is in gene microarray. Researchers are still trying to tackle technical problems stemming from interplatform variability, interlaboratory comparability, interexperiment reproducibility and intraexperimenter protocol differences. Efforts have been directed at automating the procedure and minimizing the handling of specimens to one person in the laboratory (Raymond et al. 2006). The MicroArray Quality Control consortium was created to address the issues of microarray gene expression reproducibility (Shi et al. 2006). Research institutions, federal agencies and the industry joined forces to overcome issues of reproducibility and establish a consistent framework for using this method. In the meantime, researchers have been presenting and publishing their data without major criticism. CAM basic science research would benefit from similar support to tackle similar CAM-related issues.

TOWARD STANDARDS IN CAM LABORATORY RESEARCH

Several examples of standard quality control criteria have been developed in CAM. Aside from those in the DMILS and parapsychology literature, other quality standards have been developed. Linde and colleagues (1994) applied and published standards for laboratory research in homeopathy. Jonas & Crawford (2002) adapted standard Consolidated Standards of Reporting Trials (CONSORT) criteria for the evaluation of prayer and energy medicine research. Hintz et al. have further refined these criteria (2003). Others in herbal research have been previously mentioned (Table 4.3).

CONCLUSION

The reductionist paradigm that has been dominating conventional science for decades is being revisited due to the growing body of evidence that physiological and pathophysiological processes are caused by a multitude of factors that go beyond the genetic make-up. For the last half-century biologists have been focusing on the small pieces of the puzzle rather than the holistic picture. In contrast, CAM basic research helps bring our focus back to the integrative paradigm. Psychosocial, behavioural and environmental factors are now being considered. Biology and biomedicine are opting for the approach that is currently called systems biology and systems medicine. Encouraged by the availability of extremely large databases and technological advances, biochemists, molecular biologists and geneticists are starting to connect the dots and draw maps of the multitude of molecular pathways such as protein–protein interactions (interactomes), with the

Table 4.3 ***Quality reporting of evidence***

Type of research	Quality scoring system	References	Description
Laboratory research	Modified LOVE	Sparber AG, Crawford CC, Jonas WB 2003 Laboratory research on bioenergy. In: Jonas WB, Crawford CC (eds) Healing, Intention and Energy Medicine. London: Churchill Livingstone, p. 142	Modification of standard LOVE scale developed by Crawford et al. (2003) to focus specifically on laboratory studies
	Quality evaluation score	Linde K, Jonas WB, Melchart D et al. 1994 Critical review and meta-analysis of serial agitated dilutions in experimental toxicology. Human and Experimental Toxicology 13: 481–492	Quality evaluation criteria for assessing animal studies in homeopathy
	Quality evaluation scoring	Nestmann ER, Harwood M, Martyres S 2006 An innovative model for regulating supplement products: natural health products in Canada. Toxicology 221: 50–58.	Quality evaluation criteria for assessing studies in herbal treatments

LOVE, Likelihood of Validity Evaluation.

ultimate goal that one day they will decipher the mechanism-based uniqueness of individuals for the purpose of developing better approaches to the treatment of disease.

The evidence-based approach to CAM research and the emerging systems integration of biology and biomedical research are converging in their goals and research methodology. While the dawn of the 21st century has ushered in the use of the words integrative, systems biology and personalized medicine, CAM as an integrative paradigm offers the most personalized treatment approach of all. These characteristics of CAM are now also goals of allopathic medicine and its research (Lee & Mudaliar 2009; Pene et al. 2009). Basic science researchers in CAM will advance their research agenda by taking advantage of the new developments in genomics, proteomics and metabolomics and by utilizing these high-throughput methodologies.

With accepted standards for laboratory research, it is possible to conduct valid basic research for most CAM modalities that is less reductionistic than the conventional approaches. CAM scientists may be ahead of the game because they are already working within an integrative paradigm. However, a new panoramic synthesis of the CAM paradigm needs to integrate evidence-based laboratory standards, high-throughput data-generating techniques and bioinformatics-based data analysis.

REFERENCES

Abu-Asab, M., Chaouchi, M., Amri, H., 2008a. Evolutionary medicine: A meaningful connection between omics, disease and treatment. Proteomics 2 (2), 122–134.

Abu-Asab, M.S., Chaouchi, M., Amri, H., 2008b. Phylogenetic modeling of heterogeneous gene-expression microarray data from cancerous specimens. Omics 12 (3), 183–199.

Albanese, J., Martens, K., Karanitsa, L.V., et al., 2007. Multivariate analysis of low-dose radiation-associated changes in cytokine gene expression profiles using microarray technology. Exp. Hematol. 35 (4 Suppl. 1), 47–54.

Albert, V., 2006. Parsimony, Phylogeny and Genomics. Oxford University Press, New York.

Amri, H., Ogwuegbu, S.O., Boujrad, N., et al., 1996. In vivo regulation of peripheral-type benzodiazepine receptor and glucocorticoid synthesis by ginkgo biloba extract EGb 761 and isolated ginkgolides. Endocrinology 137 (12), 5707–5718.

Amri, H., Drieu, K., Papadopoulos, V., 1997. Ex vivo regulation of adrenal cortical cell steroid and protein synthesis, in response to adrenocorticotropic hormone stimulation, by the ginkgo biloba extract EGb 761 and isolated ginkgolide B. Endocrinology 138 (12), 5415–5426.

Amri, H., Drieu, K., Papadopoulos, V., 2003. Transcriptional suppression of the adrenal cortical peripheral-type benzodiazepine receptor gene and inhibition of steroid synthesis by ginkgolide B. Biochem. Pharmacol. 65 (5), 717–729.

Barrett, T., Troup, D.B., Wilhite, S.E., et al., 2009. NCBI GEO: archive for high-throughput functional genomic data. Nucleic Acids Res. 37 (Database issue), D885–D890.

Baumans, V., 2004. Use of animals in experimental research: an ethical dilemma? Gene Ther. 11 (Suppl. 1), S64–S66.

Chen, T.R., Dorotinsky, C., Macy, M., et al., 1989. Cell identity resolved. Nature 340 (6229), 106.

Chin, L., Gray, J.W., 2008. Translating insights from the cancer genome into clinical practice. Nature 452 (7187), 553–563.

Cho, W.C., 2007. Application of proteomics in Chinese medicine research. Am. J. Chin. Med. 35 (6), 911–922.

Churchill, G.A., 2002. Fundamentals of experimental design for cDNA microarrays. Nat. Genet. 32 (Suppl.), 490–495.

Clamp, M., Fry, B., Kamal, M., et al., 2007. Distinguishing protein-coding and noncoding genes in the human genome. Proc. Natl. Acad. Sci. U. S. A. 104 (49), 19428–19433.

Clarke, J.D., Zhu, T., 2006. Microarray analysis of the transcriptome as a stepping stone towards understanding biological systems: practical considerations and perspectives. Plant J. 45 (4), 630–650.

Crawford, C.C., Sparter, A.G., Jonas, W.B., 2003. A systematic review of the quality of research on hands-on and distance healing: clinical and laboratory studies. Altern. Ther. Health Med. 9 (Suppl.), A96–A104.

DeKosky, S.T., Williamson, J.D., Fitzpatrick, A.L., et al., 2008. Ginkgo biloba for prevention of dementia: a randomized controlled trial. JAMA 300 (19), 2253–2262.

Dirks, W.G., MacLeod, R.A., Drexler, H.G., 1999. ECV304 (endothelial) is really T24 (bladder carcinoma): cell line cross-contamination at source. In Vitro Cell Dev. Biol. Anim. 35 (10), 558–559.

Dobbin, K.K., Zhao, Y., Simon, R.M., 2008. How large a training set is needed to develop a classifier for microarray data? Clin. Cancer Res. 14 (1), 108–114.

Fonnebo, V., Grimsgaard, S., Walach, H., et al., 2007. Researching complementary and alternative treatments – the gatekeepers are not at home. BMC Med. Res. Methodol. 7, 7.

Gao, Y.Z., Guo, S.Y., Yin, Q.Z., et al., 2007. An individual variation study of electroacupuncture analgesia in rats using microarray. Am. J. Chin. Med. 35 (5), 767–778.

Giordano, J., Garcia, M.K., Boatwright, D., et al., 2003. Complementary and alternative medicine in mainstream public health: a role for research in fostering integration. J. Altern. Complement. Med. 9 (3), 441–445.

Gordon, J.S., 2002. New White House report. Commission supports scientific research on CAM. Health Forum J. 45 (3), 33.

Guo, P., Ma, Z.C., Li, Y.F., et al., 2004. [Effects of siwu tang on protein expression of bone marrow of blood deficiency mice induced by irradiation.]. Zhongguo Zhong Yao Za Zhi 29 (9), 893–896.

Hagerman, A.E., Butler, L.G., 1981. The specificity of proanthocyanidin-protein interactions. J. Biol. Chem. 256 (9), 4494–4497.

Hammer, K.D., Hillwig, M.L., Neighbors, J.D., et al., 2008. Pseudohypericin is necessary for the light-activated inhibition of prostaglandin E_2 pathways by a 4 component system mimicking an *Hypericum perforatum* fraction. Phytochemistry 69 (12), 2354–2362.

Hartmann, O., 2005. Quality control for microarray experiments. Methods Inf. Med. 44 (3), 408–413.

Hayasaki, T., Sakurai, M., Hayashi, T., et al., 2007. Analysis of pharmacological effect and molecular mechanisms of a traditional herbal medicine by global gene expression analysis: an exploratory study. J. Clin. Pharm. Ther. 32 (3), 247–252.

Higuchi, A., Yamada, H., Yamada, E., et al., 2008. Hypericin inhibits pathological retinal neovascularization in a mouse model of oxygen-induced retinopathy. Mol. Vis. 14, 249–254.

Hintz, K.J., Yount, G.L., Kadar, I., et al., 2003. Bioenergy definitions and research guidelines. Altern. Ther. Health Med. 9 (Suppl. 3), A13–A30.

Holst, S., Lund, I., Petersson, M., et al., 2005. Massage-like stroking influences plasma levels of gastrointestinal hormones, including insulin and increases weight gain in male rats. Auton. Neurosci. 120 (1–2), 73–79.

Hudson, J., Altamirano, M., 2006. The application of DNA micro-arrays (gene arrays) to the study of herbal medicines. J. Ethnopharmacol. 108 (1), 2–15.

Ivetic, V., Popovic, M., Naumovic, N., et al., 2008. The effect of ginkgo biloba (EGb 761) on epileptic activity in rabbits. Molecules 13 (10), 2509–2520.

Jacobs, J., Jimenez, L.M., Malthouse, S., et al., 2000. Homeopathic treatment of acute childhood diarrhea: results from a clinical trial in Nepal. J. Altern. Complement. Med. (New York, NY) 6 (2), 131–139.

Jacobs, J., Guthrie, B.L., Montes, G.A., et al., 2006. Homeopathic combination remedy in the treatment of acute childhood diarrhea in Honduras. J. Altern. Complement Med. (New York, NY) 12 (8), 723–732.

Jonas, W.B., Crawford, C.C., 2002. Healing, Intention and Energy Medicine. Churchill Livingstone.

Jonas, W.B., 2005. Building an evidence house: challenges and solutions to research in complementary and alternative medicine. Forsch. Komplementarmed. Klass. Naturheilkd. 12 (3), 159–167.

Jonas, W.B., Crawford, C.C., 2003. Science and spiritual healing: a critical review of spiritual healing, 'energy' medicine and intentionality. Altern. Ther. Health Med. 9 (2), 56–61.

Kasper, S., Anghelescu, I.G., Szegedi, A., et al., 2006. Superior efficacy of St John's wort extract WS 5570 compared to placebo in patients with major depression: a randomized, double-blind, placebo-controlled, multi-center trial [ISRCTN77277298]. BMC Med. 4, 14.

Kasper, S., Gastpar, M., Muller, W.E., et al., 2008. Efficacy of St. John's wort extract WS 5570 in acute treatment of mild depression: a reanalysis of data from controlled clinical trials. Eur. Arch. Psychiatry Clin. Neurosci. 258 (1), 59–63.

Kunin, V., Copeland, A., Lapidus, A., et al., 2008. A bioinformatician's guide to metagenomics. Microbiol. Mol. Biol. Rev. 72 (4), 557–578. Table of Contents.

Kurakin, A., 2005. Self-organization vs Watchmaker: stochastic gene expression and cell differentiation. Dev. Genes. Evol. 215 (1), 46–52.

Kurakin, A., 2007. Self-organization versus Watchmaker: ambiguity of molecular recognition and design charts of cellular circuitry. J. Mol. Recognit. 20 (4), 205–214.

Lauber, W.M., Carroll, J.A., Dufield, D.R., et al., 2001. Mass spectrometry compatibility of two-dimensional gel protein stains. Electrophoresis 22 (5), 906–918.

Ledford, H., 2008. Drug markers questioned. Nature 452 (7187), 510–511.

Lee, C.H., Mo, J.H., Shim, S.H., et al., 2008. Effect of ginkgo biloba and dexamethasone in the treatment of 3-methylindole-induced anosmia mouse model. Am. J. Rhinol. 22 (3), 292–296.

Lee, S.S., Mudaliar, A., 2009. Medicine. Racing forward: the Genomics and Personalized Medicine Act. Science 323 (5912), 342.

Li, S.S., 2007. Commentary – the proteomics: a new tool for Chinese medicine research. Am. J. Chin. Med. 35 (6), 923–928.

Li, A., Lao, L., Wang, Y., et al., 2008. Electroacupuncture activates corticotrophin-releasing hormone-containing neurons in the paraventricular nucleus of the hypothalammus to alleviate edema in a rat model of inflammation. BMC Complement. Altern. Med. 8, 20.

Linde, K., Jonas, W.B., Melchart, D., et al., 1994. Critical review and meta-analysis of serial agitated dilutions in experimental toxicology. Hum. Exp. Toxicol. 13 (7), 481–492.

Lu, H.M., Liang, Y.Z., Wu, X.J., et al., 2006. Tentative fingerprint-efficacy study of *Houttuynia cordata* injection in quality control of traditional Chinese medicine. Chem. Pharm. Bull. (Tokyo) 54 (5), 725–730.

Lum, J.H., Fung, K.L., Cheung, P.Y., et al., 2002. Proteome of Oriental ginseng Panax ginseng C. A. Meyer and the potential to use it as an identification tool. Proteomics 2 (9), 1123–1130.

Lund, I., Lundeberg, T., Kurosawa, M., et al., 1999. Sensory stimulation (massage) reduces blood pressure in unanaesthetized rats. J. Auton. Nerv. Syst. 78 (1), 30–37.

Lund, I., Ge, Y., Yu, L.C., et al., 2002. Repeated massage-like stimulation induces long-term effects on nociception: contribution of oxytocinergic mechanisms. Eur. J. Neurosci. 16 (2), 330–338.

Marcus, W.L., 2005. Editorial: how to evaluate folk remedy data for human use: two approaches. J. Environ. Pathol. Toxicol. Oncol. 24 (3), 145–147.

Masters, J.R., Bedford, P., Kearney, A., et al., 1988. Bladder cancer cell line cross-contamination: identification using a locus-specific minisatellite probe. Br. J. Cancer 57 (3), 284–286.

McKenna, D.J., Jones, K., Hughes, K., 2001. Efficacy, safety and use of ginkgo biloba in clinical and preclinical applications. Altern. Ther. Health Med. 7 (5), 70–86 8–90.

Meyer, N., Penn, L.Z., 2008. Reflecting on 25 years with MYC. Nat. Rev. Cancer 8 (12), 976–990.

Miller, S., Stagl, J., Wallerstedt, D.B., et al., 2008. Botanicals used in complementary and alternative medicine treatment of cancer: clinical science and future perspectives. Expert. Opin. Investig. Drugs 17 (9), 1353–1364.

Moffett, J.R., Arun, P., Namboodiri, M.A., 2006. Laboratory research in homeopathy: con. Integr. Cancer Ther. 5 (4), 333–342.

NCCAM Interim Policy, 2005. Biologically Active Agents Used in Complementary and Alternative Medicine (CAM) and Placebo Materials. http://grantsnihgov/grants/guide/notice-files/NOT-AT-05–003html.

Neild, G.H., Foxall, P.J., Lindon, J.C., et al., 1997. Uroscopy in the 21st century: high-field NMR spectroscopy. Nephrol. Dial Transplant. 12 (3), 404–417.

Pene, F., Courtine, E., Cariou, A., et al., 2009. Toward theragnostics. Crit. Care Med. 37 (Suppl. 1), S50–S58.

Pontzer, C., Johnson, L., 2007. Omics and variable responses to CAM: Secondary analysis of CAM clinical trials. NCCAM publications. www.nih.gov.

Pretner, E., Amri, H., Li, W., et al., 2006. Cancer-related overexpression of the peripheral-type benzodiazepine receptor and cytostatic anticancer effects of Ginkgo biloba extract (EGb 761). Anticancer Res. 26 (1A), 9–22.

Raymond, F., Metairon, S., Borner, R., et al., 2006. Automated target preparation for microarray-based gene expression analysis. Anal. Chem. 78 (18), 6299–6305.

Sawyers, C.L., 2008. The cancer biomarker problem. Nature 452 (7187), 548–552.

Shanaiah, N., Zhang, S., Desilva, M.A., et al., 2008. NMR-based metabolomics for biomarker discovery. In: Wang, F. (Ed.), Biomarker Methods in Drug Discovery and Development. Humana Press, New Jersey, pp. 341–368.

Shi, L., Reid, L.H., Jones, W.D., et al., 2006. The MicroArray Quality Control (MAQC) project shows inter- and intraplatform reproducibility of gene expression measurements. Nat. Biotechnol. 24 (9), 1151–1161.

Sung, H.J., Kim, Y.S., Kim, I.S., et al., 2004. Proteomic analysis of differential protein expression in neuropathic pain and electroacupuncture treatment models. Proteomics 4 (9), 2805–2813.

Tiller, W.A., 1997. Science and human transformation: subtle energies, intentionality and consciousness. Pavior, Walnut Creek, California.

van der Greef, J., McBurney, R.N., 2005. Innovation: Rescuing drug discovery: in vivo systems pathology and systems pharmacology. Nat. Rev. Drug Discov. 4 (12), 961–967.

Ventura, C., 2005. CAM and cell fate targeting: molecular and energetic insights into cell growth and differentiation. Evid. Based Complement. Alternat. Med. 2 (3), 277–283.

Verhoef, M.J., Rose, M.S., White, M., et al., 2008. Declining conventional cancer treatment and using complementary and alternative medicine: a problem or a challenge? Curr. Oncol. 15 (Suppl. 2), 101s–106s.

Verpoorte, R., Crommelin, D., Danhof, M., et al., 2009. Commentary: 'A systems view on the future of medicine: Inspiration from Chinese medicine?' J. Ethnopharmacol. 121 (3), 479–481.

Wei, C., Li, J., Bumgarner, R.E., 2004. Sample size for detecting differentially expressed genes in microarray experiments. BMC Genomics 5 (1), 87.

White House Commission on CAM, 2002. http://wwwwhccamphhsgov/.

Wu, Y.Z., Li, S.Q., Zu, X.G., et al., 2008. Ginkgo biloba extract improves coronary artery circulation in patients with coronary artery disease: contribution of plasma nitric oxide and endothelin-1. Phytother. Res. 22 (6), 734–739.

Yang, S.Y., Kim, H.K., Lefeber, A.W., et al., 2006. Application of two-dimensional nuclear magnetic resonance spectroscopy to quality control of ginseng commercial products. Planta Med. 72 (4), 364–369.

Yang, Y., Zhu, M., Wu, L., et al., 2008. Assessment of data processing to improve reliability of microarray experiments using genomic DNA reference. BMC Genomics 9 (Suppl. 2), S5.

Yang, Y., Adelstein, S.J., Kassis, A.I., 2009. Target discovery from data mining approaches. Drug Discov. Today.

Yount, G., Solfvin, J., Moore, D., et al., 2004. In vitro test of external Qigong. BMC Complement. Altern. Med. 4, 5.

Yu, T., Tsai, H.L., Hwang, M.L., 2003. Suppressing tumor progression of in vitro prostate cancer cells by emitted psychosomatic power through Zen meditation. Am. J. Chin. Med. 31 (3), 499–507.

Yuan, R., Lin, Y., 2000. Traditional Chinese medicine: an approach to scientific proof and clinical validation. Pharmacol. Ther. 86 (2), 191–198.

Zhang, F., Pasumarthi, K.B., 2008. Embryonic stem cell transplantation: promise and progress in the treatment of heart disease. BioDrugs 22 (6), 361–374.

Randomized controlled trials

5

Claudia M. Witt • George T. Lewith

CHAPTER CONTENTS

INTRODUCTION

We plan to discuss the principles and concepts that underpin randomized controlled trials (RCTs). This research methodology can be employed in a number of different contexts but RCTs are usually used in clinical settings. A trial, holding other factors constant, can be run to compare performance about a number of criteria, such as: 'which treatment works better than a placebo?' or 'which device is most energy-efficient?' The fundamental principles of RCTs remain the same in whichever context they are applied and this chapter aims to outline the steps that are important in setting up an RCT and

DOI: 10.1016/B978-0-443-06956-7.00005-7

meeting the requirements of a research protocol. RCTs allow us to answer very specific questions. They set out to evaluate the effect of a particular treatment or strategy in a population where an intervention is introduced, often by comparing the outcome with a control group where no intervention, or a standard intervention, may have been used. The population must be well defined and carefully selected.

A number of implicit assumptions underpin the RCT as follows (adapted from Vickers et al. 1997):

- We have an incomplete understanding of the world and knowledge evolves and develops. It is contingent and never definitive.
- Research methods evolve and change as we continue to learn about the world. Thus any trial will be as good as we can make it at the time and the knowledge gained is likely to be modest and incremental.
- Logically, cause precedes effect, or put another way, *A* leads to *B*.
- Beliefs cannot influence random events.
- In a well-designed study, the researcher's beliefs cannot influence the outcome.
- Good research aims to minimize the effects of bias, chance variation and confounding.
- Research that investigates whether treatments do more good than harm must be a priority.

These tenets lead to the claim that the RCT provides the 'gold standard' for research. It is the best means of attributing real cause and effect and therefore adds to our stock of knowledge. Not all researchers necessarily believe all of these, but they provide a sound framework for conducting a RCT.

THE RESEARCH QUESTION

An RCT is challenging and researchers contemplating a trial must ask themselves:

- What is a good question?
- How can questions be matched to the research design?
- What is the best strategic approach to the research?
- How can we interpret the results appropriately?

The first prerequisite for refining a research question is to carry out a thorough literature search. A literature search is an iterative and developmental process that will contribute directly and indirectly to protocol development. It will help to identify whether the question one wants to ask has already been asked and also point out the strengths and weaknesses of previous research in addressing and answering the question.

A question is likely to be answerable if it is explicit, focused and feasible. In other words, it should be possible to link the effect of an intervention explicitly to a specific outcome. The research should be focused. There should be a very clear, simple primary question and a research method that will provide an answer – the trick is not to ask too many primary questions simultaneously, even in a complex study. If there are multiple questions, then the primary research question must be given priority. The primary research question must be framed so that it is both possible

Table 5.1 ***Different types of research questions and their suitability for randomized controlled trials (RCT)***

Category of question	Examples	Suitable for RCT
Attributing cause and clinical effect	Does homeopathically prepared grass pollen reduce symptoms of hayfever more than a non-active (placebo) treatment?	Y
	Is polypharmacy more effective than a single-remedy approach in the homeopathic treatment of chronic hayfever?	Y
What happens in clinical practice?	What is the cost-effectiveness of adding homeopathic treatment to a standard care package in hayfever?	Y
	What are the patterns of cross-referral between conventional and CAM practitioners in a multidisciplinary pain clinic?	N
	How common are serious neurological complications following chiropractic cervical manipulation?	N
What do people do?	How many people visit practitioners of CAM each year?	N
	What do patients tell their primary care physician about usage of CAM?	N
	How many nurses practice complementary medicine?	N
What do people believe and how do they explain it?	What do nurses believe about therapeutic touch?	N
	What is the patient's experience of the acupuncture consultation?	Y
By what mechanisms does a therapy work?	What are the effects of needling the Hoku point on the production of endogenous opiates?	Y
Does something proposed in a therapy actually exist?	Does peppermint oil reduce histamine-induced contractions of tracheal smooth muscle?	Y
	Does homeopathically prepared copper ameliorate the effects of copper poisoning in a plant model?	Y
Is a diagnostic or prognostic test accurate?	How sensitive and specific is detection of gallbladder disease by examining photos of the iris?	N
	Is tongue diagnosis reliable?	N

Reproduced from Vickers et al. (1997).

and practical to answer the question. Some examples of questions are given in Table 5.1.

The findings must be achievable within a reasonable period of time and within the bounds of the scientific and financial resources available. Randomization is designed to even out all the things we 'don't know' about the groups we are comparing. These factors may allow for misinterpretation of the study's findings and they are usually considered to be 'confounding factors'. Randomization also involves minimizing 'bias': if either confounding factors or biases are known to the researcher, then they should be introduced into the study protocol at an early stage and may result in possibly modifying the research question or trial methodology, thus allowing an appropriate trial design to emerge.

CONFIRMATORY AND EXPLORATORY STUDIES

In effect RCTs are mainly used to test a predefined hypothesis. When planning a confirmatory trial it is helpful to do a pilot trial with the aim of generating a hypothesis and to test the planned outcome measures and the study protocol for feasibility. In addition, pilot studies can be helpful in providing an idea of the effect size of the intervention and this in turn will inform the sample size for any larger, more definitive study. In these pilot trials statistics are used on an exploratory basis. The present published literature suggests that in CAM research confirmatory studies are often done without pilot trials and quite a large proportion of the confirmatory (definitive) studies seem like pilot studies and are too small to have enough power to detect a significant difference between groups. The reasons for this might be limited financial resources for CAM research and the fact that CAM has fewer qualified and experienced researchers than conventional medical research environments.

When planning a study it is important to clarify the study in more detail by considering the following aspects (Chow & Liu 2004):

- What aspects of the intervention are being studied?
- Is it important to investigate other issues that may have an impact on the intervention?
- Which control(s) or placebos might be used or considered?

Developing a hypothesis is an important issue when planning these studies. A hypothesis always consists of a null hypothesis (H_0) which assumes no effect and an alternative hypothesis (H_A) which holds the null hypothesis not to be true and consequently assumes an effect. The alternative hypothesis is more directly connected to the specific research question.

The aim of confirmatory studies is to answer research questions based on the hypothesis proposed by the researcher. Therefore, posing an adequate and answerable research question is essential as a clear, well-researched, thoughtful and specific question based on appropriate study design has a reasonable chance of providing a valid answer. One of the main reasons (other than failure to recruit) why the majority of research proposals are either unclear or fail to provide a useful answer is that the initial research question itself lacks clarity. The core elements of a precise research question for a confirmatory RCT can be summarized by PICO (patients, intervention, control intervention, outcome = primary endpoint; see example in Figure 5.1). Using PICO can be very helpful in developing your hypothesis.

(P) Patients: patients suffering from chronic low back pain
(I) Intervention: acupuncture treatment
(C) Control: patients receiving conventional non steroidal anti inflammatory drug (Diclofenac)
(O) Outcome: average pain intensity during the last 7 days on a visual analogue scale
Research question: 'Is acupuncture (I) more effective than the pain killer diclofenac (C) for pain reduction measured on a visual analogue scale (O) for treating patients with chronic low back pain (P)?'

FIGURE 5.1 An example of PICO (patients, intervention, control intervention, outcome).

STUDY HYPOTHESIS AND HYPOTHESIS TESTING

The research question and the subsequent hypothesis build the basis for hypothesis testing. If the null hypothesis can be rejected based on a predefined significance level (e.g. 5% or 1%), the alternative hypothesis will be accepted. This means that, from the example shown in Figure 5.1, if there is a significant difference on the visual analogue scale ($P < 0.05$) between the acupuncture and the diclofenac group, the null hypothesis (H_0: acupuncture = diclofenac) can be rejected and the alternative hypothesis (H_A: acupuncture ≠ diclofenac) is applicable.

If there is no significant difference between both groups this does not necessarily mean that the null hypothesis is true as there may simply not be enough evidence to reject it. For example, if the sample size is too small the study may be underpowered. The chance of the study providing a statistically significant outcome is based on assuming that a 5% (or less) chance of this event occurring randomly is significant. This could mean that, with a *P*-value of 0.04 (a 4% chance of this happening randomly), the null hypothesis would be rejected, whereas with a *P*-value of 0.06 (a 6% chance of this happening randomly) there would not be enough evidence to reject the null hypothesis. The choice of a significance level of 5% is arbitrary but applicable throughout biological science and therefore the outcome of the study needs to be interpreted with caution, particularly with respect to the number of people entered. The greater sample size or number of people entered into the study, the more statistical 'power' it has and the more its statistical conclusions can be 'trusted'.

However a significant difference between groups does not relate to the clinical importance of this finding as the statistical significance depends to a large extent on the sample size (number of people) and the variability of the condition within the study. Accordingly a large study might find a small but clinically unimportant difference between treatments, which is highly significant. Equally, a small study with few people might find a large difference that could be clinically important. Clinical importance describes a difference between two treatments that has a relevant effect size which is noticeable for, and valuable to, a patient with that condition.

Most randomized controlled studies evaluate if one intervention is superior to another. This is generally the case for treatment comparisons with a waiting list or a placebo intervention as controls. However, for some comparisons we test for similarity between two treatments (equivalence) or non-inferiority, but these equivalence studies, which include both non-inferiority and non-superiority trials, are rare in CAM. A non-inferiority hypothesis

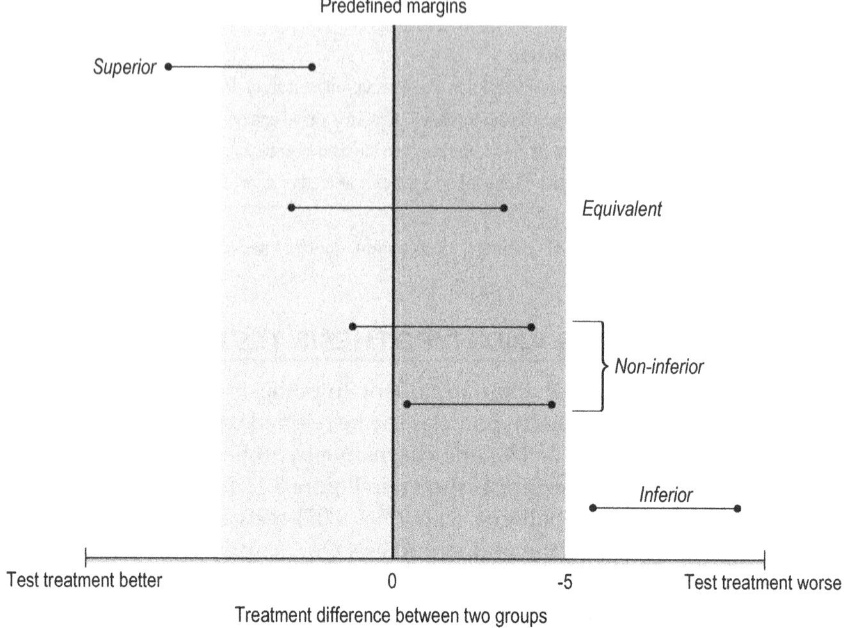

FIGURE 5.2 Confidence intervals for equivalence and non-inferiority trials.

could, however, be very useful when comparing a CAM treatment with a conventional treatment. Non-inferiority or equivalence trials have methodological features that differ from superiority trials. In an equivalence trial, the null and alternative hypotheses are reversed. This means the null hypothesis is that treatment *A* is different from treatment *B*, whereas the alternative hypothesis is that there is no difference between the treatments.

In addition the effect size of the reference treatment has to be known and the margin for the non-inferiority has to be predefined for the power calculation and subsequent sample size. This margin represents the smallest value for a clinically relevant effect and outcomes within this margin are defined as non-inferior (Piaggio et al. 2006). The interpretation of the results depends on where the confidence interval lies relative to both the margin of non-inferiority and the null effect. For two-sided evidence (equivalence trials) two margins are needed (one above zero and one below) (Figure 5.2).

DETERMINING THE SAMPLE SIZE

When planning a study probably the most important question is how many patients are needed to have enough statistical power to detect a clinically meaningful difference between the treatment groups. If the budget is limited or the medical conditions allow only a small number of patients to be included in the study, the study may fail to reach adequate power and could be of very limited value. An appropriate sample size is essential for a worthwhile study. The sample size calculation requires that the hypothesis should be clearly stated and a valid design and appropriate test statistics should be used. In hypothesis testing two errors can occur: the type I error (α) takes place when the null hypothesis is rejected although it was true and the type II error (β) is when the null hypothesis is not rejected when it was false. The probability of making a type I error is called the level of significance whereas the type II error is called power. A type I error is usually considered to be the most important of the two items this approach primarily tries to control for. To determine the sample size the investigator should provide the following information:

- the significance level
- the power
- a clinically meaningful difference
- information about the standard deviation.

In clinical studies a significance level of 5% is usually chosen to reflect 95% confidence in the conclusions and usually a power of 80% or 90% is used in conjunction with this. Estimating a clinically meaningful difference and the standard deviation for the planned trial is often difficult, especially for CAM treatments, where there may be no previous data for the outcome for the intervention being evaluated. If the expected difference is large, fewer patients will be needed than if the expected difference is small. An important influence on the sample size is the variability of the patient outcomes for the primary outcome. If a high standard deviation is expected (lots of variability) more patients are needed to detect a significant difference between treatments than if the patient outcomes are more homogeneous.

Many CAM studies are conducted with small research budgets and consequently small sample sizes; therefore the sample size which would detect a significant difference between treatment groups may not be achieved. From a methodological perspective it is bad science to perform an underpowered study. If the budget is not sufficient to perform a trial of adequate size it is better to do no study, unless it is a pilot.

THE ESSENTIAL ELEMENTS OF A RANDOMIZED CONTROLLED TRIAL

The RCT is the most reliable study design to detect whether the difference in the outcomes of two or more interventions is caused by a specific treatment. In effect it is the 'gold standard' for clinical research. With the aim for control for baseline differences, patients are allocated at random to receive one of several interventions. In addition, the treatment group is compared to at least one control group. Different control groups exist and the choice of control depends on the research question (Table 5.2). Placebo-controlled trials only tell us if the treatment is better than a placebo and we always need more information that that to inform clinical practice, where many treatments may be available for one condition.

Randomized trials can be open or blinded but it depends on the specific intervention as to which activities within a trial can be realistically blinded. Although RCTs are relatively straightforward, a lot of methodological errors have occurred in the past and no doubt will continue to appear in future

Table 5.2 *Control groups according to the research question*	
Research question	**Adequate control group**
Is the treatment effect specific?	Placebo
Is the treatment superior to no treatment?	Waiting list control
Is the treatment superior (or non-inferior) to standard therapy?	Standard treatment
Is the treatment superior (or non-inferior) to another treatment?	Other treatment
Is the treatment in addition to usual care superior to usual care alone?	Usual care

literature. Guidelines for performing RCTs have been developed to improve their quality. These include good clinical practice, which regulates the functions and processes or the reporting (Altman et al. 2001) in RCTs as well as the inclusion of a standard reporting system for trial recruitment and compliance (Moher et al. 2001). Some of the CAMs that may be evaluated also have specific reporting requirements that are associated with Consolidated Standards of Reporting Trials (CONSORT); this includes Standards for Reporting Interventions in Controlled Trials of Acupuncture (STRICTA) (MacPherson et al. 2001) and for homeopathy RedHot (Dean 2006). These standards are of great importance and improve the quality of RCTs but they require more resources and funding in order to perform the RCT.

RANDOMIZATION

Randomization is usually used to control conscious and unconscious bias as well as any unknown confounders in the allocation of patients to treatment groups. The purpose is to generate comparable patient groups with similar baseline characteristics. It is vital that the random allocation is performed properly and described in detail in the methodology, as inadequate or insecure randomization can be associated with very biased and usually positive findings (Shulz et al. 1995).

There are many examples where randomization is insufficiently performed and reported (Altman et al. 2001).

In order to avoid this criticism in planning a study the following issues need to be considered:

- Is randomization on patient or cluster level?
- How should the treatment groups be distributed (equal or unequal numbers)?
- Should you employ simple randomization or restricted randomization (blocking, stratification)?
- How will the randomization list be generated?
- How will the procedure operate so that it is appropriately concealed?

For instance, cluster randomization is used when whole social groups (families) or GP practices have to be assigned to different intervention groups. However, most trials use patient-level randomization and assignment is performed independently for each patient. In a two-armed trial with a 1:1 ratio the chance of a patient receiving either verum or control is 50%. RCTs with more arms (e.g. verum, control 1 and control 2) can also involve equal numbers in each group; for example in a three-armed trial with a 1:1:1 ratio the probability to be assigned to one of the groups is 33%. Unequal randomization with a higher chance of being assigned to the verum group can be helpful in an environment where the acceptance of the randomization process is poor from the patient's or practitioner's perspective. Patients with an interest in CAM often have clear preferences for CAM and this can be a major influence on their decision to participate in a randomized study. Therefore a 2:1 opportunity to receive their preferred treatment could improve the acceptability of randomization and improve recruitment and retention for the study. Ethics (e.g. in cancer) can also be an argument for unequal randomization. However, unequal randomization has disadvantages as the study may lose statistical power and blocking can be compromised, so it should only be used if there are very important reasons for doing so.

Simple or complete randomization is performed when a single random list is used and each patient is randomized regardless of the recruiting study centre and patient characteristics. In small trials or multicentre trials this can result in imbalances of group size and patient characteristics between the groups, but procedures for managing and restricting randomization help to solve this problem. The most frequently used methods are blocking and stratification. Both can be predefined and taken into account when generating the randomization list. Block randomization is used to ensure that the numbers of patients in the groups are comparable. In a two-armed trial with a randomization ratio of 1:1 and a block size of eight, four patients will be randomized into the verum and the other four into the control group. One important problem of blocked randomization is that allocation becomes predictable if the size of the blocks is known by the person who assigns and treats the patient, so this information must remain secure. This can be solved either by variable block size or blinding the study personnel to the block size. Stratified randomization is used to ensure that groups are comparable for important characteristics such as the provider of the treatment or the disease stage. This is done by doing separate randomization for 'strata' such as study centres or asthma staging. Stratification requires blocking within the 'strata', otherwise it too can become ineffective (Altman et al. 2001). Blocking and randomization should be used carefully. Figure 5.3 provides an example for stratification of study centres and using a variable block design.

One can adjust the probability of assignment of new patients to treatments during the study (Chow & Liu 2004). This is called adaptive randomization. Patient outcomes can be used as they become available to adjust the randomization assignment for future patients, perhaps assigning more of them to the 'better, more effective treatment'. This allows one to improve expected patient outcomes during the experiment, while still being able to utilize the best available statistical decisions in a timely fashion. This type of randomization does not require the randomization list to be generated before the study starts.

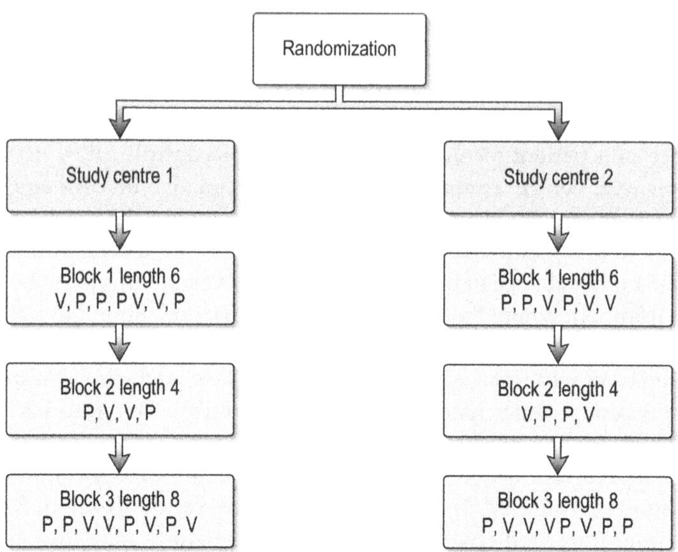

FIGURE 5.3 Randomization with stratification for centres and variable block length. V, verum; P, placebo.

The random assignment is generated directly when the current patient is randomized, usually by a computer-based algorithm.

There are many ways to generate a random list prior to study start (Jadad & Enkin 2007). Older methods such as flipping a coin or throwing dice have been replaced by a number of validated software packages (e.g. SPSS, SAS, STATA) which ensure the quality and rigour of the random sequence.

Empirical investigations have shown that concealment is the most critical element of randomization (Schulz 1995). It is absolutely essential to ensure a concealed randomization procedure or the study loses rigour. The study personnel must not be able to predict the group to which a participant will be allocated and they should not be in a position to modify this allocation. The ideal strategy for concealment depends on the intervention. In drug trials identically packaged, consecutively numbered drug containers can be used based on the randomization list. For other interventions, central randomization, using a telephone hotline or an online database, is suitable. The physician who includes a patient contacts an external clinical trial unit by phone or via the web and they inform the physician about the group allocation if the trial is single-blind. In a double-blind trial neither the physician nor the patient should know which intervention the patients get. They might get the group code or in drug trials only the code number for the blinded drug containers.

If online databases are used, a safer approach is combining two independent databases (Vickers 2006) to ensure concealment. One database is used to register the new patient. The information is then forwarded to a second database which is only accessed by an independent person and the information is then sent to the appropriate person to ensure the patient has the correct, randomized treatment. In small studies where setting up an online database or a central telephone hotline is too complex and expensive, sequentially numbered, opaque, sealed envelopes can be used. However, here it should be ensured that the envelopes really are opaque and that they are sealed so that cheating is impossible.

BLINDING

Randomization only ensures that patients in the groups are comparable for baseline characteristics, thus avoiding unknown confounders that may influence outcome, but will then be equally distributed to all the interventions in the study. This is vital and allows us to avoid bias. If patients were randomized to a group for which they had no preference they might be disappointed. This could influence how they rate the treatment outcome or result in more co-interventions. The same can occur in the provider rating; if they have special interest in one of the treatments their bias can influence the outcome. If a study does not use blinding it is classified as an open-label study, with all the disadvantages and bias that entails.

A single-blind trial is a study in which either the patient or the provider is unaware of the assignment of the patient. In reality it is mainly the patient who is blind. In a double-blind trial neither the patient nor the provider is aware of the patient's treatment assignment. Sometimes trials are described as double-blind if patients and outcome assessors (not the provider) are blinded and this can be very misleading. Triple- and quadruple-blind trials are possible when, in addition to patients and providers, the outcome assessors and statisticians are blinded. To minimize potential biases treatment providers, patients and outcome assessors and even the statisticians should be blinded for the group allocation before the analysis is completed. This is possible in most pharmaceutical research; however if two clearly distinguishable treatments are compared patients and providers cannot be blinded. This occurs when comparing non-pharmacological intervention such as acupuncture or relaxation exercises with conventional treatment.

The issue of placebo is also much more complex and involved in CAM than it is in a simple drug trial; it is always more difficult to provide a real and convincing placebo which imitates the smell and the taste of a herbal medicine product or the visual and sensory effect of an acupuncture needle (Dube et al. 2007). However, even in CAM, when the verum and the placebo are indistinguishable, blinding might influence the providers' treatment decisions. This is often discussed as a problem for trials of individualized homeopathy. In this type of homeopathy the provider prescribes an individual homeopathic remedy which should cover a whole range of symptoms for an individual patient (Witt et al. 2005). An option for the follow-up visits is usually to change the homeopathic remedy if no improvement is reported by the patient. This decision is based on an additional patient consultation, which can easily be influenced by the uncertainty of the provider (the homeopath) not knowing if there is no effect because the patient was allocated to the placebo group or whether the lack of response is due to the prescription of the wrong homeopathic remedy.

A vitally important factor for the success of blinding is to maintain it throughout the entire course of the trial. To assess if blinding is maintained throughout the study, patients, providers and assessors should be asked to guess the group allocation of each patient and the frequency of correct guesses can be compared between groups. However, if the verum is much more effective than the placebo, due to the effect of treatment, unblinding may happen. Asking these questions about blinding at an earlier stage does not solve the problem. We want to know if the patients were blinded at the time point when the primary outcome was assessed.

It is also helpful to assess the credibility of a treatment but this evaluates a slightly different dimension to blinding. Scales like this which have been used by Vincent (1990), are helpful and should be used in the early stages of the treatment.

CONTROLS

In general there are four types of treatment that the patient can receive in the control group (Chow & Liu 2004): (1) placebo; (2) no treatment; (3) other active treatments; and (4) different dose or regime of the verum intervention.

PLACEBO CONTROLS

Placebo is used to detect the assumed specific effect of treatment, for example, in the case of pharmaceutical research, the true pharmacological activity of the active chemical treatments. Shapiro (1964) suggests that 'A placebo is any therapy (or that component of any therapy) that is intentionally or knowingly used for its nonspecific, psychological, therapeutic effect, or that is used for a presumed specific therapeutic effect on a patient, symptom or illness but is without specific activity for the condition being treated [...] The placebo effect is the nonspecific psychological or psycho-physiological therapeutic effect produced by a placebo.' A full chapter in this text is devoted to a deeper understanding of the placebo effect and its implications for CAM research (see Chapter 16).

When using placebo controls in clinical trials, ethical aspects have to be taken into account. The decision to use a placebo control in a trial may be unethical but to some extent this depends on the severity of the disease and available options for conventional treatment. One of the key elements for the success of a placebo-controlled clinical trial is whether a placebo treatment can be made to match the active treatment in all aspects, such as size, colour, coating, texture and taste of a medicine or herbal decoction. This will be more difficult for herbal medicine, especially Chinese herbal medicine, where strong-tasting decoctions are used. It may be simpler for a homeopathic pill but may make the context of the homeopathic consultation very complicated and diminish the context validity or generalizability of homeopathic practice in this environment. For interventions such as massage, yoga and qigong, a true placebo intervention may be almost impossible as we have no real idea about the exact mechanisms involved in these therapies and therefore we cannot realistically design a specific placebo if the active ingredient is unknown. In acupuncture there is still an ongoing discussion as to whether there is an inert placebo intervention that is convincing and can be used in an RCT (see Chapter 11).

NO-TREATMENT CONTROL

A no-treatment group can quantify one part of non-specific effects that includes regression to the mean during the normal course of disease. This can be very helpful when performing studies in CAM interventions such as acupuncture, particularly if the sham-control response rates are high and well described. The response in the no-treatment group will always be lower than in a placebo group so the decision as to whether a no-treatment control group can be used requires both practical and ethical consideration as well as careful reference to the specific research question addressed by the study.

ACTIVE TREATMENT CONTROL

The use of other active treatments as control groups can not only solve ethical problems, but is also helpful in providing data for decision-making in usual care. The active treatment control can be a standard treatment, or at least a treatment which already has a known efficacy. The advantage of this kind of control is that it should have shown superiority over placebo in previous well-designed trials so if the verum treatment is superior to the standard intervention, superiority over placebo might be assumed. However, we have limited evidence for many conventional treatments used in routine conventional medical care, so the choice of the active treatment control should be considered carefully. In spite of this, conventional routine medical care has been used as a control in several acupuncture studies (Vickers et al. 2004; Witt et al. 2006a, b, c, 2008) and can be very helpful in decision-making for health care purchasers who want to select the best, cheapest and safest treatment available. Superiority over placebo cannot be assumed in such a heterogenic active treatment control group so outcomes must be interpreted with caution.

DIFFERENT DOSES OR REGIMES OF THE VERUM INTERVENTION AS CONTROLS

To characterize the dose–response relationship one really needs a phase II study in which different doses or regimes of the verum intervention are used. Phase II studies allow us to identify the minimum effective and the maximum tolerable dose. They are usually four-armed trials which involve three different doses of the intervention and a placebo group, but such studies are very rare in the area of CAM. The type of trial that we have been discussing in this chapter is usually referred to as a phase III clinical trial.

THE INFLUENCE OF EXPECTATION

The influence of patient expectations on outcomes is related to both within-group changes (from baseline to follow-up) and between-group differences (between the 'real' treatment and placebo). These suggestions are supported by two systematic reviews (Crow et al. 1999; Mondloch et al. 2001).

If patients included in a trial have higher expectations of a positive outcome than the 'average' patient then this could result in within-group changes which are larger than in a more representative sample. High expectations might also be associated with high response rates and improved outcomes in the placebo control group. This could result in a ceiling effect, making it more difficult to detect a significant difference between verum and placebo if everyone improves because they expect and believe the treatment will work for them. By pooling data from four acupuncture trials we were able to show a significant association between greater improvement and high outcome expectations (Linde et al. 2007).

In order to account for patient expectations and to relate this to the main outcomes, patient expectations should be assessed at baseline before randomization. A reliable and valid, yet simple, tool for measuring aspects of expectations in clinical trials is still needed. Meanwhile simple questions such as: 'How effective do you consider the treatment in general?' with responses such as 'very effective, effective, slightly effective, not effective, don't know' should be used routinely in trials involving the assessment of chronic pain and other chronic benign conditions where expectation and belief may be important predictors of treatment outcome.

STUDY DESIGNS

PARALLEL GROUP DESIGNS

The most commonly used study design for RCTs is the parallel group design in which each patient receives only one treatment in a randomized fashion. Compared to other designs, such as cross-over designs, a parallel group design is easy to implement, widely accepted and the analysis and interpretation of the results are less complicated. It is also the most appropriate for CAM as we are usually unsure about the duration of any treatment effect so designs like cross-over may result in confusion and carry-over effects when using interventions such as acupuncture. The simplest type of parallel group design is a two-arm study, as illustrated in Figure 5.4.

A parallel group design can have three or four treatment (intervention) or comparison groups and patients can be allocated to the groups in equal or unequal numbers. A run-in period with no active treatment and perhaps an appropriate control can be useful to wash out the effects of previous therapy and encourage compliance (particularly with the trial outcome measures) as well as obtaining baseline data against which to compare posttreatment outcome.

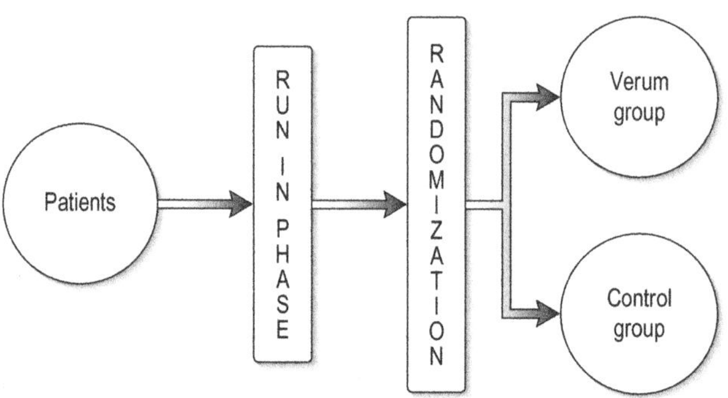

FIGURE 5.4 Two-group parallel design.

CROSS-OVER DESIGNS

A cross-over design is a modified randomized block design where patients receive more than one treatment at different preagreed time periods during the study. It is a complete cross-over design if each group in this design, in a randomized sequence, receives all treatments under investigation. The simplest cross-over design includes a two-group cross and two treatment periods (Figure 5.5).

A cross-over can involve more treatment groups and the allocation to the groups can involve equal or unequal numbers of people.

The advantages of a cross-over design are that it allows within-patient comparison between treatments. Each patient in effect acts as his or her own control, which removes interpatient variability from the comparisons between treatments and provides good unbiased estimates for the difference between treatments (Chow & Liu 2004). To prevent carry-over effects, washout phases can be included in the design but the main problem with CAM treatments is that the washout periods are debatable and unclear for almost all the CAM interventions that have been studied. These designs are almost impossible to interpret if treatment effects are maintained for an indefinite period. Consequently this design is more suitable for drug trials than for interventions such as acupuncture. A good example for a cross-over design in CAM is that of Frei et al. (2005), who investigated the use of homeopathy in children with attention deficit hyperactivity disorder. In this study, patients received verum or placebo for 6 weeks and were then crossed over to receive placebo or verum for a second period of 6 weeks.

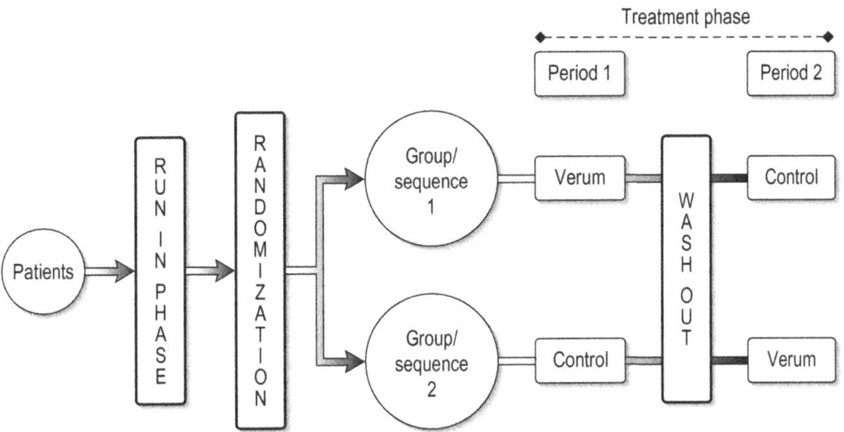

FIGURE 5.5 Cross-over design with two groups and two treatment periods.

GROUP SEQUENTIAL DESIGNS

We may be investigating a treatment that is of possible benefit but may also be harmful to the patients entered. In these situations a group sequential design is valuable as it divides patient entry into a number of equal-sized groups. This allows for some interim analysis and the early identification of adverse reactions so that any decision to stop the trial is based on repeated significance tests of the accumulated data after each group is evaluated (Pocock 1977). These designs are based on sequential testing and other adaptive rules. The literature in this area is huge (Chow & Liu 2004) and the problem of multiple testing has to be taken into account.

PRAGMATIC VERSUS EXPERIMENTAL STUDIES

Pragmatic studies aim to evaluate whether an intervention is effective under the sort of conditions that a patient might find in a clinic. These trials have model validity as far as the intervention is concerned. For instance, an acupuncture or herbal treatment may be adapted to suit some trial conditions in a very rigorous, placebo-controlled experiment and this may not really reflect good clinical practice. The resulting study may be of high scientific quality, but in effect is of little use to clinicians and health care providers, as one may not be able to generalize to the wider population from the results obtained. Pragmatic studies use wide inclusion criteria, allow flexibility in the treatment regimen and often focus on patient-centred outcomes such as quality of life or self-recorded pain (Zwarenstein 2008). Experimental or explanatory studies address whether an intervention works under controlled conditions. These studies typically use placebos or standardized interventions as controls. Experimental studies can have a high internal validity whereas pragmatic studies may have less internal validity but are more generalizable and relevant to clinical practice (see Chapter 1). The external validity of a study depends on the following aspects: (1) study participants; (2) interventions; and (3) outcome measures.

The generalizability of the study results depends on whether the group of study participants is representative of the usual type of patients with this specific condition. In experimental studies homogeneous patient groups are preferred, with the aim of reducing bias and enlarging internal validity. These patients are rarely representative of the people suffering from the disease under investigation, for example elderly patients over 70 years of age often suffer from cardiovascular diseases but because of their comorbidity they are often excluded from experimental studies on cardiovascular drugs. Within the context of health service research and decision-making it makes sense to investigate a treatment in a representative manner and as it is used in routine clinical care (Witt 2009). Therefore if you wished to evaluate whether acupuncture should be reimbursed by health insurance companies it would be better to assess the broad range of acupuncture styles likely to be found in practice instead of using a standardized treatment protocol.

This tension remains unresolved within the context of clinical trials in CAM and indeed conventional medicine; there are many studies in which CAM treatments have been applied in an inadequate manner and without model validity in order to improve rigour, reduce bias or increase feasibility. Such trials are very difficult to interpret and may be very of little value in the context of clinical practice and health care decision-making.

Using patient-centred outcomes should include taking relevant and valid measures that are appropriate to the condition being studied and ideally incorporating follow-up periods which are long enough to provide information about long-term effects. In pragmatic studies more subjective symptom-oriented outcomes such as symptom diaries or disease-specific quality-of-life questionnaires are often used. In contrast, more conventionally structured experimental studies may involve 'hard' outcome parameters such as laboratory measurements, if the condition within the study allows these measures to be usefully employed.

Most CAM trials in chronic benign diseases such as migraine and osteoarthritis have study observation periods of about 6 months at the most. Long-term follow-up in these trials is rare. This is unfortunate as health care providers would ideally like to be able to make thoughtful decisions that take into account the long-term effects of an intervention.

In reality there is often a compromise between internal and external validity in the design of any trial and this is usually and sensibly based on the study or research question. If the aim of the study is to give guidance to health service purchasers, a more population-based and 'pragmatic' approach is needed. If the aim is to develop a new intervention and determine its efficacy over placebo, an experimental study is more likely to produce the most valuable results. As mentioned in Chapter 1, CAM treatments are in general very diverse, widely used and widely available before they are evaluated scientifically. Consequently pragmatic studies can provide helpful information enabling medical decision-making. Ideally it would be best to have information from both experimental and pragmatic studies for all treatments, but this is not usually possible.

ANALYSING RANDOMIZED CONTROLLED TRIALS

STUDY POPULATIONS

There are different types of study populations. The intention-to-treat (ITT) population includes all patients who were randomized at the beginning of the trial with the intention that they should receive one of the study interventions. This means that even data from patients who did not follow the protocol, or who dropped out without receiving any treatment, need to be analyzed. The ITT analysis represents a conservative but widely used statistical approach and enhances the external validity of the study. The per protocol population (PP) represents the other side of this equation and includes only patients who followed the study protocol; this group of people should be predefined before analysing the data. For trials with a superiority hypothesis the ITT analysis is the primary analysis and the PP analysis can be performed as a secondary, but much less convincing, dataset. However in studies that have a non-inferiority hypothesis the converse may be true.

ATTRITION RATES AND MISSING DATA

In studies with longer follow-up periods patients may drop out prematurely or not follow the study protocol, perhaps by not completing the outcome questionnaires. The outcomes for these patients might differ considerably from those remaining in the study. Patients who dropped out might have been non-responders or might have experienced more severe side-effects. It is therefore important to keep attrition rates as low as possible in order to increase the study rigour. There are statistical methods that can reduce the impact of missing data, but these are far from perfect. If the amount of missing data is small, statistical methods are helpful in estimating the impact of the missing data and several such statistical methods exist. The commonest one is the 'last value carried forward'. This means that the values from an earlier measurement are transferred to the following one. However, if a disease is progressive, these values will be positive and a more appropriate method is to use imputation techniques. These substitute a missing data point or a missing component of a data point with some value. Once all missing values have been imputed, the dataset can be analysed using standard techniques for complete data. There are different imputation techniques available (Twisk & de Vente 2002; Donders et al. 2006).

BASELINE DIFFERENCES BETWEEN GROUPS

Randomization does not always generate groups which are comparable for all baseline characteristics. If studies are small baseline differences between groups can often occur just by chance. A treatment is only independently associated with the outcome after all confounders have been taken into account. There is some evidence that the baseline value of the outcome can influence the outcome after treatment (Vickers 2004). Because of this, the use of analysis of covariance (ANCOVA) with the baseline values as a covariate is the most simple recommended analytical approach for all RCTs, even if baseline differences are not found. This method accounts for any variability in baseline values between the two or more groups in the study.

CONCLUSION

This chapter describes the main principles of RCT design, particularly with respect to CAM. RCTs were developed for the pharmaceutical industry, ideally to test the specific effects of drugs. They can usefully be adapted to evaluate a variety of different CAM techniques but this needs to be done thoughtfully and appropriately. The most important issue with respect to the design of an RCT is the research question. If you want to consider an RCT design, do you have a specific question that is best answered through an RCT? The advent of the RCT is both a blessing and a curse; it has certainly improved our understanding of medical evidence, but inevitably it is limited in its scope. Good science and clinical relevance do not always go hand in hand, and attempting to achieve both simultaneously requires clear thinking and the ability to work within a research team.

REFERENCES

Altman, D.G., Schulz, K.F., Moher, D., et al., 2001. The revised CONSORT statement for reporting randomized trials: explanation and elaboration. Ann. Intern. Med. 134 (8), 663–694.

Chow, S.C., Liu, J.P., 2004. Design and Analysis of Clinical Trials second ed. John Wiley, Hoboken, US, pp. 101 142, 167, 179, 422.

Crow, R., Gage, H., Hampson, S., et al., 1999. The role of expectancies in the placebo effect and their use in the delivery of health care: a systematic review. Health Technol. Assess. 3 (3), 1–96.

Donders, A.R., van der Heijden, G.J., Stijnen, T., et al., 2006. Review: a gentle introduction to imputation of missing values. J. Clin. Epidemiol. 59 (10), 1087–1091.

Dube, A., Manthata, L.N., Syce, J.A., 2007. The design and evaluation of placebo material for crude herbals: *Artemisia afra* herb as a model. Phytother. Res. 21 (5), 448–451.

Dean EM, Coulter, M.K., Fisher, P., et al., 2006. Report data on homeopathic treatments (RedHot): a supplement to CONSORT. Forsch. Komplementarmed. (13)368–371.

Frei, H., Everts, R., von, A.K., et al., 2005. Homeopathic treatment of children with attention deficit hyperactivity disorder: a randomised, double blind, placebo controlled crossover trial. Eur. J. Pediatr. 164 (12), 758–767.

Jadad, A., Enkin, M.W., 2007. Randomised controlled trials. second ed. Blackwell BMJ Books, London.

Linde, K., Witt, C.M., Streng, A., et al., 2007. The impact of patient expectations on outcomes in four randomized controlled trials of acupuncture in patients with chronic pain. Pain 128 (3), 264–271.

MacPherson, H., White, A., Cummings, M., et al., 2001. Standards for reporting interventions in controlled trials of acupuncture: the STRICTA recommendations. Complement. Ther. Med. (9)246–249.

Moher, D., Schulz, K.F., Altman, D., 2001. The CONSORT Statement: revised recommendations for improving the quality of reports of parallel group randomised trials. JAMA 285 (15), 1987–1991.

Mondloch, M.V., Cole, D.C., Frank, J.W., 2001. Does how you do depend on how you think you'll do? A systematic review of the evidence for a relation between patients' recovery expectations and health outcomes. CMAJ 165 (2), 174–179.

Piaggio, G., Elbourne, D.R., Altman, D.G., et al., 2006. Reporting of noninferiority and equivalence randomized trials: an extension of the CONSORT statement. JAMA 295 (10), 1152–1160.

Pocock, S.J., 1977. Group sequential methods in the design and analysis of clinical trials. Biometrika 64 (2), 191–199.

Schulz, K.F., 1995. Subverting randomization in controlled trials. JAMA 274 (18), 1456–1458.

Schulz, K.F., Chalmers, I., Hayes, R.J., et al., 1995. Empirical evidence of bias. Dimensions of methodological quality associated with estimates of treatment effects in controlled trials. JAMA 273 (5), 408–412.

Shapiro, A.K., 1964. Etiological factors in placebo effect. JAMA 187, 712–714.

Twisk, J., de Vente, W., 2002. Attrition in longitudinal studies. How to deal with missing data. J. Clin. Epidemiol. 55 (4), 329–337.

Vincent, C., 1990. Credibility assessments in trials of acupuncture. Complement. Med. Res. 4, 8–11.

Vickers, A.J., 2004. Statistical reanalysis of four recent randomized trials of acupuncture for pain using analysis of covariance. Clin. J. Pain 20 (5), 319–323.

Vickers, A.J., 2006. How to randomize. J. Soc. Integr. Oncol. 4 (4), 194–198.

Vickers, A., Cassileth, B., Ernst, E., et al., 1997. How should we research unconventional therapies? A panel report from the conference on Complementary and Alternative Medicine Research Methodology, National Institutes of Health. Int. J. Techno. Assess. Health Care 13 (1), 111–121.

Vickers, A.J., Rees, R.W., Zollman, C.E., et al., 2004. Acupuncture for chronic headache in primary care: large, pragmatic, randomised trial. BMJ 328 (7442), 744.

Witt, C.M., 2009. Efficacy, effectiveness, pragmatic trials–guidance on terminology and the advantages of pragmatic trails. Forsch Komplementmed 16 (5), 292–294.

Witt, C.M., Lüdtke, R., Baur, R., et al., 2005. Homeopathic medical Practice: Long-term results of a cohort study with 3981 patients. BMC Public Health 5, 115.

Witt, C.M., Jena, S., Selim, D., et al., 2006a. Pragmatic randomized trial of effectiveness and cost-effectiveness of acupuncture for chronic low back pain. Am. J. Epidemiol. 164, 487–496.

Witt, C.M., Jena, S., Brinkhaus, B., et al., 2006b. Acupuncture in Patients with Osteoarthritis of the Knee and the Hip. Arthritis Rheum. 54 (11), 3485–3493.

Witt, C.M., Jena, S., Brinkhaus, B., et al., 2006c. Acupuncture for patients with chronic neck pain. Pain 125, 98–106.

Witt, C.M., Jena, S., Brinkhaus, B., et al., 2006d. Acupuncture for patients with chronic neck pain. Pain 125, 98–106.

Witt, C.M., Reinhold, T., Brinkhaus, B., et al., 2008. Acupuncture in patients with dysmenorrhea: a randomized study on clinical effectiveness and cost-effectiveness in usual care. Am. J. Obstet. Gynecol. 198 (2), 166–168.

Zwarenstein, M., Treweek, S., Gagnier, J.J., et al., 2008. CONSORT group; Pragmatic Trials in healthcare (Practic) group. Improving the reporting of pragmatic trials: an extension of the CONSORT statement. BMJ 337, a 2390.

FURTHER READING

Saks, M., Allsop, J. (Eds.), 2007. Researching Health. Sage Publications, London.

Schulz, K.F., Schulz, D.A., Grimes, 2002. Allocation concealment in randomised trials, defending against deciphering. Epidemiology Series. Lancet pp. 359.

Systematic reviews and meta-analyses in CAM: contribution and challenges

6

Klaus Linde • Ian D. Coulter

CHAPTER CONTENTS

INTRODUCTION

Every year more than two million articles are published in over 20 000 biomedical journals (Mulrow 1995). Even in speciality areas it is impossible to keep up to date with all relevant new information. In this situation systematic reviews hold a key position to summarize the state of the current knowledge. A review is called systematic if it uses predefined and explicit methods for identifying, selecting and assessing the information (typically research studies) deemed relevant to answer the particular question posed. A systematic review is called a meta-analysis if it includes an integrative statistical analysis (pooling) of the included studies.

Within complementary medicine systematic reviews are of major relevance. This chapter aims to give an introduction on how to read and how to do a systematic review or a meta-analysis, and discusses advances and limitations of this method.

Most available systematic reviews on complementary medicine have focused on treatment effects. Therefore, most of the content of this chapter refers to such reviews. But of course, it is possible to do systematic reviews on other topics, for example the validity and reliability of diagnostic methods (for example, on iridology: Ernst 1999), side-effects (for example, on side-effects

DOI: 10.1016/B978-0-443-06956-7.00006-9

and interactions of St John's wort: Knüppel & Linde 2004), on surveys (for example, on reasons for and characteristics associated with complementary and alternative medicine (CAM) use among adult cancer patients: Verhoef et al. 2005), observational studies of association of risk or protective factors with major diseases (for example, whether the consumption of green tea is associated with a lower risk of breast cancer: Seely et al. 2005), or even on other systematic reviews (for example, a review of reviews of acupuncture: Linde et al. 2001a). The principles are the same as for reviews of studies on treatment effects but details in the methodological steps can differ.

THE PROTOCOL

A systematic review is, in principle, a retrospective study. The unit of investigation is the original research study (primary study), for example, a randomized controlled trial (RCT). The retrospective nature limits the conclusiveness of systematic reviews. Nevertheless, the methods of retrospective studies should be defined as far as possible in advance.

The protocol of a systematic review should have subheadings similar to those in this article. For writing a feasible and useful protocol it is necessary to have at least some basic ideas what and how much primary research is available. Therefore, in practice the protocol of a systematic review often has to be developed in a stepwise approach where the methods are defined rather loosely in the early screening phase and then become increasingly specific.

Examples of detailed protocols of systematic reviews can be found in the Cochrane Library (www.cochrane.org), the electronic publication of a worldwide network for systematic reviews of health care interventions.

THE QUESTION

As in any research a clear and straightforward question is a precondition for a conclusive answer. A clearly defined question for a systematic review on a treatment is, for example, whether extracts of St John's wort (*Hypericum perforatum*) are more effective than placebo in reducing the clinical symptoms of patients with major depression (Linde et al. 2008). A question of this type already predefines the group of patients (those with major depression), the type of experimental (extracts of St John's wort) and control intervention (placebo) as well as the outcome of interest (clinical symptoms of depression). Systematic reviews on such narrowly defined questions make sense, particularly when a number of similar studies are available but their results are either not widely known or contradictory, or if the number of patients in the primary studies is too small to detect relevant differences with sufficient likelihood.

In complementary medicine the number of studies on a particular topic is often small. If the question is very narrow it may be that only a few or even no relevant trials can be identified. For example, a systematic review has been performed to assess whether there is evidence from randomized trials that acupuncture is effective for treating swallowing difficulties in patients with stroke (Xie et al. 2008). Only one trial met the inclusion criteria. While it can be easily concluded from such a review that there is very little evidence, this is not very satisfying for reviewers or readers.

Sometimes it may be useful to ask broader questions, for example: 'Is there evidence that acupuncture can reduce symptoms associated with acute stroke?' Such a review will give a more descriptive overview of inhomogeneous studies (regarding study design, outcomes, prevention or treatment). It will be more hypothesis-generating than hypothesis-testing.

SEARCHING THE LITERATURE

An obvious precondition for a good systematic review is that the relevant literature is covered comprehensively. Until the late 1990s the majority of studies in the area of complementary medicine were published in journals that were not covered by the most important electronic databases such as PubMed/Medline or Embase. This has changed over the last 15 years. Several journals focusing on research in CAM are now included in these databases, and many studies are published in 'conventional' medical journals. Studies published in journals not listed in these major databases tend to have lower quality (Linde et al. 2001b). However, literature searches restricted to the major databases might miss relevant high-quality studies. Therefore, depending on the subject it will be necessary that reviewers should search more specialized databases, and in any case they should use additional search methods.

A very effective and simple method is checking the references of identified studies and reviews relevant to the topic. This method often also identifies studies which are published only as abstracts, in conference proceedings or books. The problem of this method can be that studies with 'undesired' results are systematically undercited. Contacting persons, institutions or industry relevant to the field can help both in identifying new sources to search (for example, a specialized database which was unknown to you before) and obtaining articles directly. Finally, handsearching of journals and conference proceedings is a possibility, although this often surpasses the time resources of reviewers.

A problem that has to be kept in mind is that specific complementary therapies and research activities might be concentrated in certain countries. For example, thousands of randomized trials on traditional Chinese medicine have been performed in China. These articles have been published almost exclusively in Chinese journals and in Chinese language. While western researchers are often reluctant to search and include studies from China due to their generally low quality (Wang et al. 2007), the almost exclusively positive results, raising fundamental doubts about their reliability (Vickers et al. 1998) and the need of resources for search and translation, this practice will have to change in the future.

In practice, the scrutiny of the literature search will depend strongly on the resources available. Reviews which are based on literature searches in only one or two of the mentioned sources should, however, be interpreted with caution, keeping in mind that a number of relevant studies might have been missed.

A major problem pertinent to systematic reviews is publication bias (Dickersin et al. 1987; Kleijnen & Knipschild 1992). Publication bias occurs when studies with undesired results (mostly negative results) are published less often than those with desired results (mostly positive results). Especially small negative or inconclusive studies are less likely to be published. Sometimes authors do not submit such studies; sometimes journal editors reject them. Publication bias typically leads to overly optimistic results and conclusions in systematic reviews.

Reviewers should try to find out whether unpublished studies exist. Informal contacts with researchers in the field are an effective way of achieving this. However, it is often difficult to get written reports on these studies. Handsearching the abstract books and proceedings of research meetings is another potential method of identifying otherwise unpublished studies. Recently, there have been developments that randomized clinical trials are registered beforehand (http://clinicaltrials.gov/ or http://www.controlled-trials.com/). Such registers will probably become the best way in the future to check for unpublished or ongoing studies, but even today many small trials do not become registered.

There are no foolproof ways to detect and quantify publication bias (see section on checking the robustness of results, below, for a method of estimating the influence). Every reviewer and all readers should always be aware of this risk.

SELECTING THE RELEVANT STUDIES

Selecting the studies for detailed review from the often large number of references identified from the search is the next crucial step in the review process. Readers should check carefully whether this process was transparent and unbiased. Readers should be aware that minor changes in inclusion criteria can result in dramatic differences in the number of included studies in reviews addressing the same topic (Linde & Willich 2003).

A good systematic review of studies on diagnosis or therapy should explicitly define inclusion and exclusion criteria (Box 6.1). It has been outlined above that 'the question' of the review already crudely predefines these criteria. In the methods section of a systematic review these criteria should be described in more detail. For example, in a review on garlic for treating hypercholesterinaemia (such as Stevinson et al. 2000), it should be stated at which cholesterol level patients were considered as hypercholesterinaemic. Garlic can be applied in quite different ways (fresh, dried preparations, oil) and we need to know whether all of them were considered (this was not reported explicitly in this specific review).

BOX 6.1 Inclusion and exclusion criteria for primary studies in systematic reviews should be defined on the following levels:

- Type of patients/participants (for example, patients with serum cholesterol > 200 mg/dl)
- Type of studies (for example, randomized double-blind studies)
- Type of intervention (for example, garlic mono-preparations in the experimental group and placebo in the control group)
- Type of outcomes (for example, trials reporting total cholesterol levels as an endpoint)
- Eventually other restrictions (for example, only trials published in English, published in a peer-reviewed journal, no abstracts)

Another selection criterion typically applies to the type of studies considered. For example, many reviews are limited to randomized trials. The measurement and reporting of predefined outcomes as inclusion criteria are of particular relevance when a meta-analysis is planned. This often leads to the exclusion of a relevant proportion of otherwise relevant studies and the reader has to consider whether this might have influenced the findings of the review. Some reviews have language restrictions. This might not only result in the exclusion of a relevant proportion of trials but also change the results (Pham et al. 2005).

In practice the selection process is mostly performed in two steps. In the first step all the obviously irrelevant material is discarded, for example, all articles on garlic which are clearly not clinical trials in patients with cardiovascular problems. To save time and money this step is normally done by only one reviewer in a rather informal way. The remaining articles should then be checked carefully for eligibility by at least two independent reviewers (so that one does not know the decision of the other). In the publication of a systematic review it is advisable to list the potentially relevant studies which were excluded and give the reasons for exclusion. A consensus paper on how meta-analyses should be reported recommends the use of flow charts displaying the number of papers identified, excluded and selected at the different levels of the review and assessment process (Moher et al. 2009). This makes the selection process transparent for the reader.

EXTRACTING INFORMATION

Finally if a number of eligible studies have been identified, obtained and have passed the selection process, relevant information has to be extracted. If possible the extraction should be standardized, for example, by using a pretested form. The format should allow one to enter the data into a database and to perform basic statistical analyses. Another efficient method is to enter the data directly into a prestructured table. Regardless of what method is used, reviewers have to have a clear idea of what information they need for their analysis and what readers will need to get their own picture. Extraction and all assessments should be done by at least two independent reviewers. Coding errors are inevitable and personal biases can influence decisions in the extraction process. The coded information of the reviewers must be compared and disagreements discussed.

ASSESSING QUALITY

A major criticism of sceptics towards meta-analysis (and, to a lesser extent, also to non-meta-analytic systematic reviews) is the garbage-in, garbage-out problem. The results of unreliable studies do not become more reliable by lumping them together. It has been shown in conventional and complementary medicine that less rigorous trials tend to yield more positive results (Schulz et al. 1995; Lijner et al. 1999; Linde et al. 1999). Sometimes it may be better to base the conclusions on a few, rigorous trials and discard the findings of the bulk of unreliable studies. This approach has been called 'best-evidence synthesis' (Slavin 1986). While it is sometimes considered as an alternative, it is in principle a subtype of systematic reviews in which defined quality aspects are used as additional inclusion criteria (see White et al. 1997, as an example from complementary medicine).

However, the assessment of quality is difficult. The first problem is that quality is a complex concept. Methodologists tend to define quality as the likelihood that the results of a study are unbiased. This dimension of quality is sometimes referred to as internal validity or methodological quality. But a perfectly internally valid study may have fundamental flaws from a clinician's point of view if, for example, the outcomes measured are irrelevant for the patients or patients are not representative of those commonly receiving the treatment.

A second problem is that quality is difficult to operationalize in a valid manner. An experienced reviewer will find a lot of subtle information giving an indication on the quality of the study 'between the lines' from omissions and small details. However, subjective global ways to assess quality are not transparent and prone to subjective biases.

Many systematic reviews on treatment interventions include some standardized assessments of internal validity. There is agreement that key criteria for the internal validity of treatment studies are random allocation, blinding and adequate handling of dropouts and withdrawals. In the past these and other criteria have typically been combined in scores (see Moher et al. 1995, 1996 for overviews). But the validity of such scores is doubtful (Jüni et al. 1999). Today it is clearly preferred to assess single validity items without summarizing them in a score, and to investigate whether quality has an impact on findings. Currently, the most important tool is the Cochrane Collaboration's 'risk of bias' assessment (Higgins & Altman 2008). Whether the criteria are combined in scores or applied separately, the problems remain that the formalized assessment is often crude and the reviewers have to rely on the information reported.

In conclusion, assessments of methodological quality are necessary but need to be interpreted with caution. The assessment of other dimensions of quality is desirable, but the problems in the development of methods for this purpose (which have to regard the specific characteristics of the interventions and conditions investigated) are even greater than for internal validity.

SUMMARIZING THE RESULTS

The clinical reader of a systematic review is mainly interested in its results. While the majority of readers will only look on the abstract and meta-analytic summary, the review also has to provide sufficient information for those who want to get their own idea of the available studies and their results. For example, in a review of acupuncture in headache it will be relevant for the specialist to know what type of headache was studied in each primary study, to have information on the sex and age of the patients, and where they were recruited. Regarding the methods readers should know what the design was, whether there was some blinding, how long the patients were followed and whether follow-up was complete. They need details on the nature of the experimental (which acupuncture points, how many treatments) and the control interventions (type of sham acupuncture). And, of course, readers want to know which outcomes have been measured and what the results were. This detailed information is typically summarized in a table.

If the primary studies provide sufficient data the results are summarized in effect size estimates. Table 6.1 lists some of the most common measures.

Tables including a graphical display of the results are extremely helpful. Table 6.2 shows the standard display from a meta-analysis from the Cochrane Library, in this case on randomized trials comparing hypericum extracts and standard antidepressants (separated in the subgroups older antidepressants and selective serotonin reuptake inhibitors (SSRIs)) in patients with major depression (Linde et al. 2008). For each single study the results in the groups (the number of patients responding and the number of patients allocated to the group) compared are listed in columns two to five. In columns seven and eight the effect size estimates (in this case the ratio between the proportion of patients responding in treatment and control groups) and their respective confidence intervals are presented for each study numerically and graphically. The boxes in the graph indicate the effect size estimates of the single trials while the horizontal lines represent the respective 95% confidence intervals. The diamonds represent the pooled effect size estimates for all trials comparing hypericum extracts and older antidepressants (first diamond), SSRIs (second diamond) and all trials analysed together (third diamond). In the example, effect estimates right of the vertical line (which represents equal responder rates in treatment and control group) indicate superiority of hypericum, those on the left superiority of the control treatment. However, the side representing superiority depends on the outcome measure in other meta-analyses. If the 95% confidence interval does not include the vertical line the difference between treatment and control is statistically significant ($P < 0.05$).

Table 6.1 ***Commonly used estimates to summarize the results of controlled trials***

Estimate	Calculation	Advantages/disadvantages
For dichotomous data (e.g. response, death etc.)		
Odds ratio	$\frac{a \times d}{b \times c}$	Most widespread estimate in epidemiology/intuitively difficult to understand
Relative risk (rate ratio)	$\frac{a/(a+b)}{c/(c+d)}$	Easy to understand/problematic in case of very low or high control group event rates
For continuous data (e.g. blood pressure, enzyme activity etc.)		
Weighted mean difference	$x_e - x_c$ weighted by 1 / variance	Easy to interpret/only applicable if all trials measure the outcomes with the same scale
Standardized mean difference	$\frac{x_e - x_c}{SD}$	Applicable over different scales/clinically difficult to interpret

a = number of patients with an event in the experimental group
b = number of patients without event in the experimental group
c = number of patients with an event in the control group
d = number of patients without event in the control group
x_e = mean experimental group
x_c = mean control group
SD = standard deviations (either of the control group or pooled for both groups)

Table 6.2 *Example for the presentation of results in systematic reviews: treatment responders and risk ratios (proportion of responders in the hypericum group/proportion of responders in the control group) of randomized controlled trials comparing hypericum extracts and standard antidepressants in patients with major depression*

Study or subgroup	Hypericum		Standard			Risk ratio M-H, random, 95% CI	Risk ratio M-H, random, 95% CI
	Events	Total	Events	Total	Weight		
4.1.1. vs. older antidepressants							
Harrer 1993	27	51	28	51	4.3%	0.96 [0.67, 1.38]	
Philipp 1999	76	106	70	110	12.2%	1.13 [0.94, 1.36]	
Vorbach 1997	36	107	41	102	4.4%	0.84 [0.59, 1.20]	
Wheatley 1997	40	87	42	78	5.7%	0.85 [0.63, 1.16]	
Woelk 2000	68	157	67	167	7.6%	1.08 [0.83, 1.40]	
Subtotal (95% CI)		**508**		**508**	**34.2%**	**1.02 [0.90, 1.15]**	
Total events	247		248				
Heterogeneity: $Tau^2 = 0.00$; $Chi^2 = 3.97$, df = 4 (P= 0.41); $I^2 = 0\%$							
Test for overall effect: Z = 0.30 (p = 0.77)							
4.1.2 vs. SSRIs							
Behnke 2002	16	35	21	35	2.9%	0.76 [0.49, 1.20]	
Bjerkenstedt 2005	22	54	20	54	2.6%	1.10 [0.68, 1.77]	
Brenner 2000	7	15	6	15	0.9%	1.17 [0.51, 2.66]	
Fava 2005	17	45	14	47	1.8%	1.27 [0.71, 2.26]	
Gastpar 2005	70	123	72	118	10.2%	0.93 [0.76, 1.15]	
Gastpar 2006	71	131	71	127	9.6%	0.97 [0.78, 1.21]	
Harrer 1999	50	77	57	84	9.6%	0.96 [0.77, 1.19]	
HDTSG 2002	46	113	55	109	6.2%	0.81 [0.60, 1.08]	
Moreno 2005	4	20	11	20	0.7%	0.36 [0.14, 0.95]	
Schrader 2000	57	125	39	113	5.3%	1.32 [0.96, 1.82]	
Szegedi 2005	86	122	73	122	12.2%	1.18 [0.98, 1.42]	
van Gurp 2002	25	45	23	45	3.8%	1.09 [0.74, 1.60]	
Subtotal (95% CI)		**905**		**889**	**65.8%**	**1.00 [0.90, 1.12]**	
Total events	471		462				
Heterogeneity: $Tau^2 = 0.01$; $Chi^2 = 15.43$, df = 11 (P = 0.16); $I^2 = 29\%$							
Test for overall effect: Z = 0.06 (P = 0.95)							
Total (95% CI)		**1413**		**1397**	**100.0%**	**1.01 [0.93, 1.09]**	
Total events	718		710				
Heterogeneity: $Tau^2 = 0.00$; $chi^2 = 19.37$, df = 16 (P = 0.25); $I^2 = 17\%$							0.1 0.2 0.5 1 2 5 10
Test for overall effect: Z = 0.14 (P = 0.89)							favours standard favours hypericum

Events, number of patients with response; M-H, Mantel–Haenszel method; 95% CI, 95% confidence interval; see text for further explanations.
Modified from Linde et al. (2008).

Column six gives the weight of each study in the pooled estimate, which depends on sample sizes and variances. The line 'heterogeneity' gives indication whether the results of the trials vary more than expected by chance alone. Three measures are given: tau^2, the chi^2 statistic and I^2. For the average reader and researcher I^2 is by far the easiest to interpret. An I^2-value of 0%, for example, indicates that the differences in the findings of the single trials might well be due to chance while a value above 50% indicates that the trials probably differed in some relevant aspects. Possible reasons for heterogeneity are bias in some trials and variable patient characteristics. Meta-analyses with indication of heterogeneity have to be interpreted with special caution. The *P*-values in the test of the overall effect are similar to the *P*-values in trials.

A number of computer programs for systematic reviews and meta-analysis are available. Depending on the type of data and other characteristics of the data (for example, heterogeneity) different statistical techniques are adequate. Although some computer programs allow the novice to perform meta-analyses it is recommended to get guidance or advice from a statistician or an experienced reviewer if pooling of independent studies is an issue.

CHECKING THE ROBUSTNESS OF RESULTS

If possible, a systematic review should include sensitivity analyses to check the robustness of the results. For example, one can check whether the conclusions would be altered if only studies meeting defined quality criteria were included. Subgroup analyses (for example, on a specific group of trials) can be of value, too, but should be interpreted with caution, particularly if they were not predefined. Unfortunately, a considerable number of primary studies are needed to perform sensitivity and subgroup analyses in a meaningful manner.

Textbooks on systematic reviews recommend to use funnel plots as another means of investigating empirically for biases. A precondition for a funnel plot is a sufficiently large and clinically reasonably homogeneous group of studies (so that a single 'true' effect size is a plausible expectation). In funnel plots effect sizes of single studies are plotted against a measure of precision or sample size. The basic idea is that larger studies provide the more reliable estimates of treatment effects as they are less prone to random error (chance variation), within-study bias (larger studies tend to have better internal validity) and publication bias (larger studies are more expensive, known to more people and therefore more likely to be published regardless of the results). If the results of the small studies differ only due to chance variation the resulting graph should resemble an inverted funnel. An asymmetric plot has long been interpreted as an indication of publication bias. However, the concept of 'small-study effects', including both elements of publication and within-study bias, is more accurate (Sterne et al. 2001). In any case, both the reviewer and the reader should consider an asymmetric funnel plot a red flag: the findings of the review might be biased!

WHO SHOULD DO SYSTEMATIC REVIEWS?

Many people grossly underestimate the amount of time needed to perform a rigorous systematic review. Protocol development, literature search, extraction, discussion of disagreements in coding and assessments, obtaining missing data from authors and analysing are all time-consuming steps, and a realistic timeline from start to completion of the final report is 12–24 months with repeated periods of intensive work. Of course, it is also possible to make systematic reviews faster but this will probably result in rather superficial work that is of doubtful usefulness.

Until recently, many systematic reviews on complementary medicine have been performed by research methodologists with limited experience on the interventions and conditions investigated. Preferably, the research team for a systematic review should have competency in methodology, intervention and condition under scrutiny to ensure that the results will be both methodologically sound and clinically relevant. As complementary therapies are often controversial and prejudices strong it is desirable to include persons with different prejudices to make the review as balanced as possible. Many steps in retrospective studies like systematic reviews include rather arbitrary decisions which leave space for personal biases to infect the results.

The Cochrane Collaboration is a worldwide network of researchers aimed to perform, regularly update and disseminate systematic reviews of health care interventions (Ezzo et al. 1998). Within the collaboration there is a group focusing on complementary medicine. Researchers who plan to do a systematic review should consider contacting that group (http://www.cochrane.org/). The main challenge for the Cochrane Collaboration is that the resources available for doing reviews are limited and those working on the reviews are to a large extent volunteers. This limits the reviews in several ways. The first is in the number of languages which can be searched and the publications that are evaluated by someone both fluent in the language and expert in systematic reviews. Secondly it limits the resources available both to attain databases to search and in their actual search. Thirdly it greatly affects the amount of grey literature that can be searched. This includes written work such as degree theses, unpublished results from trials, negative results from trials and data collected from agencies such as the US Food and Drug Administration.

An alternative to the Cochrane Collaboration is found in the Evidence-based Practice Centers (EPC) administered by the US Agency for Healthcare Research and Quality (AHRQ) but funded by other agencies, such as the National Center for Complementary and Alternative Medicine (NCCAM). Each EPC is constructed slightly differently and each must compete annually for contracts to produce evidence reports for the government agency, or on occasions, for third-party organizations (Coulter 2007). From 2000 to 2003 NCCAM through AHRQ established an EPC for CAM.

The greatest difference between these centres and the Cochrane Collaboration is in resources such as funding. Coulter (2007) has shown that, in their study of Ayurvedic medicine for the treatment of diabetes mellitus, done at the Southern California EPC, the project was able to visit the major research centres in India, access and purchase Indian journals, and review theses in their native language. In the final systematic review, 35 studies came from the western literature and 27 came from the Indian literature. Of those on which statistical analysis was performed 12 were from India and only eight from western literature. So the Indian literature had a great influence on the systematic review. This is not unusual for CAM where many of the systems (traditional Chinese medicine, Ayurvedic medicine, homeopathy, yoga, acupuncture) are not systems that originated in the west and often have a very long published history in languages other than English. So systematic reviews that confine their reviews to English only run the risk of missing important evidence. However it is not practical to expect that the EPCs will be able to conduct the number of systematic reviews that are produced by the Cochrane collaboration and by other means. The work of the EPCs is available online at (http://www.ahrq.gov/clinic/epcix.htm) as evidence reports.

HOW TO IDENTIFY EXISTING SYSTEMATIC REVIEWS

The most relevant sources to identify existing systematic reviews are PubMed (http://www.ncbi.nlm.nih.gov/sites/entrez?db=pubmed) and the Cochrane Library (http://www.cochrane.org/). By using the term 'systematic reviews' as 'subset' in the menu 'limits' or the term 'meta-analysis' as 'publication type' in the same menu, and combining it with the clinical problem of interest, PubMed can be searched efficiently. The search for the 'subset systematic reviews' will identify a larger number of articles (for example, a search for hypericum yielded 72 hits in January 2010), including meta-analyses, systematic reviews without pooling and a number of other papers resembling systematic reviews. The search for the 'publication type meta-analysis' will yield a more selected group of systematic reviews and meta-analyses but may miss a few relevant articles (in case of the hypericum search it yielded 18 hits).

The Cochrane Library an online resource (http://www.thecochranelibrary.com) produced by the above-mentioned Cochrane Collaboration. It contains the full text of all reviews performed by the network as well as references and abstracts of a large number of other systematic reviews.

LIMITATIONS OF SYSTEMATIC REVIEWS

Clearly, although systematic reviews are of utmost importance, they are prone to a number of biases. Even the best systematic review will be of limited value if the primary studies are flawed. It has been shown that the findings of very large clinical trials (which are considered as the ultimate gold standard to assess the merit of a treatment) differ in a considerable number of cases from those of meta-analyses on the same topic (Lelorier et al. 1997). The large number of decisions in a systematic review can also have a relevant impact on the results. As a consequence it should not be surprising that systematic reviews performed by different research groups sometimes come to conflicting conclusions (see Linde & Willich 2003 for a review).

Readers should check reviews carefully. Guidelines for critical appraisal are available (see references for further reading). Box 6.2 lists a number of questions to consider when reading systematic reviews. Systematic reviews cannot replace original research. Particularly in complementary medicine, their conclusiveness will remain limited unless new, reliable primary studies become available.

As this article has noted, each step of the systematic review poses questions that must be asked by the reader to assess whether the review was rigorous, comprehensive, inclusive and valid (Coulter 2006). The search and hence the conclusions can be biased at many points and, like many other methods, with systematic reviews, if you put garbage in, you get garbage out.

BOX 6.2 Questions to consider when reading a systematic review

- Was there a clearly defined question?
- Was the literature search comprehensive?
- Were inclusion and exclusion criteria defined and adequate?
- Was bias avoided in the process of selecting studies for inclusion in the review from the body of literature identified?
- Was the quality of the included studies assessed using relevant criteria?
- Have patients, methods, interventions and results of the included studies been described in sufficient detail?
- If the review included a meta-analysis, were the methods used adequate and the primary studies sufficiently comparable?
- Have the shortcomings of the review been discussed?
- Are the results relevant to clinical practice?

But there are other major issues that must caution the current use of systematic reviews for CAM. Maybe the most important issue is their often questionable external validity and clinical relevance. Most available CAM reviews are restricted to RCTs and exclude observational studies. However, RCTs of CAM interventions often reflect very little how the treatment is actually used in practice. For example, in homeopathy three-quarters of the available randomized trials investigate standardized treatment interventions, although individualization is a cornerstone of this therapy (Shang et al. 2005). Traditional healing systems like Chinese medicine normally use complex interventions such as a combination of acupuncture, moxibustion, herbal medicines, and manipulative or relaxation techniques, whereas randomized trials in this area are typically limited to one component such as acupuncture or a standardized combination of herbs. Furthermore, many trials use sham or placebo controls to investigate 'specific' effects in often artificial conditions. Randomized trials investigating whole systems in a pragmatic manner and comparing with realistic alternatives are extremely rare.

Furthermore, for the foreseeable future the number of RCTs done in CAM will continue to lag well behind those in allopathic medicine. For much of CAM there is no interest in, or profit in, pharmaceutical companies funding such trials. Issues such as property rights for indigenous healing traditions have made this less attractive for such research. Moreover, the practice of CAM does not favour the development and use of the 'magic bullets' of single active drugs and allopathic medicine has shown some antipathy to using CAM products. The amount of public research funding for CAM is miniscule. The USA is spending by far the most of all western countries for CAM research, but still the budget of the relevant institute (the NCCAM) for 2006 was only 0.42% of the total National Institutes of Health budget (National Institutes of Health 2007). Simply put, there is neither enough funding nor enough effort being put into conducting RCTs on CAM and there will not be for some time to come.

High-quality observational studies could greatly contribute to the evidence base on CAM, and discrediting such studies in favour of randomized trials is inappropriate. There is an expanding body of literature on studies examining

RCTs and observational studies for the same disease and intervention. Earlier studies concluded that non-randomized studies overestimated treatment benefits. More recently, the studies show that both randomized and non-randomized studies yield very similar results (for example, Benson & Hartz 2000; Concato et al. 2000; Linde et al. 2007). Some studies have found little evidence of a difference in the treatment effects between RCTs and observational studies when the comparisons were made for the same treatment. The results of well-designed observational studies did not systematically exaggerate the magnitude of the effects of treatment compared to the RCTs for the same topic (Coulter 2006).

While efficacy is important, ultimately it is effectiveness that we wish to know about in truly evidence-based practice. It is effectiveness, not efficacy, studies that provide evidence of how a therapy will work in real practice. In fact there is an urgent need to put the practice back into practice-based medicine (Coulter 2007). The very studies that improve the quality of systematic reviews, that is, placebo-controlled RCTs, deal with efficacy and not effectiveness. Because they tend to be conducted under artificial conditions they seldom provide the type of information needed to make a decision vis-à-vis an individual patient. Well-designed observational studies could provide much better information in this regard.

In some areas of CAM most studies are observational. While randomized trials in CAM often suffer from relevant shortcomings, the quality of many observational studies is even worse. There is a clear need to improve and develop observational studies in CAM. The challenge for reviewers is to develop standards for judging the quality of observational studies. Reviewers should also follow guidelines for reporting meta-analyses of observational studies (Stroup et al. 2000).

We can also note that whole areas of evidence, such as health services research and programme evaluation, tend to be left out of systematic reviews (Coulter & Khorsan 2008). Such work, which is based on real-world practice, adds an element of reality to evidence-based research.

We would be incomplete if we did not mention other approaches to systematic review and meta-analysis besides those described here. Of particular interest may be those from the educational and behavioural literature that also evaluate complex interventional treatments and research. These methods may provide a better approach to heterogeneous studies that allow for valid conclusions (see Jonas et al. 2001 for an example). The value of this approach is that it can manage complex and heterogeneous aspects of interventional research, and yet still come up with what is considered valid conclusions. These should be considered and further developed in CAM and whole systems research.

HOW SHOULD WE USE SYSTEMATIC REVIEWS IN CAM?

Clearly the answer is: cautiously but, that being noted, systematic reviews can provide some very useful functions for CAM. Firstly they are excellent sources for reviewing the state of the science. They can and do draw attention to methodological weaknesses in the quality of evidence which arises from the quality of the research. They have established the lack of good-quality, rigorous trials in CAM. Such studies have also shown that some of the attributed 'quality differences' arise when you compare CAM and whole systems research with approaches to drug research. This is not simply differences in quality but differences in research methodology which make it inappropriate to use terms such as 'superior' or 'inferior'. They are simply different (Crawford et al. 2009). Secondly they do review adverse events (usually through case reports) and make risk/benefit assessments. Thirdly they provide a clearing ground for basic questions and allow us to move on to more important second-order questions. So, for example, if systematic reviews can establish that acupuncture, manipulation, yoga and homeopathy have some efficacy, then the research agenda can be moved to the more significant questions of: for what type of patients, for what health problems and in whose hands does the therapy achieve the best results? In a metaphorical sense this could be considered the equivalent of a gardener clearing the undergrowth to get at the good plants.

In those areas where good systematic reviews of CAM are available we can move towards more evidence-based practice but also move towards determining clinical applications and to new research questions such as the rate of appropriate and inappropriate practice. The early work at RAND on manipulation for low-back pain (Coulter et al. 1995) led to a systematic review and a meta-analysis. An expert panel was then set up and a set of indications based on both the systematic review and clinical experience was created for the use and non-use of manipulation for low-back pain. This in turn led to a field study in which the rate of chiropractic appropriate and inappropriate manipulation for low-back pain was established (Coulter 2001). While it showed on the one hand that 27% of patients were inappropriately manipulated, it also showed that 41% were candidates for manipulation but were not manipulated (Coulter et al. 1995; Coulter 2001). Such research, if repeated across CAM, could establish whether or not inappropriate care (one of the dominant concerns by allopathic medicine and funding health care agencies about CAM) is a problem. Furthermore, systematic reviews are often precursors to the development of consensus conferences and guidelines.

In summary, systematic reviews are somewhat like the curate's egg: parts of it are excellent, the rest, not so good. More training and application of a variety of systematic review approaches should be developed and applied to CAM.

REFERENCES

Benson, K., Hartz, A.J., 2000. A comparison of observational studies and randomized, controlled trials. N. Engl. J. Med. 342, 1878–1886.

Concato, J., Shah, N., Horwitz, R.I., 2000. Randomized, controlled trials, observational studies, and the hierarchy of research designs. N. Engl. J. Med. 342, 1887–1892.

Coulter, I.D., 2007. Evidence based complementary and alternative medicine: promises and problems. Forsch. Komplementarmed. 14, 102–108.

Coulter, I.D., 2001. Evidenced-based practice and appropriateness of care studies. J. Evid. Based Dent. Pract. 1, 222–226.

Coulter, I.D., 2006. Evidence summaries and synthesis: necessary but insufficient approach for determining clinical practice of integrated medicine? Integr. Cancer Ther. 5, 282–286.

Coulter, I.D., 2007. Putting the practice into evidence-based dentistry. CDAJ 35, 45–49.

Coulter, I.D., Khorsan, R., 2008. Is health services research the holy grail of CAM

research? Altern. Ther. Health Med. 14, 40–45.
Coulter, I.D., Shekelle, P., Mootz, R., et al., 1995. The use of expert panel results: The RAND Panel for Appropriateness of Manipulation and Mobilization of the Cervical Spine. J. Topics in Clinical Chiropractic 2 (3), 54–62.
Crawford, C.C., Huynh, M.T., Kepple, A., et al., 2009. Assessment of the quality of research studies of conventional and alternative treatment(s) of primary headache. Pain Physician 12, 461–470.
Dickersin, K., Chan, S., Chalmers, T.C., et al., 1987. Publication bias and clinical trials. Contr. Clin. Trials 8, 343–353.
Ernst, E., 1999. Iridology: a systematic review. Forsch. Komplementärmed. 6, 7–9.
Ezzo, J., Berman, B.M., Vickers, A.J., et al., 1998. Complementary medicine and the Cochrane Collaboration. JAMA 280, 1628–1630.
Higgins, J.P.T., Altman, D.G. (Eds.), 2008. Chapter 8: Assessing risk of bias in included studies. In: Higgins, J.P.T., Green, S. (Eds.), Cochrane Handbook for Systematic Reviews of Interventions Version 5.0.1 (updated September 2008). The Cochrane Collaboration. Available from www.cochrane-handbook.org.
Jonas, W.B., Anderson, R.L., Crawford, C.C., et al., 2001. A systematic review of the quality of homeopathic clinical trials. BMC Complement. Altern. Med. 1: Document 12.
Jüni, P., Witschi, A., Bloch, R., et al., 1999. The hazards of scoring the quality of clinical trials for meta-analysis. JAMA 282, 1054–1060.
Kleijnen, J., Knipschild, P., 1992. Review articles and publication bias. Arzneim-Forsch/Drug Research 42, 587–591.
Knüppel, L., Linde, K., 2004. Adverse effects of St. John's wort: a systematic review. J. Clin. Psychiatry 65, 470–479.
LeLorier, J., Grégoire, G., Benhaddad, A., et al., 1997. Discrepancies between meta-analysis and subsequent large randomized, controlled trials. N. Eng. J. Med. 337, 536–542.
Lijner, J.G., Mol, B.W., Heisterkamp, S., et al., 1999. Empirical evidence of design-related bias in studies of diagnostic tests. JAMA 282, 1061–1066.
Linde, K., Willich, S., 2003. How objective are systematic reviews? Differences between reviews on complementary medicine. J. R. Soc. Med. 96, 17–22.
Linde, K., Schulz, M., Ramirez, G., et al., 1999. Impact of study quality on outcome in placebo-controlled trials of homeopathy. J. Clin. Epdemiol. 52, 631–636.
Linde, K., Vickers, A., Hondras, M., et al., 2001a. Systematic reviews of complementary therapies - an annotated bibliography. Part I: Acupuncture. BMC Complement. Altern. Med. 1: Document 3.
Linde, K., Jonas, W.B., Melchart, D., et al., 2001b. The methodological quality of randomized controlled trials of homeopathy, herbal medicine and acupuncture. Int. J. Epidemiol. 30, 526–531.
Linde, K., Streng, A., Hoppe, A., et al., 2007. Randomized trial vs. observational study of acupuncture for migraine found that patient characteristics differed but outcomes were similar. J. Clin. Epidemiol. 60, 280–287.
Linde, K., Berner, M., Kiston, L., 2008. St John's wort for major depression. Cochrane Database Syst. Rev. (4), CD000448.
Moher, D., Jadad, A.R., Nichol, G., et al., 1995. Assessing the quality of randomized controlled trials: an annotated bibliography of scales and checklists. Control. Clin. Trials 16, 62–73.
Moher, D., Jadad, A.R., Tugwell, P., 1996. Assessing the quality of randomized controlled trials – current issues and future directions. Int. J. Technol. Assess. Health Care 12, 196–208.
Moher, D., Liberati, A., Tetzlaff, J., et al., 2009. Preferred reporting items for systematic reviews and meta-analyses: the PRISMA statement. PLoS Med. 6, e1000097.
Mulrow, C.D., 1995. Rationale for systematic reviews. In: Chalmers, I., Altman, D.G. (Eds.), Systematic reviews. BMJ Books, London, p. 1.
National Institutes of Health. Summary of the FY, 2007. In: Presidents Budget. p. 9. http://officeofbudget.od.nih.gov/pdf/Press%20info%20final.pdf.
Pham, B., Klassen, T.P., Lawson, M.L., et al., 2005. Language of publication restrictions in systematic reviews gave different results depending on whether the intervention was conventional or complementary. J. Clin. Epidemiol. 58, 769–776.
Schulz, F.K., Chalmers, I., Hayes, R.J., et al., 1995. Empirical evidence of bias: dimensions of methodological quality

associated with estimates of treatment effects in controlled trials. JAMA 273, 408–412.
Seely, D., Mills, E.J., Wu, P., et al., 2005. The effects of green tea consumption on incidence of breast cancer and recurrence of breast cancer: a systematic review and meta-analysis. Integr. Cancer Ther. 4, 144–155.
Shang, A., Huwiler-Müntener, K., Nartey, L., et al., 2005. Are the clinical effects of homoeopathy placebo effects? Comparative study of placebo-controlled trials of homoeopathy and allopathy. Lancet 366, 726–732.
Slavin, R.E., 1986. Best-evidence synthesis: an alternative to meta-analysis and traditional reviews. Educational Research 15, 9–11.
Sterne, J.A.C., Egger, M., Davey Smith, G., 2001. Investigating and dealing with publication and other bias. In: Egger, M., Davey Smith, G., Altman, D.G. (Eds.), Systematic reviews in healthcare: meta-analysis in context. BMJ Books, London, pp. 189–208.
Stevinson, C., Pittler, M.H., Ernst, E., 2000. Garlic for treating hypercholesterinemia. A meta-analysis of randomized controlled clinical trials. Ann. Intern. Med. 133, 420–429.
Stroup, D.F., Berlin, J.A., Morton, S.C., et al., 2000. Meta-analysis of observational studies in epidemiology: a proposal for reporting. Meta-analysis Of Observational Studies in Epidemiology (MOOSE) group. JAMA 283, 2008–2012.
Verhoef, M.J., Balneaves, L.G., Boon, H.S., et al., 2005. Reasons for and characteristics associated with complementary and alternative medicine use among adult cancer patients: a systematic review. Integrat. Cancer Ther. 4, 274–286.
Vickers, A., Goyal, N., Harland, R., et al., 1998. Do certain countries produce only positive results? A systematic review of controlled trials. Control. Clin. Trials 19, 159–166.
Wang, G., Mao, B., Xiong, Z.Y., et al., 2007. The quality of reporting of randomized controlled trials of traditional Chinese medicine: a survey of 13 randomly selected journals from mainland China. Clin. Ther. 29, 1456–1467.
White, A.R., Resch, K.L., Ernst, E., 1997. Smoking cessation with acupuncture? A 'best evidence synthesis'. Forsch. Komplementärmed. 4, 102–105.
Xie, Y., Wang, L., He, J., et al., 2008. Acupuncture for dysphagia in acute stroke. Cochrane Database Syst. Rev. (3), CD006076.

FURTHER READING

Borenstein, M., Hedges, L.V., Higgins, J.P.T., et al., 2009. Introduction to Meta-Analysis. Wiley, Chichester.
Cooper, H., Hedges, L.V. (Eds.), 1994. The handbook of research synthesis. Russel Sage Foundation, New York.
Egger, M., Davey Smith, G., Altman, D.G. (Eds.), 2001. Systematic reviews in healthcare: meta-analysis in context. BMJ Books, London.
Higgins, J.P.T., Green, S. (Eds.), 2008. Cochrane Handbook for Systematic Reviews of Interventions Version 5.0.1 (updated September 2008). The Cochrane Collaboration. Available online from www.cochrane-handbook.org.
Leandro, G., 2005. Meta-analysis in Medical Research: The handbook for the understanding and practice of meta-analysis. BMJ Books, London.

Health services research as a form of evidence and CAM

7

Ian D. Coulter • Raheleh Khorsan

CHAPTER CONTENTS

INTRODUCTION

> *Health services research (HSR), an Association for Health Services Research (AHSR) lobbyist once said, was as difficult to sell as a dead fish wrapped in newspaper*
> (Gray et al. 2003, pp.W3–287).

> *HSR methods may be used to improve clinical, patient-centred, and economic outcomes across both allopathic and complementary and alternative medicine (CAM) systems of care…HSR has much to contribute to CAM, and conventional HSR has much to discover from addressing the broader range of issues required by CAM*
> (Herman et al. 2006).

These two statements represent the range of opinions concerning the use of HSR and CAM. Perhaps the truth lies somewhere between the two. As stated by Coulter & Khorsan (2008), 'So it would seem that HSR is neither a panacea nor the Holy Grail. It clearly has an important contribution to make, but as with all research paradigms, it addresses only one way of knowing. It may be a truth but not the only truth and certainly not the whole truth. To the CAM community "proceed with caution" might be the appropriate guideline.'

In this chapter we will explore the nature of HSR and outline what it could contribute to the researching of CAM.

DOI: 10.1016/B978-0-443-06956-7. 00007-0

WHAT IS HEALTH SERVICES RESEARCH?

In a previous paper Coulter described HSR. He states:

> *WITHOUT an HSR component, the move towards evidence-based dentistry will remain more a promise than a reality. The major concerns of HSR – such as linking structure, process, and outcome; measuring quality of care; evaluating access, cost, services, and utilization of care; measuring health care need and health risks; accessing patient measures such as satisfaction and health-related quality of life; and appropriateness research – are all crucially important to evidence-based dentistry*
>
> (Coulter 2001 pp. 720–721).

HSR was defined by the Institute of Medicine, in a major report in 1979, as the investigation of the relationship between social structure, process and outcomes for personal health services. The last involves a transaction between a client and a provider to promote health. Andersen et al. (1994) state that this definition requires that HSR includes structure and/or process. The structural component includes personnel, facilities, services available, organizational features and financing. Process is the transaction that occurs between the provider and the patient. Under this definition of HRS the focus goes beyond the disease and interventions of clinical studies to include the total organization of the care delivery.

HSR involves four levels: (1) the clinical level; (2) the institutional level; (3) the systemic level; and (4) the contextual level (Andersen et al. 1994). The structure and process across organization types can affect effectiveness and clinical outcomes. At the systemic level the way in which health care is organized (e.g. a nationally funded and organized health care system) clearly has an impact on the patient–provider transaction. At the contextual level other policies (i.e. welfare policy) also have an impact.

A key structural component of HSR is finances. While HSR has made numerous contributions to understanding health care, its focus on outcomes and linking these to structure and process makes it a core consideration in any discussion of health services. Health policy should involve adopting the most efficacious, effective therapies with the best outcomes within real practices and within the resources available. Cost-effectiveness and cost–benefit analyses are an essential part of that determination (Clancy & Kamerow 1996; Kay & Blinkhorn 1996). The ultimate objective of HSR is to improve the quality of care (Brown et al. 2000).

Steinwachs & Hughes (2008) note that it is largely HSR that is drawn upon by decision-makers and informs policy decisions and tends to be the primary source for information on how well health systems, at least in the USA, are functioning. This fact in itself should make it of prime interest to the CAM community.

The field was defined by the Academy of Health as follows:

> *HSR is the multidisciplinary field of scientific investigation that studies how social factors, financing systems, organizational structures and processes, health technologies, and personal behaviors affect access to health care, quality and cost of health care, and ultimately our health and well-being. Its research domains are individuals, families, organizations, institutions, communities, and populations*
>
> (Lohr & Steinwachs 2002).

Clearly then health services research covers a huge swathe of health concerns. In fact the challenge might be to identify what is not included. Herman et al. (2006) summarize HSR research by stating that it's the 'study of the effect of various components of healthcare system (e.g. social factors, financing systems, organizational structures and process, delivery of care, health technologies, personal behaviors) on healthcare outcomes (e.g. access, quality, cost, patient health and well-being)'(p. 79).

They also note that only three areas are excluded: (1) demonstration projects; (2) studies of efficacy done in laboratories or on animals; and (3) randomized controlled trials (RCTs) using strict protocols and defined patient groups. 'In short, HSR is based on the assumption that efficacious treatments exist. It then evaluates the various components of treatment delivery (e.g. policy, structures, processes) with respect to outcomes to make healthcare more efficient, effective, and cost-effective' (Herman et al. 2006, p. 79).

It is clear therefore why the CAM community might be interested in HSR. Firstly, its major concerns do dovetail very well with the types of concerns the CAM community is worried about, including access, utilization, funding, cost and outcomes. Secondly, because it is the field that is used by policy-makers it does have a significant role in shaping both the health care debates and health care delivery. Few other fields have as much potential to have an impact on the system organization and delivery of health as opposed to, say, impacting on specific therapy and treatment. Thirdly, but by no means least, it employs research methodologies that seem more appropriate to assessing CAM than the traditional RCTs so prevalent in biomedicine. There is therefore much for CAM to relate to in HSR.

Unfortunately, until quite recently, CAM has not very frequently been the subject in HSR. One feature that HSR does share with CAM is that, relatively speaking, in the USA it receives one of the lowest amounts of funding from the National Institutes of Health (NIH) (in 2005 about 5% of the budget) (Herman et al. 2006). Of course that greatly exceeds the budget for the National Center for Complementary and Alternative Medicine (NCCAM), which was 0.42% of the total NIH budget in 2006, which might help explain why investigating CAM has not constituted a large part of HSR (Coulter 2007).

WHAT KIND OF EVIDENCE DOES HSR COLLECT AND WHAT KIND OF METHODS DOES IT USE?

The most dominant feature of HSR is that it is very multidisciplinary. It is done by statisticians, epidemiologists, sociologists, psychologists, anthropologists, economists, behavioural scientists, management/organizational studies, medicine, nursing, dentists, chiropractors, acupuncturists, and other health professions. Because of this it uses multimethods. The hierarchy of evidence that characterizes systematic reviews and meta-analysis does not make sense in this area (Coulter 2006).

While health planners may give more weight to economic factors such as cost, these may not be the most significant variables determining the outcomes of the health care. The relevance of any form of evidence in HSR will be dictated by both the purpose for which the information is being used and the context in which it is gathered. In the house of evidence, as outlined by

Jonas (2005), HSR falls into the category he labels 'use testing'. This is in contrast to what he terms 'effects testing'. As Jonas notes, HSR research can provide information about the relevance and utility of practices whether they are proven or unproven in terms of efficacy. HSR represents a pluralistic approach to evidence.

There is no single methodology or research design for conducting HSR. This is a point also made by Walach et al. with regard to CAM: 'More specifically we will argue that there is no such thing as an inherently ideal methodology. There are different methods to answer different questions' (Walach et al. 2006 p. 2).

They suggest that instead of a hierarchical model of evidence the more appropriate model is a circular one. Under this approach there are a multiple of optimal methods and the most powerful method might be triangulation. This occurs when two distinct methodological and independent approaches are used to investigate the same phenomenon. So, for example, RCTs may need to be supplemented by long-term observational studies to see if therapies have the same effect in clinical practice that they have in controlled trials.

Steinwachs & Hughes (2008) note that the report *Crossing the Quality Chasm: A New Health Care Systems for the 21st Century* (Committee on the Quality of Care in America 2001) identified six critical elements: (1) patient safety; (2) effectiveness; (3) timeliness; (4) patient-centred care; (5) efficiency; and (6) equity. It is HSR that provides the measurement tools for evaluating these goals.

THE MARRIAGE OF CAM AND HSR

In two recent articles by Herman et al. (2006) and Coulter & Khorsan (2008), the merits of the match between CAM and HSR have been examined. In their paper Herman et al. (2006) identify 355 studies in the field of HSR and CAM therapies. But this represented only 2% of studies identified in the search (up to 2005) as HSR. Of those with abstracts that clearly identified the nature of the study, the bulk was surveys of CAM users which often included their reasons for using CAM. The next most frequent were descriptive surveys of providers 'to obtain their characteristics, the characteristics of their patients, and the specific therapies they prescribe' (p. 80). There was one study looking at the economic impacts of CAM, eight on research needs and five on research methods. Their paper therefore is more focused on what HSR research can bring to CAM (and the reverse). They suggest that studies of integrative medicine (IM), health insurance coverage, effectiveness, cost-effectiveness, practice guidelines and whole-systems research are all areas of potential work for HSR in CAM. Because of the way the literature search was conducted (and that only those studies with abstracts were reviewed), the number of studies probably represents a very incomplete list. In two earlier papers focusing just on chiropractic, the number of studies listed in HSR and social sciences was 105 (Mootz et al. 1997) and 81, respectively (Mootz et al. 2006).

Coulter & Khorsan (2008) for their part make the case that one of the significant contributions of HSR to CAM is in the area of descriptive studies. Despite the fact we now have numerous studies on the utilization of CAM we still have very little good empirical data on what is done in CAM practices. From the studies we can tell you the percentage of the population using various CAM professionals but not what they are being treated for, what they are being treated with, what it costs and what the outcomes are. As they note, until we know more about the practice, the scope of practice, patient characteristics, utilization rates, patient numbers, patient health problems, therapies being used, cost and funding, it is difficult to design appropriate studies, including whole-systems research. 'The studies on epidemiology, insurance, and cost effectiveness can all contribute to our understanding of CAM' (Coulter & Khorsan 2008 p. 40). In the case of chiropractic there is now a large body of descriptive studies as well as other HSR studies. The latter has included studies on workman's compensation, comparisons of chiropractic and medical care, evaluation by patients, the testing of various hypotheses about chiropractic utilization using empirical data, studies of the efficacy of chiropractic in clinical trials, meta-analysis of studies on manipulation, field studies on the appropriateness of chiropractic manipulation and the economic cost of chiropractic. Therefore, there exists for chiropractic 'an extensive body of data that describes the practice, the patients, and the providers of chiropractic' (Coulter & Khorsan 2008 p. 42).

Because HSR focuses on existing practices and programmes in the real world as opposed to the artificial world created under RCTs, it speaks to a major concern of CAM – effectiveness. As Coulter & Khorsan note, 'in this way HSR introduces a badly needed dose of realism into the evidence-based practice movement' (Coulter & Khorsan 2008 p. 41). Steinwachs & Hughes (2008) observe that effectiveness research is undertaken in community settings and with patients who are not subjected to inclusion or exclusion criteria and who can be given multiple interventions.

Steinwachs & Hughes (2008) identify key areas where they feel HSR can make major contributions to CAM: studies evaluating the quality of health care; studies of the structure of health care; studies of the process of health care; studies of the outcomes of care; and public health studies focusing on preventive health services.

Coulter & Khorsan (2008) add to this list two other major areas: studies on the health-related quality of life and studies on the appropriateness of care.

However we wish to focus on its potential in another area – whole-systems research and programme evaluation.

WHOLE-SYSTEMS RESEARCH

Numerous commentators have noted that, in studying CAM, and more recently IM, we need to move away from the reductionist model used in RCT to study the whole system. The favoured theoretical models for doing this have been systems theory (Beckman et al. 1996; Bell et al. 2002; Verhoef et al. 2005) and/or complexity theory (Kernick 2006).

Originally systems theory grew out of work in biology but was later applied in the field of cybernetics, information theory and computers. Beckman et al. (1996) identify the following features of systems theory. First, it posits a multilevelled structure in which the whole cannot be reduced to its parts or the sum of its parts. A change in any subpart has an impact on all the other parts. Second, it posits an ecological view of systems in which a system interacts constantly with its environment and where the results are processes rather than final structures so that health becomes a process, not an endproduct. Third, it posits non-linear causality. Fourth, it sees systems as self-organizing and with emergent properties which cannot be found in the constituent parts. Fifth, the systems are therefore self-transcendent, meaning they can transcend any one state and create new structures and processes. Sixth, the mind represents the dynamics of self-organization and is characteristic not only of individuals but also of social, cultural and ecological systems.

For Bell et al., systems theory provides a 'rational conceptual framework within which to evaluate CAM systems, integrative medicine' (Bell et al. 2002 p. 13). As they note, the classic view of health care looks at structure, process and outcome. But all of these present a challenge to CAM and IM. If we acknowledge that CAM and IM represent multiple systems we need scientific methods that can assess 'multi-causal illnesses, multiple interventions, and multi-dimensional outcomes (bio-psycho-social)' (Bell et al. 2002 p. 137). As they further note, there are new analytical and statistical methods for doing this kind of assessment.

Verhoef et al. (2005) make a similar case for whole-systems research and CAM. They further note that in whole-systems research both the patient–practitioner relationship and the therapeutic environment would not be ignored (what the present authors would term the health encounter). Furthermore systems research would include what they term 'model validity'; that is, it would research the unique healing theory and the therapeutic context (Jonas & Linde 2002). They note, as does Bell and her colleagues (2002), that this approach will require both quantitative and qualitative methods, especially the use of observational methods.

Kernick (2006) feels that one of the reasons HSR has not been more influential (and therefore its results less implemented) is because its research models have been too simplistic to reflect the real health care environment. The assumptions underlying the major research model (the RCT) have been linearity in causal effects, reductionism, determinism, impartiality of the observer, and that the natural state of systems is equilibrium. In contrast he sees that in complexity theory (1) there are complex systems that consist of a large number of interacting elements; (2) there are reiterative loop backs and that these non-linear instabilities lead to innovation and unpredictable behaviour; (3) small changes on one area can cause large changes across the whole system; (4) the system is different than the sum of its parts; (5) the behaviour of complex systems can result from emergent properties; (6) systems may operate away from equilibrium, there may be multiple equilibria and equilibrium states are invariably suboptimal; (7) complex systems do not have clear boundaries; and (8) history is important in complex systems and the past will influence the present. Given these features of systems, breaking them down into component parts may destroy the very thing you are trying to understand. Patterns of order evolve and self-organize: the important focus is on the interactions between the elements and not the elements themselves.

IS HSR WHOLE-SYSTEMS RESEARCH?

The answer to this question is: yes and no. Coulter & Khorsan (2008) in their paper looked at the view one can get from HSR of chiropractic and from the social sciences such as anthropology and sociology. Their conclusion is that HSR research provides a distinctly different picture of chiropractic. In that picture chiropractic looks like a neuromusculoskeletal specialty whose focus is overwhelmingly on the spine and the neuromuscolskeletal system of the body. Chiropractic appears narrow in the scope of both its therapies (dominantly manipulation) and in terms of the health problems it treats (back and back-related problems). However in the case of chiropractic there is a fairly extensive body of ethnographic observation studies by social scientists (Coulter 2004). This allows us then to make a comparison of the view from both.

In the social science literature chiropractic appears as a holistic practice with a broad focus on wellness. While manipulation may be the major therapy it is given within a framework of a very broad philosophical paradigm characterized by vitalism. Although the patients may present a very narrow range of initial health problems, the care is expanded to include posture, stress, exercise, weight, diet, nutrition and lifestyle counselling. As noted by Coulter (2004), if you only looked at the quantitative data from HSR on chiropractic (and, as noted earlier, there is an extensive body of that) you miss all the information that you get from qualitative observation and, more importantly, miss understanding what the chiropractic health encounter is about. If we pose the question: what elements contribute to the effectiveness of chiropractic? you would not be able to answer that question just using the current HSR data.

But is this the result of abstinence (the absence of action) or impotence (the inability to perform the action)? While the outcome of these two may be the same the cause is quite different. We would like to suggest that it is the result of abstinence. We would further suggest that it is in the area of programme evaluation that we can find a solution to both this issue and the issue of whole-system research because the failure with regard to chiropractic is a failure to conduct whole-systems research.

CASE STUDIES AND PROGRAMME EVALUATION

For the most part programme evaluation is about effectiveness, not efficacy, and about total programmes, not simple therapeutic interventions. But because they are about programmes they are often combined with a case study methodology (Yin 1994) and use both qualitative and quantitative methods to examine how the programmes function (Jinnett et al. 2002).

CASE STUDIES

Case study methods are particularly appropriate for studying new and emergent programmes and have been used successfully to evaluate programmes in medical centers (Yin & Heald 1975; Patton 1990). Case studies are particularly strong at discovering the key factors that facilitate and inhibit desired outcomes and understanding the process and mechanisms through which these factors interact. Case studies are also one of the few techniques that provide indepth information about how programs are working (or not working) within the larger social and organizational contexts in which they are embedded (Coulter et al. 2007).

Case study methodology relies on a two-step sampling procedure. Investigators first decide what case (or cases) they will examine (case-based sampling), and then decide what kinds of data will be collected from each case (within-case sampling). The power of case studies does not depend on the number of cases but instead comes from the range and diversity of the within-case sample of people and data collection techniques.

By using stakeholder analysis, the cases will yield a rich description of how the programmes grapple with the challenge of providing CAM or for patients within various settings (e.g. hospitals). An example of this type of study is the study of a hospital-based IM program by Coulter et al. (2007).

Such studies can collect quantitative data about the programme's organization, costs and patient loads to understand how such a programme fits into a larger care network. Coulter et al. (2007) used stakeholder analysis to describe beliefs, behaviours and vested interests of at least five groups: (1) key administrators; (2) providers of care in the programmes; (3) clinicians within the larger medical centre who may or may not have referred patients; (4) CAM providers, when they were used; and (5) patients.

The aim of the qualitative component is to elucidate issues that cannot be answered by the quantitative analyses and to explore additional areas that are difficult to address in a quantitative work (Van Maanen 1979; Miles & Huberman 1994).

PROGRAMME EVALUATION

Programme evaluation traditionally involves three levels of evaluation: (1) structural evaluation; (2) process evaluation; and (3) outcome evaluation. The point of such evaluations is to determine the merit, worth and significance of the programme and hopefully assist those who may wish to expand, change or replicate it in other facilities.

An evaluation strategy will usually include contextual (Israel et al. 1995), formative process (Scheirer 1994; Brindis et al. 1998) and summative elements (Rossi et al. 1999).

Contextual evaluation is used to assess and compare the environments and the population characteristics of the programme. An evaluation here will focus on the influence of these factors on the intervention structures, processes and outcomes.

In the initial phases of a programme, formative evaluation can be used to collect data on intervention structures and processes. Process evaluation is used to assess the extent to which the intervention components are implemented as planned. Summative evaluation measures the extent to which programme goals and objectives were achieved and the intermediate and longer-term impact of the programme. The programme evaluation should be a combination of qualitative and quantitative methods, allowing triangulation of the data.

Structural evaluation

Structural evaluation is used to determine the structure of the organization and will often use both institutional documents, such as organizational charts (business plans, financial information on resources), staffing (staffing ratios) and interviews with key personnel. Structure involves official descriptions of the programme and the environment. It will also involve the logic of the programme, the goals/milestones and values (Scriven 1991). It would include a description of the structure and facilities of a clinic, the staffing, the equipment, support services, location and appearance of the clinic (Rossi et al. 1999).

Process evaluation

Process evaluation moves from what is stated on paper to what actually occurs in practice. Here evaluators will often make extensive use of one-on-one qualitative interviews with the participants in the programme (staff) but also with other key stakeholders at each site. They might also use ethnographic observation. The key is to distinguish what people say – the rhetoric – from what they do – the reality.

Often it will involve a two-stage process evaluation. It begins with an initial assessment to identify how the programme really operates (the lived programme as opposed to the programme on paper) and to establish a baseline to evaluate change over the life of the programme. This can be followed with a more expansive evaluation to identify potential mechanisms that may help account for why the programme has been more or less successful, why it has achieved the outcomes it has or the barriers that interfere with its success.

Process evaluation also includes 'the interactions between the health care providers and patients over time' (Steinwachs & Hughes 2008 p. 5). It can look at treatment over time, relate treatment to complaints/diagnoses, look at the number of services and 'provides insights into the timeliness of care, organizational responsiveness, and efficiency' (Steinwachs & Hughes 2008 p. 5). As these authors note:

> *evaluation of the process of care can be done by applying the six goals for health care quality. Was the patient's safety protected (i.e. were there adverse events due to medical errors or errors of omission)? Was care timely and not delayed or denied? Were the diagnosis and treatments provided consistent with scientific evidence and best professional practice? Was the care patient-centered? Were services provided efficiently? Was the care provided equitable?*
>
> (Steinwachs & Hughes 2008 p. 5).

Outcome evaluation

Outcome programme evaluation will involve both quantitative measures (such as repeated use of a programme; satisfaction scores; spending patterns; functional patient measures; health status outcomes; health-related quality of life; biological markers) and qualitative data from interviews with participants (patients) and staff (stakeholders). The outcomes measured will be highly dependent on the type of programme and its objectives.

Outcome measures will often involve comparing what the original objectives were, particularly if these were related to needs assessment, with what has been achieved. Wherever possible this should be done with objective measures but it will also involve qualitative measures. For each objective or goal it is necessary to operationalize an indicator that can act as a measurement that would represent the successful achievement of the objective/goal. This would also incorporate the earlier comment about including the philosophical model of the program. If this model subscribes to holistic health care, to what extent is the care delivered holistic? If it claims to be IM, to what extent is it integrated?

Two types of outcomes that are frequently included in outcome assessments, in contrast to clinical outcomes, are changes in beliefs/attitudes/perceptions versus changes in behaviour. In the area of CAM and IM both would be considered significant measures, as would be spiritual health.

Within the field of programme evaluation there are numerous models of what outcomes are important to measure. One approach stresses determining the merit, worth and significance of the programme (Scriven 1991). Outcomes here would include direct and indirect outcomes, intended and unintended, immediate or long-term, side-effects and economic outcomes (cost verses benefits). Some approaches assess the outcomes from the point of view of policy (Henry & Melvin 2003). Still others use a theory-driven evaluation (Donaldson & Scriven 2002). Fetterman (2002) evaluates outcomes in terms of empowerment.

At its best, outcome evaluation should be useful to those in the programme (Donaldson 2001). A method which is used to help participants build a better programme is appreciative enquiry (Fetterman 2002). Such an approach is based on discovering the unique factors within a programme (leadership, relationships, culture, structure, rewards) that bring about the outcomes and envisaging a different outcome or programme but building on the current one.

CONCLUSION

It is clear that there is much in HSR that commends it to those who are either involved in, or want to see, more rigorous research on CAM but who find the current evidence-based practice model, with its hierarchy of knowledge and its reliance on efficacy studies and the RCT, as either an incomplete or inadequate model for CAM research. For those who are interested in a whole-systems model and systems theory and complexity theory, while it is clear at a theoretical level this is a fruitful way to go, no one has yet delineated a simple analytical model for applying it so that variables as diverse as biological markers to ethnographic observations can be included within the one model. We are suggesting here that programme evaluation offers an already established, very pragmatic way of moving towards whole-systems research (Jonas et al. 2006). It is an established field with a variety of theoretical models at its disposal; it combines both quantitative and qualitative data; it looks at the three crucial elements of structure, process and outcomes and under those categories can capture all the elements that CAM providers have identified as important and look at their interactions; its ultimate purpose is better outcomes for patients; it captures the contextual data necessary for replicating programmes; it deals with the real world of clinical practice; it studies effectiveness, not efficacy; it has a track record of applications; and it is used by decision-makers to make health policy.

We are left with the question of how we evaluate the evaluations themselves. Are there ways in which we can judge rigorous evaluations from less rigorous evaluations? Djulbegovic et al. (2006) suggest that Wilson's term 'consilience' provides a way of conceptualizing the bringing together of knowledge to overcome the fragmentation of knowledge in contemporary science. 'The consilience is a test of truth of the theory or interpretation of evidence. The "consilience test" takes place when findings obtained from one class of facts coincide with findings obtained from a different class of observations' (Djulbegovic et al. 2006 p. 105). In the social sciences this would be termed triangulation, the use of bodies of data from independent sources and/or using different methodologies. So, within a single case study we can compare the data collected from qualitative methods with those collected from qualitative sources and compare data from medical records with data collected from questionnaires or interviews. Across case studies we can compare the findings to determine if consistent linkages between, say, structures and outcomes are being found.

Gartlehner et al. (2006) have devised a set of criteria that can be used to evaluate effectiveness studies to distinguish between efficacy and effectiveness trials. The latter measures the degree of benefit under real-world clinical practice. They recommend seven criteria for effectiveness trials: (1) populations in effectiveness studies should reflect the initial care facilities to a diverse population; (2) eligibility criteria must allow the population to reflect the homogeneity of the actual population (i.e. their comorbidities, compliance rates, use of other medications or therapies); (3) health outcomes that are relevant to the condition of interest should be the principal measures; (4) study duration should mimic a minimum length of treatment in a clinical setting to allow the assessment of outcomes and compliance should be an outcome measures, not an inclusion/exclusion criterion; (5) adverse event assessments should be limited to critical issues; (6) the sample size should be sufficient to detect at least a minimally important difference on a health-related quality of life scale; and (7) statistical analysis should not exclude patients with protocol deviations, compliance issues, adverse events, drug regimens, comorbidities and concomitant treatments. In testing these criteria the authors found an interrater reliability of 78.3% using experts from the North American-funded Evidence-based Practice Centers to judge both efficacy and effectiveness studies. This work demonstrates that formal criteria can be established to rate the quality of effectiveness and/or evaluation studies (see Chapter 1 for quality criteria scales for evaluating effectiveness research). Thus, HSR has an important role in understanding CAM and needs more emphasis in health care.

REFERENCES

Andersen, R.M., Davidson, P.L., Ganz, P.A., 1994. Symbiotic relationships of quality of life, health services research and other health research. Qual. Life Res. 3 (5), 365–371.

Beckman, J.F., Fernandez, C.E., Coulter, I.D., 1996. A systems model of health care: a proposal. J. Manipulative Physiol. Ther. 19 (3), 208–215.

Bell, I.R., Caspi, O., Schwartz, G.E., et al., 2002. Integrative medicine and systemic outcomes research: issues in the emergence of a new model for primary health care. Arch. Intern. Med. 162 (2), 133–140.

Brindis, C., Hughes, D.C., Halfon, N., et al., 1998. The use of formative evaluation to assess integrated services for children. The Robert Wood Johnson Foundation Child Health Initiative. Eval. Health Prof. 21 (1), 66–90.

Brown, G.C., Brown, M.M., Sharma, S., 2000. Health care in the 21st century: evidence-based medicine, patient preference-based quality, and cost effectiveness. Qual. Manag. Health Care. 9 (1), 23–31.

Clancy, C.M., Kamerow, D.B., 1996. Evidence-based medicine meets cost-effectiveness analysis. JAMA. 276 (4), 329–330.

Committee on the Quality of Care in America, 2001. Crossing the Quality Chasm: A New Health Care System for the 21st Century. Institute of Medicine National Academy Press, Washington, DC.

Coulter, I.D., 2001. Evidence-based dentistry and health services research: is one possible without the other? J. Dent. Educ. 65 (8), 714–724.

Coulter, I.D., 2004. Competing views of chiropractic: health services research versus ethnographic observation. In: Oths, K.S., Hinojosa, H.Z. (Eds.), Healing by Hand: Manual Medicine and Bonesetting in Global Perspective. AltaMira Press, Walnut Creek, CA.

Coulter, I.D., 2006. Evidence summaries and synthesis: necessary but insufficient approach for determining clinical practice of integrated medicine? Integr. Cancer Ther. 5 (4), 282–286.

Coulter, I.D., 2007. Evidence based complementary and alternative medicine: promises and problems. Forsch. Komplementmed. 14 (2), 102–108.

Coulter, I.D., Khorsan, R., 2008. Is health services research the Holy Grail of complementary and alternative medicine research? Altern. Ther. Health Med. 14 (4), 40–45.

Coulter, I.D., Ellison, M.A., Hilton, L., et al., 2007. Hospital-Based Integrative Medicine: A Case Study of the Barriers and Factors Facilitating the Creation of a Center. RAND MG-591-NCCAM. RAND Health, Santa Monica, CA.

Djulbegovic, B., Morris, L., Lyman, G., 2006. Evidentiary Challenges to Evidence-based Medicine. J. Eval. Clin. Pract. 2, 99–100.

Donaldson, S.I., 2001. Overcoming our negative reputation: Evaluation becomes known as a helping profession. American Journal of Evaluation 22, 355–361.

Donaldson, S.I., Scriven, M., 2002. Evaluating social programs and problems: Visions for the new millennium. Erlbaum, Mahwah, NJ.

Fetterman, D.M., 2002. Empowerment evaluation: building communities of practice and a culture of learning. Am. J. Community Psychol. 30 (1), 89–102.

Gartlehner, G., Hansen, R.A., Nissman, D., et al., 2006. A simple and valid tool distinguished efficacy from effectiveness studies. J. Clin. Epidemiol. 59 (10), 1040–1048.

Gray, B.H., Gusmano, M.K., Collins, S.R., 2003. AHCPR and the changing politics of health services research. Health Aff. (Millwood). (Suppl) Web Exclusives, W3-283–307.

Henry, G.T., Melvin, M.M., 2003. Beyond Use: Understanding Evaluation's Influence on Attitudes and Actions. American Journal of Evaluation. 24 (3), 293–314.

Herman, P.M., D'Huyvetter, K., Mohler, M.J., 2006. Are health services research methods a match for CAM? Altern. Ther. Health Med. 12 (3), 78–83.

Institute of Medicine, 1979. Health Services Research: Report of a Study. No. 78-06 National Academy of Sciences Press, Washington, DC.

Israel, B.A., Cummings, K.M., Dignan, M.B., et al., 1995. Evaluation of health education programs: current assessment and future directions. Health Educ. Q. 22 (3), 364–389.

Jinnett, K., Coulter, I., Koegel, P., 2002. Cases, context and care: the need for grounded network analysis. In: Levy, J.A., Pescosolido, B.A. (Eds.), Advances in Medical Sociology, vol. 8. Social Networks and Health. Elsevier Science, Oxford, UK.

Jonas, W.B., 2005. Building an evidence house: challenges and solutions to research in complementary and alternative medicine. Forsch. Komplementarmed. Klass. Naturheilkd. 12 (3), 159–167.

Jonas, W.B., Linde, K., 2002. Conducting and Evaluating Clinical Research in Complementary and Alternative Medicine. In: Gallin, J.I. (Ed.), Principles and Practice of Clinical Research. Academic Press, New York, pp. 401–426.

Jonas, W.B., Beckner, W., Coulter, I.D., 2006. Proposal for an integrated evaluation model for the study of whole systems health care in cancer. Integr. Cancer Ther. 5 (4), 315–319.

Kay, E., Blinkhorn, A., 1996. Dental health services research: what is it and does it matter? Br. Dent. J. 180 (3), 116–117.

Kernick, D., 2006. Wanted–new methodologies for health service research. Is complexity theory the answer? Fam. Pract. 23 (3), 385–390.

Lohr, K.N., Steinwachs, D.M., 2002. Health services research: an evolving definition of the field. Health Serv. Res. 37 (1), 7–9.

Miles, M.B., Huberman, A.M., 1994. Qualitative Data Analysis: An expanded sourcebook, second ed. Sage Publications, Thousand Oaks, CA.

Mootz, R.D., Coulter, I.D., Hansen, D.T., 1997. Health services research related to chiropractic: review and recommendations for research prioritization by the chiropractic profession. J. Manipulative Physiol. Ther. 20 (3), 201–217.

Mootz, R.D., Hansen, D.T., Breen, A., et al., 2006. Health services research related to chiropractic: review and recommendations for research prioritization by the chiropractic profession. J. Manipulative Physiol. Ther. 29 (9), 707–725.

Patton, M.Q., 1990. Qualitative evaluation and research methods, second ed. Sage Publications, Newbury Park, CA.

Rossi, P.H., Freeman, H.E., Lipsey, M.W., 1999. Evaluation: A Systematic Approach. Sage Publications, Thousand Oaks, CA.

Scheirer, M.A., 1994. In: Designing and Using Process Evaluation. Handbook of Practical Program Evaluation. Jossey-Bass, San Francisco, pp. 40–68.

Scriven, M., 1991. Evaluation Thesaurus. Sage Publication, Newbury Park, CA.

Steinwachs, D.M., Hughes, R.G., 2008. Chapter 8: Health Services Research: Scope and Significance. In: Hughes, R.G. (Ed.), Patient safety and quality: An evidence-based handbook for nurses. AHRQ Publication No 08-0043. Agency for Healthcare Research and Quality, Rockville, MD, pp. 1–15.

Van Maanen, J., 1979. Qualitative Methodology. Sage Publications, Beverly Hills, CA.

Verhoef, M.J., Lewith, G., Ritenbaugh, C., et al., 2005. Complementary and alternative medicine whole systems research: beyond identification of inadequacies of the RCT. Complement. Ther. Med. 13 (3), 206–212.

Walach, H., Falkenberg, T., Fonnebo, V., et al., 2006. Circular instead of hierarchical: methodological principles for the evaluation of complex interventions. BMC Med. Res. Methodol. 6, 29.

Yin, R.K., 1994. Case Study Research. Design and Methods, second ed. Sage, Newbury Park, CA.

Yin, R.K., Heald, K.A., 1975. Using The Case Survey Method To Analyse Policy Studies. Adm. Sci. Q. 20, 371–381.

SECTION II
SPECIAL ISSUES IN ESTABLISHING CAM RESEARCH QUALITY

SECTION CONTENTS

Research in herbal medicine

8

Simon Y. Mills

CHAPTER CONTENTS

INTRODUCTION

Although herbal or plant-based remedies are extremely popular treatments around the world, their use in developed countries invokes complex regulatory and academic issues. In some parts of the world, notably the USA, they are supplied as dietary supplements with relatively few regulatory or scientific standards. In other countries they may hold default medicinal status. In Europe particularly, where herbal remedies are referred to as 'herbal medicinal products', 'phytomedicines' or 'plant drugs', they are regulated alongside conventional medicines, at least as far as standards of quality and safety are concerned. In some countries phytomedicines are actually orthodox pharmaceuticals, prescribed by doctors and dispensed or supplied primarily by pharmacists.

Herbal medicines are perhaps the most tangible targets among complementary treatments for research and investigation. The leading manufacturers in Europe have a long history of providing clinical data in the orthodox forum and there is a relatively good stock of scientific literature. Herbs can also be the origin of new synthetic medicines. They may even be the basis of

DOI: 10.1016/B978-0-443-06956-7.00008-2

patentable extracts. All this means that research into their activity can be commercially justified. There is a vast record of scientific papers in which plants or their constituents have been subject to laboratory studies to investigate their prospects for leads in pharmaceutical research. Even though the trend in pharmaceutical research is moving away from plant leads and the long-term prospects here are not promising, the levels of published papers show no signs of reducing.

However, there is a difference between plants as leads for pharmaceutical development and as herbal medicines used by humans. Unfortunately the clinical evidence base for the use of plants as medicines has at best been patchy. The use of herbal medicines as elements in considered clinical strategies, as applied by qualified herbal practitioners for example, has as poor a publication record as any other complementary discipline. Establishing efficacy of herbal products in law has usually been a pragmatic exercise. Undemanding requirements in lieu of clinical evidence have recently been adopted in Europe and the future prospect for research investment by herbal medicine manufacturers has unfortunately been diminished.

Experience of herbal remedies within a modern medical culture does confirm that they have distinguishing features. They have been used continuously for many decades or centuries, often in ways much different from those of modern prescription. Their modern and traditional descriptions are often very different. Plants consist of many chemical constituents with inherent variability and with complex pharmacological effects on the body. There are different issues of both efficacy and safety and it is unwise to compare them directly to medicines made up of single chemical entities. To be consistent to this difference the research methods employed should also be adapted.

One research area of promise is the massive human experience of herbal remedies. Even today the World Health Organization considers that the majority of remedies consumed by humans around the world are plant-based in a traditional context, and historically the dominance of plants in medicine must have been overwhelming. The vast majority of this human use is unrecorded and most of the available data are not rigorously collated. However, there is still a rich vein of material to be mined and proposals are outlined here.

THE EVIDENCE FRAGMENTS

There are four major types of research data on medicinal plants or their constituents (Table 8.1). As these are more than are available for other complementary treatments it is fair to subject them to a robust test of relevance. They may be reviewed from the perspective of a herbal remedy user, whether through self-prescription or in herbal practice. Do they help to make an informed decision about the safe and beneficial use of a herbal remedy? Most of these sources of data fail this test and remain barely useful fragments.

FRAGMENT 1: CONTROLLED CLINICAL TRIALS

In the case of clinical trial evidence, the literature is mixed. There are increasing well-conducted random-assigned, double-blind controlled studies, and even systematic reviews of these. The literature on ginkgo (*Ginkgo biloba*)

Table 8.1 *Fragments in the herbal research literature*		
Fragment	**Positives**	**Problems**
Controlled clinical trials	Highest-quality evidence of the specific effects of a remedy Particularly relevant to the remedy and to the main use of herbs for self-medication	Economics not suited to trials in non-proprietary products Methodological challenges for herbal remedies Clinical trial findings may be inappropriate for self-medication Reduced incentives of new legislation
Animal studies	Prominent in herbal scientific literature May allow insight into pharmacological and physiological processes	Ethically unacceptable to many who might choose the herbal option Many trials compromised by unrealistic dosing Interspecies differences in metabolism of key plant constituents
In vitro studies	Vast proportion of literature, linked mainly to pharmaceutical development May allow insight into cellular processes, particularly where plant products are administered externally or by injection	Cannot account for the fact that most plant constituents are metabolically altered on oral consumption Usually other unrealistic dosage regimens Distorting effects of using glassware on plant materials chosen for research
Traditional use evidence	Overwhelming human medical experience through history Relates to actual dose and human use of herbs With systematic organization collective experiences may be extracted and linked to evidence in other fragments	Uncontrolled observations masked by non-specific and cultural effects and observer bias Records usually of poor quality

(The European Scientific Cooperative on Phytotherapy 2003), which has been among the most widely prescribed of all drugs in continental Europe, and on St John's wort (*Hypericum perforatum*) (The European Scientific Cooperative on Phytotherapy 2003), many hundreds of papers in each case, with dozens of these being full clinical trials.

There is little doubt that orthodox evidence requirements are potentially appropriate for most herbal medicines consumed by the public. Over-the-counter (OTC) herbal use in Europe far outstrips practitioner prescription, probably by a factor of more than 20:1 (IMS/PhytoGold 1998). For researching OTC label indications for discrete medicinal products, in which individual responses to remedies are not the critical issue, the double-blind controlled clinical trial is clearly the most applicable method. In addition, as the 'patient' is in many cases not being diagnosed professionally and is determining his or her own treatment and prognosis, self-assessment questionnaires are often an appropriate measure of progress. These are not expensive to administer. As this is often 'outpatient' medicine research, costs can be saved as close clinical supervision need not be always be necessary throughout the trial.

There are however practical problems in pursuing good clinical research in herbal medicine:

1. Herbal medicine in the west can boast few teaching hospitals or research institutes, nor support from public resources. Industrial investment has been limited to a few larger manufacturers used to working in a pharmaceutical culture. In most parts of the sector the necessary infrastructure is lacking. Neither can the costs of undertaking research studies easily be commercially justified: it is difficult to patent herbs and the size of the market for any individual product is only occasionally comparable to that for any patentable conventional drug. Commercial investment in clinical trials costing many hundreds of thousands of euros per product can only be justified if manufacturers can recover their investment in the market. A crude herbal is free for anyone to copy. Leading phytomedicine manufacturers therefore produce new extracts from plants that they can commercially protect. For example, there are almost no clinical trial data for ginkgo leaves as such: the research has been conducted on patented extracts of ginkgo (notably one known as EGb761) (Kressman et al. 2002). The same is largely true for black cohosh, saw palmetto, St John's wort, horse chestnut and kava. It is difficult for the wider herbal community to claim efficacy for non-standardized products based on these clinical data. The very high and rapidly escalating costs of conducting clinical trials to modern ethical standards and regulatory requirements put off all but the most promising prospects.
2. The indications often claimed for herbal medicines include many without robust outcome measures. Most are destined for the self-medication OTC market so are by definition directed at lesser degrees of morbidity where hard measures are elusive. By contrast, most synthetic OTC medicines on the market have 'switched' from prescription status and have acquired their efficacy evidence on harder clinical indications and in hospital or similar settings. Without hard or acceptably validated outcome measures, with more variable and lower-grade symptoms among the patient population, and with a greater likelihood of self-limiting or other spontaneously changing conditions, clear treatment effects are harder to establish. The result is that it is usually particularly necessary to recruit large patient samples and to devise tight exclusion criteria to constrain variation in the sample. All this places extra logistical demands on those wishing to set up effective clinical trials for these products.
3. Herbs are compound medicines, occupying an unusual position as being medicines with many of the characteristics of foods. As a complex of pharmacologically active chemicals, the whole package will have different properties from that of any single constituent acting alone. Knowing the action of the latter will not itself be predictive on the effect of the former, particularly if the experimental evidence is based on work done on laboratory animals (see below). It is therefore rare to find the satisfactory preclinical evidence often required by ethics committees for the approval of major clinical studies.
4. There are some instances in herbal research where blinding will be difficult. For example, bitter remedies, potentially mediated by the effects

on digestive functions of stimulation of the bitter taste buds, have played an important part in the claims of traditional herbal medicine: this is almost impossible to blind. There will as always be a role for the good single-blind study, especially if other elements are rigorously controlled.

5. In the past clinical studies in the use of herbal medicines have often been of indifferent methodological quality. Modern studies, even those otherwise highly rated, can be undermined because they neglect basic precautions against the very variable quality of herbal products. In a surprising proportion of clinical trial papers the herbal product used is not quantified, stabilized or verified (Wolsko et al. 2005). Other studies may not relate to the herbal remedy as such but to its chemically defined ingredients. For example, the well-claimed benefits of horsechestnut (*Aesculus hippocastanum*) on the venous system are actually based on studies of a major constituent, aescin. Many studies on kava-kava (*Piper methysticum*) are actually of the pyrone kavain. It may be even more misleading: the reputation that the greater celandine (*Chelidonium majus*) has in liver conditions is based on commercially sponsored studies on a semisynthetic derivative Ukrain.
6. There are other unintended consequences of clinical research that can limit their benefits to manufacturers. It is surprising how even the best track record of research has failed to lead to medicine registrations outside central Europe: St John's wort, ginkgo and hawthorn (*Crataegus* spp.) are prescription medicines in Germany but have no medicinal status at all in the UK and USA. In part this is linked to the indications established by such studies. In all three cases the studies point to uses that are not appropriate for unsupervised self-medication – depression, cardiovascular disease and heart disease respectively. Because self-medication is generally permitted only for minor self-limiting conditions, in those countries where herbs are more likely to be chosen by the public clinical research may actually be counterproductive.

Looking ahead there are new reasons for concern. In Europe, where so much of the herbal clinical literature has been generated, there is a new regulatory regime. The Directive on Traditional Herbal Medicinal Products permits the registration (rather than licensing) as medicines of herbal products on the basis of their traditional use rather than on proven efficacy (Directive 2004). Such products still have to comply with pharmaceutical good manufacturing practice (GMP) and safety monitoring, but there is no longer any incentive to prove their efficacy in clinical trials. In fact, as the Directive does not apply 'where the competent authorities judge that a traditional herbal medicinal product fulfils the criteria for authorization', any such data may bar a herbal product from the less expensive registration option and lead to a requirement that it be licensed as a full medicine. There is a concern that the new Directive will lead to a progressive devaluing of herbal medicines and a drying up of clinical research activity.

The herbal practitioner, or phytotherapist, has other reasons to note the limitations of the controlled clinical study. Herbal practitioners emphasize the individuality of their treatments; they most often mix a number of individual herbs in a prescription and in many cases construct a unique mixture. Like other complementary practitioners they might also point out that conventional clinical trials involve the homogenization of the patient population so that only an average effect is confirmed and genuinely important benefits for a minority of the population will be overlooked. Clinical trial data will help with, but still not answer, the fundamental question: 'is this remedy going to be good for this patient?'

Nevertheless the controlled clinical trial is a notably flexible instrument and clinical trial data at least involve rigorous observations of human use of plants: of the forms of research available they are by far the most valuable in making clinical judgements. Perhaps better hopes lie with the moves towards sustainable economic development in countries around the world. Renewed interest in the potential of indigenous medical traditions, in some cases linked to emerging economies, has increased research activities in a wider range of plants (Blumenthal & Cavaliere 2006). At best standards developed for herbal research in Europe can be exported to improve the quality of investigation elsewhere and new products linked to sustainable 'freetrade' arrangements. There is still a hunger for beneficial natural medicines. If there is any substance in the promise, new ways will be found to service that demand.

FRAGMENT 2: EVIDENCE FROM ANIMAL STUDIES

Investigations of medicinal activity in animals raise particular concerns among those who would otherwise be amenable to using herbal approaches and are therefore often discouraged in the herbal industry. However it is salutary to note that the international scientific literature on plant remedies and their constituents is still dominated by in vivo studies.

As well as challenging moral and ethical sensibilities such studies have other shortcomings. They are always undermined by interspecies differences and often by therapeutically inappropriate mode of application. Observations often relate to unrealistically high doses, and particularly to intraperitoneal or intravenous injection rather than oral administration. In the case of plants, whose constituents are usually transformed by digestive action and hepatic first-pass effect, these latter factors seriously undermine any projection to the effect of the whole plant on oral consumption in humans. Differences in liver processing among animal species add a particular extra uncertainty for complex chemical entities like plants. It has been established, for example, that critical P450 cytochrome metabolic pathways differ significantly in laboratory animals compared to humans (Blumenthal & Cavaliere 2006).

At best oral administration of plants in realistic doses to animals may help to explore some basic pharmacological processes. In most cases these data should be ruthlessly marginalized in projecting clinical effects in humans.

FRAGMENT 3: EVIDENCE FROM IN VITRO STUDIES

In laboratory experiments it is extremely difficult to reproduce the balance of plant constituents that will actually reach internal tissues after digestion, absorption and the hepatic first-pass effects. In cell and tissue cultures concentrations of active principles at cell membranes and receptors usually far exceed those ever reached in vivo.

Most in vitro studies are on isolated fractions of the plant. It is very doubtful that the action of the whole plant can be determined by knowing the effects of individual constituents. Interaction between dozens or even hundreds of these limits the inferences that can be drawn. There have been some calculations demonstrating the synergistic effects of plant constituents in the whole plant which reinforce this point (Bogaards et al. 2000).

One particular hurdle arises from the historical choice of glass ('vitro') to conduct these experiments. Some key plant constituents are adherent to glass surfaces and quickly coat glassware, so compromising observations. Plants therefore have to be 'cleaned up' before being tested, leaving out important principles like resins, tannins, gums and mucilages.

The best that can be claimed for this work is that it may suggest pharmacological mechanisms. It can have almost no impact on judgements in clinical practice.

FRAGMENT 4: EVIDENCE FROM TRADITIONAL USE AND PRACTITIONER EXPERIENCE

Accounts of other people's use of medicines, particularly by observers outside the culture concerned, are vulnerable to observer error and usually relate to isolated cases or reputations in which non-specific influences on efficacy may be overwhelming. Without some form of confirmation any such report is at best an anecdote and when the additional cultural contexts are added it is difficult to generalize to the wider human community. Organized traditional records, as in the classic texts from earlier cultures, may be more systematized but suffer from *'shibboleth'* status: they are very rarely subject to rigorous review and have usually been transmitted didactically in a way that may enhance the powerful impact of suggestion on efficacy. Nevertheless, even with these caveats, clinical experience is the prime source of information on which most practitioners in any tradition base their judgements. Although personal perceptions of treatment benefit are obscured by non-specific effects, including placebo, collective impressions have great potency in determining the therapeutic profile of any remedy. Indeed it has been proposed that herbal texts may provide resources for modern data-mining techniques to identify novel pharmacotherapeutic leads for bioactive compounds (Williamson 2001; Buenz et al. 2006). Substantial accounts, for example as seen in systematic compilations of ethnobotanic records (Moerman 1998; Allen & Hatfield 2004; Buenz et al. 2004), can provide valuable sources for processing and distillation. Organized pre-modern physician texts, such as those of Eclectic physicians of 19th-century North America (Perry 1980), have relevance in modern clinical experience and should not be dismissed. The vast classical literature from China, India, Islamic and other regions is still the basis of medical practice and education in these countries today. There is potential – largely unexplored – scope for a distillation of such experiences. One form of correlation between traditional use and pharmacological research is outlined in Table 8.2 and referred to on page 161.

Table 8.2 ***Phytochemical groups in traditional and modern use***

Phytochemical subgroup and common sources	Subjective impact and application in traditional medicine of plants rich in this subgroup	Observed pharmacological activity
Acrid, 'pungent' principles (hot spices), e.g. in cayenne, ginger, peppers	Hot, heating, increasing warmth to diseased tissues, preventing food poisoning in hot climates, sustaining febrile response in fever management, topical to arthritis and other subdermal inflammations	Thermogenic[1] and metabolic stimulant,[2] involving catecholamine release and possibly reflex irritation, e.g. from vanilloid receptors on C-fibres,[3] increased gastric secretions,[4] propylactic against some food poisoning, pain relief,[5–9] increase in absorption of other nutrients and agents[10,11]
Anthraquinone and other laxatives, e.g. in senna, cascara, aloes	Laxative, topically anti-inflammatory	Laxative,[12–14] anti-inflammatory[15,16]
Aromatic (essential) oils, e.g. in cinnamon, cardamon, fennel, rosemary and other kitchen spices	Aromatic and warming, settling digestion, stimulating digestion in debilitated states, warming treatment for bronchial congestions	Carminative,[17] spasmolytic,[18] anti-inflammatory [19], antiparasitic,[20] antifungal,[21] mouthwashes,[22] antisenescence[23] and improved cognition,[24] antiseptic,[25–27]; wound healing,[28] expectorant,[29] diuretic[30]
Bitters, e.g. in wormwood, chicory, hops, coffee, angostura, quinine bark, condurango	Bitter, stimulant to appetite and digestion, choleretic, cooling effect in fever management, prevention and treatment of enteric infections, tonic	A property of many phytochemicals with pharmacological interest;[31] perhaps evolving as a protective against harm,[32] leads to systemic or local[33,34] gastric responses shown possibly leading to cholecystokinin, gastrin, secretin and other endogenous hormone release[35,36] digestive stimulant[37,38]
Fibre, e.g. in flaxseed, psyllium	Bulking, bowel regulator, demulcent (like mucilages)	Bulking laxative,[39] hypocholesterolaemic,[40] improving glucose tolerance[41]
Fixed oils, e.g. in olive oil, seed oils	Nutritive and anti-inflammatory	Potential anti-inflammatory effect on endocannabinoid receptors,[42] especially in dermatitis[43] and rheumatoid arthritis[44]; potential benefits in schizophrenia[45] and in lowering blood cholesterol[46].
Mucilages, e.g. in slippery elm. marshmallow, plantains	Slimy, emollient, demulcent, soothing to wounds and abrasions, reducing coughing due to dry irritability, soothing upper digestive inflammations	Physical basis for soothing properties demonstrated,[47,48] antitussive[49]

Continued

Table 8.2 *Phytochemical groups in traditional and modern use—Cont'd*		
Phytochemical subgroup and common sources	**Subjective impact and application in traditional medicine of plants rich in this subgroup**	**Observed pharmacological activity**
Resins, e.g. in myrrh, Tolu balsam, balm of Gilead, mastic, propolis, dragon's blood	Sticky, antiseptic, stimulating defensive activity on exposed mucosa	Anti-inflammatory,[50,51] antiseptic, anaesthetic, and antitumour and wound-healing properties[52]
Saponins, e.g. in ginseng, liquorice, astragulus, helonias root, wild yam	Lather in water, sweet taste, emetic-expectorant, tonics and gynaecological remedies	Antimicrobial[53] and disease-preventive[54] roles in plant molecules with various competitive, modulating effects on steroidal receptors and functions postulated[55,56]; they are consistently natural surfactants and detergents[57] with cleansing properties[58]; various saponins or sapogenins have demonstrated membrane-permeabilizing, antiprotozoal,[59] immunostimulant,[60] expectorant,[61] hypocholesterolaemic,[62,63] neuroprotective,[64] anticarcinogenic,[65] antitumour,[66,67] sweetening,[68] radioprotective,[69] anticoagulant,[70] anticariogenic, hypolipidaemic effects and are effective in reducing urinary stones[71] and aid digestion of nutrients[72]
Tannins, e.g. in oak, witchhazel	Astringent, making leather, wound cautery, anti-inflammatory in upper digestive tract, reducing reflex diarrhoea in gastroenteritis	Tannins precipitate proteins, so wound healing,[73] astringent cross-links exposed protein molecules,[74] styptic,[75] protective,[76,77] antidiarrhoeal,[78] antisecretolytic, antiphlogistic, antimicrobial and antiparasitic effects,[79] though may also inhibit digestive enzymes and depress growth rate,[80] some other polyphenolic health benefits possible[81]

[1]Kawada T, Sakabe S, Watanabe T et al. Some pungent principles of spices cause the adrenal medulla to secrete catecholamine in anesthetized rats. Proceedings of the Society for Experimental Biology and Medicine 1988; 188(2): 229–233

[2]Doucet, E., Tremblay, A. Food intake, energy balance and body weight control. European Journal of Clinical Nutrition 1997; 51(12): 846–855.

[3]Biro, T., Acs, G., Acs, P., et al. Recent advances in understanding of vanilloid receptors: a therapeutic target for treatment of pain and inflammation in skin. Journal of Investigative Dermatology Symposium Proceedings 1997; 2(1): 56–60

Continued

Table 8.2 ***Phytochemical groups in traditional and modern use—Cont'd***

[4]Desai, H.G., Venugopalan, K., Philipose, M., et al. Effect of red chilli powder on gastric mucosal barrier and acid secretion. Indian Journal of Medical Research 1977; 66(3): 440–448

[5]Towheen TE, Hochberg MC. A systematic review of randomized controlled trials of pharmacological therapy in osteoarthritis of the knee, with an emphasis on trial methodology. Seminars in Arthritis and Rheumatism 1997; 26(5): 755–770

[6]Kingery WS. A critical review of controlled clinical trials for peripheral neuropathic pain and complex regional pain syndromes. Pain 1997; 73(2): 123–139

[7]Rains C. Bryson HM. Topical capsaicin. A review of its pharmacological properties and therapeutic potential in post-herpetic neuralgia, diabetic neuropathy and osteoarthritis. Drugs and Aging 1995; 7(4): 317–328

[8]Hautkappe M, Roizen MF, Toledano A et al. Review of the effectiveness of capsaicin for painful cutaneous disorders and neural dysfunction. Clinical Journal of Pain 1998; 14(2): 97–106

[9]Baron R, Wasner G, Lindner V. Optimal treatment of phantom limb pain in the elderly. Drugs and Aging 1998; 12(5): 361–376

[10]Johri RK, Thusi N, Khajuria A et al. Piperine-mediated changes in the permeability of rat intestinal epithelial cells. The status of gamma-glutamyl transpeptidase activity, uptake of amino acids and lipid peroxidation. Biochemical Pharmacology 1992; 43(7): 1401–1407

[11]Bano G, Raina RK, Zutshi U et al. Effect of piperine on bioavailability and pharmacokinetics of propranolol and theophylline in healthy volunteers. European Journal of Clinical Pharmacology 1991; 41(6): 615–617

[12]Mascolo N, Capasso R, Capasso F. Senna. A safe and effective drug. Phytotherapy Research 1998; 12: S143–S145

[13]Nijs G, de Witte P, Geboes K et al. In vitro demonstration of a positive effect of rhein anthrone on peristaltic reflex of guinea pig ileum. Pharmacology 47 (supp 1): 40–48

[14]Leng-Peschlow E. Sennoside-induced secretion is not caused by changes in mucosal permeability or Na+,K(+)-ATPase activity. Journal of Pharmacy and Pharmacology 1993; 45(11): 951–954

[15]Anton R, Haag-Berrurier M. Therapeutic use of natural anthraquinone for other than laxative actions. Pharmacology 1980; 20 (supp 1): 104–112

[16]Spencer CM, Wilde MI. Diacerein. Drugs 1997; 53(1): 98–106

[17]Anonymous. Herbal remedies for dyspepsia: peppermint seems effective. Prescrire Int. 2008 Jun;17(95):121–3

[18]Cavanagh HM, Wilkinson JM. Biological activities of lavender essential oil. Phytother Res. 2002 Jun;16(4):301–8

[19]Albring, M., Albrecht, H., Alcorn, G., et al. The measuring of the antiinflammatory effect of a compound on the skin of volunteers. Meth Find Exp Clin Pharmacol 1983; 5: 575–7

[20]Anthony JP, Fyfe L, Smith H. Plant active components – a resource for antiparasitic agents? Trends Parasitol. 2005 Oct;21(10):462–8

[21]Martin KW, Ernst E. Herbal medicines for treatment of fungal infections: a systematic review of controlled clinical trials. Mycoses. 2004 Apr;47(3–4):87–92

[22]Claffey N. Essential oil mouthwashes: a key component in oral health management. J Clin Periodontol. 2003;30 Suppl 5:22–4

[23]Thorgrimsen L, Spector A, Wiles A, et al. Aroma therapy for dementia. Cochrane Database Syst Rev. 2003(3):CD003150

[24]Perry NS, Bollen C, Perry EK, et al. Salvia for dementia therapy: review of pharmacological activity and pilot tolerability clinical trial. Pharmacol Biochem Behav. 2003;75(3): 651–9

[25]Carson CF, Hammer KA, Riley TV. *Melaleuca alternifolia* (tea tree) oil: a review of antimicrobial and other medicinal properties. Clin Microbiol Rev. 2006 Jan;19(1):50–62.

[26]Luqman S, Dwivedi GR, Darokar MP, et al. Potential of rosemary oil to be used in drug-resistant infections. Altern Ther Health Med. 2007 Sep-Oct;13(5):54–9

[27]Pattnaik S, Subramanyam VR, Bapaji M et al. Antibacterial and antifungal activity of aromatic constituents of essential oils. Microbios 1997; 89(358): 39–46

[28]Woollard AC, Tatham KC, Barker S. The influence of essential oils on the process of wound healing: a review of the current evidence. J Wound Care. 2007 Jun;16(6):255–7

[29]Dorow P, Weiss Th, Felix R et al. Effect of a secretolytic and a combination of pinene, limonene and cineole on mucociliary clearance in patients with chronic pulmonary obstruction. Arzneimittel-Forschung 1987; 37(12): 1378–1381

[30]Stanic G, Samarzija I, Blazevic N. Time-dependent diuretic response in rats treated with juniper berry preparations. Phytotherapy Research 1998; 12: 494–497

[31]Lesschaeve I, Noble AC. Polyphenols: factors influencing their sensory properties and their effects on food and beverage preferences. Am J Clin Nutr. 2005 Jan;81(1 Suppl):330S–5S.

[32]Behrens M, Meyerhof W. Bitter taste receptors and human bitter taste perception. Cell Mol Life Sci. 2006 Jul;63(13):1501–9

[33]Rozengurt E. Taste receptors in the gastrointestinal tract. I. Bitter taste receptors and alpha-gustducin in the mammalian gut. Am J Physiol Gastrointest Liver Physiol. 2006 Aug;291(2):G171–7

Table 8.2 ***Phytochemical groups in traditional and modern use*—Cont'd**

[34]Sternini C, Anselmi L, Rozengurt E. Enteroendocrine cells: a site of 'taste' in gastrointestinal chemosensing. Curr Opin Endocrinol Diabetes Obes. 2008 Feb;15(1):73–8.

[35]Wolf S, Mack M. Experimental study of the action of bitters on the stomach of a fistulous human subject. Drug Standards 1956; 24(3): 98–101

[36]Gebhardt R. Stimulation of acid secretion by extracts of *Gentiana lutea* L. in cultured cells from rat gastric mucosa. Pharmaceutical and Pharmacological Letters 1997; 7(2–3): 106–108

[37]Wegener T. Anwendung eines Trockenextraktes Augentianae luteae radix bei dyspeptischem Symptomkomplex. Zeitschrift für Phytotherapie 1998; 19: 163–164

[38]Moorhead LD. Contributions to the physiology of the stomach. XXVIII Further studies on the action of the bitter tonic on the secretion of gastric juice. Journal of Pharmacology and Experimental Therapeutics 1915; 7: 577–589

[39]Morcos SR, El-Baradie AA. Fenugreek mucilage and its relation to the reputed laxative action of this seed. Egyptian Journal of Chemistry 1959; 2(1): 163–168

[40]Roberts DCK, Truswell AS, Bencke A et al. The cholesterol-lowering effect of a breakfast cereal containing psyllium fibre. Medical Journal of Australia 1994; 161: 660–664

[41]Frati-Munari AC, Flores-Garduno MA, Ariza-Andraca R et al. Effect of different doses of *Plantago psyllium* mucilage on the glucose tolerance test. Archives of Investigative Medicine (Mexico) 1989; 20(2): 147–152

[42]Hansen HS, Artmann A. Endocannabinoids and nutrition. J Neuroendocrinol. 2008; 20 Suppl 1: 94–9

[43]Morse NL, Clough PM. A meta-analysis of randomized, placebo-controlled clinical trials of Efamol evening primrose oil in atopic eczema. Where do we go from here in light of more recent discoveries? Curr Pharm Biotechnol. 2006; 7(6): 503–24

[44]Belch JJ, Hill A. Evening primrose oil and borage oil in rheumatologic conditions. Am J Clin Nutr. 2000; 71 (1 Suppl): 352S–6S

[45]Joy CB, Mumby-Croft R, Joy LA. Polyunsaturated fatty acid (fish or evening primrose oil) for schizophrenia. Cochrane Database Syst Rev. 2000(2):CD001257

[46]Feldman EB. The scientific evidence for a beneficial health relationship between walnuts and coronary heart disease. J Nutr. 2002; 132(5): 1062S–1071S

[47]Obolentseva GV, Khadzhai Yal, Vidyukova AI et al. Effect of some natural substances on ulceration of the rat stomach caused by acetylsalicylic acid. Bulletin of Experimental Biology and Medicine 1974; 77: 256–257

[48]Blackburn NA, Johnson IT. The influence of guar gum on the movements of insulin, glucose and fluid in rat intestine during perfusion in vivo. Pflügers Archiv 1983; 397: 144–148

[49]Nosalova G, Strapkova A, Kardosova A et al. Antitussive Wirkung des Extraktes und der Polysaccharide aus Eibisch (*Althaea officinalis* L., var. *robusta*). Pharmazie 1992; 47: 224–226

[50]Al-Habbal, M.J., Al-Habbal, Z., Huwezi, F.U. A double-blind controlled clinical trial of mastic and placebo in the treatment of duodenal ulcer. Clinical and Experimental Pharmacology and Physiology 1984; 11: 541–544

[51]Al-Said, M.A., Ageel, A.M., Parmar, N.S. et al. Evaluation of mastic, a crude drug obtained from *Pistacia lentiscus* for gastric and duodenal anti-ulcer activity. Journal of Ethnopharmacology1986; 15: 271–278

[52]Nomicos EY. Myrrh: medical marvel or myth of the Magi? Holist Nurs Pract. 2007; 21(6): 308–23

[53]Osbourn AE. Saponins in cereals. Phytochemistry. 2003 Jan;62(1):1–4

[54]Salminen A, Lehtonen M, Suuronen T, et al. Terpenoids: natural inhibitors of NF-kappaB signaling with anti-inflammatory and anticancer potential. Cell Mol Life Sci. 2008 65:2979–2999

[55]Milanov, S., Maleeva, E., Taskov, M. Tribestan: Effect on the concentration of some hormones in the serum of healthy volunteers. MBI: Medicobiologic Information 1985; 4: 27–29

[56]Baker, M.E. Endocrine activity of plant-derived compounds: an evolutionary perspective. Proceedings of the Society for Experimental Biology and Medicine 1995; 208: 131–138

[57]Williams JR, Gong H. Biological activities and syntheses of steroidal saponins: the shark-repelling pavoninins. Lipids. 2007 Feb;42(1):77–86

[58]Kurtz ES, Wallo W. Colloidal oatmeal: history, chemistry and clinical properties. J Drugs Dermatol. 2007 Feb;6(2):167–70

[59]Francis G, Kerem Z, Makkar HP, et al. The biological action of saponins in animal systems: a review. Br J Nutr. 2002 Dec;88(6):587–605.

[60]Rajput ZI, Hu SH, Xiao CW, et al. Adjuvant effects of saponins on animal immune responses. J Zhejiang Univ Sci B. 2007 Mar;8(3):153–61

[61]Boyd, E.M., Palmer, M.E. The effect of quillaia, senega, squill, grindelia, sanguinaria, chionanthus and dioscorea upon the output of respiratory tract fluid. Acta Pharmacologica 1946; 2: 235–246

[62]Oakenfull, D., Sidhu, G.S. Could saponins be a useful treatment for hypercholesterolaemia? European Journal of Clinical Nutrition 1990; 44: 79–88.

[63]Matsuura H. Saponins in garlic as modifiers of the risk of cardiovascular disease. J Nutr. 2001 Mar;131(3s):1000S–5S

[64]Rausch WD, Liu S, Gille G, et al. Neuroprotective effects of ginsenosides. Acta Neurobiol Exp (Wars). 2006;66(4):369–75

Continued

Table 8.2 ***Phytochemical groups in traditional and modern use*—Cont'd**

[65]Kerwin SM. Soy saponins and the anticancer effects of soybeans and soy-based foods. Curr Med Chem Anticancer Agents. 2004 May;4(3):263–72
[66]Setzer WN, Setzer MC. Plant-derived triterpenoids as potential antineoplastic agents. Mini Rev Med Chem. 2003 Sep;3(6):540–56
[67]Bachran C, Bachran S, Sutherland M, et al. Saponins in tumor therapy. Mini Rev Med Chem. 2008 Jun;8(6):575–84
[68]Kinghorn AD, Kaneda N, Baek NI, et al. Noncariogenic intense natural sweeteners. Med Res Rev. 1998 Sep;18(5):347–60
[69]Lee TK, Johnke RM, Allison RR, et al. Radioprotective potential of ginseng. Mutagenesis. 2005 Jul;20(4):237–43
[70]Rao AV, Gurfinkel DM. The bioactivity of saponins: triterpenoid and steroidal glycosides. Drug Metabol Drug Interact. 2000;17(1–4):211–35
[71]Shi J, Arunasalam K, Yeung D, et al. Saponins from edible legumes: chemistry, processing, and health benefits. J Med Food. 2004 Spring;7(1):67–78
[72]Gee, J.M., Johnson, I.T. Interactions between hemolytic saponins, bile salts and small intestinal mucosa in the rat. Journal of Nutrition 1988; 118: 1391–1397.
[73]Sen CK, Khanna S, Gordillo G, et al. Oxygen, oxidants, and antioxidants in wound healing: an emerging paradigm. Ann N Y Acad Sci. 2002 May;957:239–49
[74]Lamaison JL, Carnat A, Petitjean-Freytet C. Teneur en tanins et activité inhibitrice de l'élastase chez les Rosacae. Annales de Pharmaceutiques Françaises 1990; 48(6): 335–340
[75]Root-Bernstein RS. Tannic acid, semipermeable membranes and burn treatment. Lancet 1982; 2: 1168
[76]Maity S, Vedasiromoni JR, Ganguly DK. Anti-ulcer effect of the hot water extract of black tea (*Camellia sinensis*). Journal of Ethnopharmacology 1995; 46: 167–174
[77]Murakami S, Isobe Y, Kijima H et al. Inhibition of gastric H+,K+-ATPase and acid secretion by ellagic acid. Planta Medica 1991; 57: 305–308
[78]Palombo EA. Phytochemicals from traditional medicinal plants used in the treatment of diarrhoea: modes of action and effects on intestinal function. Phytother Res. 2006 Sep;20(9):717–24
[79]Westendarp H. [Effects of tannins in animal nutrition.] Dtsch Tierarztl Wochenschr. 2006; 113(7): 264–8.
[80]Bennick A. Interaction of plant polyphenols with salivary proteins. Crit Rev Oral Biol Med. 2002; 13(2): 184–96
[81]Koleckar V, Kubikova K, Rehakova Z et al. Condensed and hydrolysable tannins as antioxidants influencing the health. Mini Rev Med Chem. 2008; 8(5): 436–47

PROSPECTS FOR HERBAL RESEARCH

There may however be ways in which we can make better sense of the available information. In the remainder of this chapter a series of research prospects are discussed which could be suitable for eliciting useful information about the effects of herbal medicine.

HERBAL RESEARCH PROSPECT 1: THE MEASUREMENT OF TRANSIENT CLINICAL EFFECTS

There is an application of the controlled clinical trial that could be particularly appropriate for assessing the impact of traditional herbal treatments: observing physiological responses to treatments in human subjects rather than direct effects on morbidity.

Traditional views of herbal remedies emphasize their primary influence on transient body functions, e.g. they are classed as diaphoretics, expectorants, circulatory stimulants, diuretics, digestive stimulants, laxatives and so on. In other words, contrary to common belief, many herbs may have almost immediate results on the body. It is possible to devise methods by which such effects can be detected. Activity on biological markers, physiological functions and tissue or fluid constitution can be monitored directly in healthy or morbid populations and could provide much useful information on the effects on the body of herbal products. With advances in non-invasive monitoring technologies it is possible to conceive of important trials in human subjects, both in observational and controlled studies.

Against such ideas it has been pointed out that measures of efficacy tend to be based on a medicine's effects on morbidity or mortality. 'Surrogate parameters' may restrict possible indications as labelled claims for herbal products. It would need to be argued in each individual case, with the support of other medical evidence, that a verified effect in changing some physiological parameter would be likely to have an effect on morbidity or mortality.

HERBAL RESEARCH PROSPECT 2: OBSERVATIONAL STUDIES

The observational study design has emerged as a research tool to complement controlled clinical trials (Dobre et al. 2007). It is more suited to establish benefit in the real world ('effectiveness') (McKee et al. 1999) and may help to assess such effectiveness in subgroups not studied in controlled trials, or over the long term. In some cases, careful observations of non-controlled clinical events may be the best or even only practicable source of evidence. These include circumstances where controlled studies are difficult, for example: (1) rare diseases; (2) where there are many clinical complexities; and (3) for cases where blinding is impossible.

Observational studies may be a particularly appropriate method for the study of herbal medicines. A persistent tradition is that these medicines may support self-corrective functions in the body, perhaps more readily than synthetic pharmaceuticals. New insights into complex dynamic systems suggest that there may be benefits in observing humans as ecosystems. It is apparent in this case that different research methodologies are required. These should: (1) have regard to the widest range of symptoms and signs together rather than particular variables in isolation; (2) aim to measure quantifiable components of health, rather than of morbidity; and (3) involve minimal intervention.

Non-invasive monitoring of physiological functions may be applied (as above), perhaps coupled with patient self-rated questionnaires, clinical observations of overall behaviour and epidemiological methods, to establish as far as possible what actually happens to individual patients when they seek treatments.

Routine collection of patient and clinical data may be practicable at a teaching clinic, for example. These could include self-rating questionnaires, for general health and for target conditions, perhaps combined with a number of other non-invasive observations, compared with general remission rates. With computer technology it is possible to accrue considerable quantities of useful observational data by involving patients and practitioners in simultaneous recording of treatments and questionnaire-derived outcomes (using simple touch-screen check-box entry forms, for example).

Although it is difficult to establish cause and effect in observational or field studies, or specifically to separate specific from non-specific treatment effects, there are a number of ways that observational studies could productively be used in herbal research. For example:

- to service controlled studies by monitoring matched groups where blinding or other ideals are impracticable

- to have individual practitioners generating longitudinal case studies, with standardized report forms, to address the question usually ignored in controlled clinical studies – the effect of long-term treatments
- to audit clinical practice and generate new hypotheses – with computerized data input (as above) and sufficient quantities of data even complex and multiple prescription patterns can be evaluated
- to generate safety data.

Such information however suffers from one clear problem: it is rarely subject to independent validation or review, so includes partisan judgements. Its use without supporting controlled data in determining efficacy of treatment is therefore limited. Nevertheless there is some evidence that good observational studies generate similar results to controlled clinical trials (Radford & Foody 2001), and in combination with other studies could provide very useful information.

HERBAL RESEARCH PROSPECT 3: SINGLE CASE STUDIES

The main charge against single case studies is that they cannot credibly select out real effects from confusing variables, and specific from non-specific treatment effects. Further investigation of such research however shows both that it can have more credibility than might be supposed, and that it is not a soft option.

The criteria for validity of such trials have been well reviewed by Aldridge (1991): a good single case study design can be very rigorous. It includes providing as many points of view on the event as possible, clarifying operational definitions and recycling observed data around the researchers (including the patient as co-researcher) for checking and possible refutation. It is possible to conduct double-blind, placebo-controlled studies in a series of such individual case studies with each patient being his or her control. These could allow for a useful database of reliable case histories to be assembled over the years, as both an educational and research exercise.

Perhaps most importantly, the single case study is the raw caseload of each practitioner. A routine of rigorously collating studies is a commendable continuing education exercise that may encourage practitioners to become more active in the generation of efficacy data.

An effective methodology for clinical studies could usefully combine elements of all three research designs above.

HERBAL RESEARCH PROSPECT 4: USING TRADITIONAL EVIDENCE

The persistent theme running through any discussion on the efficacy of herbal medicine is that it has been used over centuries and millennia. It is claimed with some justification that at least some value will have been distilled out by this vast store of human bioassay data, especially as there would have been little room for sentiment and idealism in the life-and-death situations that prevailed through most of herbal use.

However without a rigorous screening the record of traditional use can appear as little more that a motley and primitive hotchpotch of folk fancies. The review of historical methodologies highlights some limitations, but the power of cultural placebo alone renders any individual observation almost worthless. What is needed is the identification of themes, a structure for assessing traditional claims. Fortunately this may be possible.

Clinical insight into the traditional record leads to the realization that from the very earliest and most primitive accounts of herb use, humans classified the plant material into relatively consistent pharmaceutical categories. The classification was based on subjective properties of taste or appearance and the immediate impact they made on consumption. These categories, encountered repeatedly in the ethnobotanical records, became the basis of core therapeutic principles in the classic texts of China, India, Greco-Roman Europe, Islam and almost all other written traditions. Many of these categories survive today as recognizable phytochemical groups. They constitute a primal pharmaceutics of surprising potency. It had to be: there was usually no other choice. Going to a traditional herbal practitioner was often a very robust experience!

The pharmaceutical principles of traditional medicine provide a potentially robust correlation with modern herbal research, provided the latter can be linked to these phytochemical subgroups; in other words, provided both the scientific and the traditional data relate to the same common elements in comparable contexts (it is important for example that dosage and pharmacokinetic criteria in the scientific studies are consistent with traditional application).

Some of the most consistently encountered pharmaceutical categories in history are listed in Table 8.2, with the traditional experience of the category as a whole followed by the established modern pharmacological assessment. There are as many variations on these themes as there are plants included within them, but the properties listed predominate across each category. Modern ethnopharmacological studies show countless examples where pharmacological activity can be demonstrated in traditional remedies and practices. Such correlations are clearly interesting; in effect the early reputation provides the 'human bioassay data', the clinical evidence before the preclinical studies, rather than the other way around, as is usual in modern pharmaceutical research. These correspondences lift the findings of laboratory research into a real clinical context.

HERBAL RESEARCH PROSPECT 5: APPROPRIATE PRECLINICAL STUDIES

In addition to providing a second guess on the veracity of traditional reputations, laboratory studies can cast light on some of the persistent puzzles in herb use. Some of the more relevant questions follow.

Pharmacokinetic issues

Any rationale for herbal medicine is likely to be based on the activity of many plant chemical constituents. There are fundamental technical questions raised in building a rational case for herbal therapeutics. The following might usefully form the basis of relevant research questions which in turn could provide important information for quantifying efficacy and underpinning clinical research proposals.

- In what ways are plant constituents likely to interact, in the gut and body tissues, to affect bioavailability and activity? (Obvious interactions are between essential oils, mucilages, tannins, resins, alkaloids, saponins, minerals and complex carbohydrates.)
- What is known of hepatic action on plant constituents, both in terms of the results of the first-pass effect, as plant constituents move into the tissues from the digestive tract, and the impact of enterohepatic recycling?
- Following from both the above, what plant-derived constituents are likely to reach the systemic circulation (an answer to this question is an essential requisite for meaningful tissue culture experiments: see below)?
- How do changes in pharmaceutical preparation affect the bioavailability and activity of plant constituents? For example, do alcoholic extracts have significantly different actions from the aqueous extracts generally dominant in traditional practice?

With biochemical monitoring technology it is feasible that some of these answers could be obtained non-invasively in healthy human subjects. This would provide more useful answers than the traditional reliance on animal experiments.

Cell and tissue cultures

As part of the modern move to find alternatives to animal experimentation, increasing attention is being paid to techniques for assessing the effects of drugs on cultures of cells, tissues and organs in vitro. Conventional drug research is moving in this direction for preliminary screening in drug discovery programmes, and there is also a move for at least initial toxicological testing.

The advantages are in the opportunity for the direct observation of the action of an agent on target cells with some reduced ethical difficulties (although the sacrifice of animals is often necessary to supply short-lived organ and tissue samples).

The problems are the limited application of such observations to the in vivo situation and the need to confirm any in vitro findings anyway; from the point of view of herbal research there is the additional problem that it is impossible at this stage to reproduce that balance of plant constituents that will actually reach internal tissues (after digestion, absorption and the first-pass hepatic effect). Difficulties are increased by the desirability of using tissues most closely mimicking the real situation, i.e. mammalian organ cultures rather than the easier-to-culture amphibian tissues or the less sophisticated cell lines.

Nevertheless, in vitro techniques could provide valuable supplementary information to other research, as in the following suggested projects:

- the influence of herbal extracts on epithelial tissue cultures (e.g. gastric, enteric and tracheal tissues); such findings could inform pharmacokinetic calculations for herbal dosage

- observations on the biotransformation of plant constituents using liver cultures
- alteration in the migratory behaviour and internal metabolism of macrophages as a result of exposure to herbal extracts
- non-specific observations (as in gerontological research) on cell migrations, length of interphase, longevity and other pointers to in vitro cell health.

CONCLUSIONS AND RECOMMENDATIONS

There is potentially a uniquely effective evidence base for the use of herbal medicines. The materials so far available are already more extensive than in other complementary disciplines and range over many scientific modalities. However they have so far been poorly suited to clinical decisions. The research data have mostly been generated to find pharmaceutical leads and are fragmentary. Nevertheless there is scope for integration of the evidence and better research in the future, though only if two conditions are met:

1. Observations of actual human use, previously marginalized, should become central. This is already the case when establishing safety but it should be acknowledged as the key element in determining benefit as well. Human experience is all that counts in the end. In the case of herbal medicine this experience is already more extensive than in other forms of complementary medicine and it would be unrealistic to ignore it and insist that herbs are only used if proved de novo. Traditional and clinical experience should be rigorously assessed and clearly articulated to make the opening case for efficacy. It can then be refuted or amended by research in other areas. In some cases it can be seen that pharmacological or clinical research supports traditional use (for example, in Table 8.2) and in this case the latter is reinforced. In others modern findings discredit received wisdoms and these should be adjusted or discarded. It may also be possible by meta-assessment of the traditional use data to see recurrent patterns of pharmacology or therapeutics that are themselves reinforcing. It has been shown that much current research does not address clinical questions: a more useful role could be in refuting, validating or illuminating the issues and answers suggested by human experience.
2. Herbs need to remain as medicines. The great part of clinical trial research has been in support of herbal products that are prescribed and dispensed as medicines in central Europe. Although there have been some admirable clinical trials in the USA and elsewhere, these have been in publicly funded research programmes that are generally reactive to public use rather than strategically innovative. The major risks to the future funding of herbal research are regulatory regimes that classify herbs as food supplements or as second-class medicinal products with a status dependent only on traditional use. If manufacturers cannot develop a therapeutic use for a herbal product they will be unlikely to invest in researching one. If the research-funding bodies do not consider herbal remedies as serious contributors to health care they will not set aside precious resources to develop their potential. Unfortunately, the political

and market trends are set to diminish the medicinal status of herbs and there is thus a real threat to the future of good herbal research.

Good clinically relevant controlled clinical trials will always be the best measure of benefit. However, it will be a very long time before these are available for many potentially useful remedies and pragmatic alternatives should be sought in the meantime. There are two vast resources of evidence: data on human use and pharmacological evidence. Each can enrich the other and provide connections among the fragments to make better clinical judgments. It is this work we are engaged upon at www.plant-medicine.com.

REFERENCES

Aldridge, D., 1991. Single-case research designs for the clinician. J. R. Soc. Med. 84 (5), 249–252.

Allen, D.E., Hatfield, G., 2004. Medicinal Plants in Folk Tradition: An Ethnobotany of Britain and Ireland. Timber Press, Cambridge.

Blumenthal, M., Cavaliere, C., 2006. NCCAM funds new African and Chinese herbal research programs. Herbalgram 71, 20–22.

Bogaards, J.J., Bertrand, M., Jackson, P., et al., 2000. Determining the best animal model for human cytochrome P450 activities: a comparison of mouse, rat, rabbit, dog, micropig, monkey and man. Xenobiotica 30 (12), 1131–1152.

Buenz, E.J., Schnepple, D.J., Bauer, B.A., et al., 2004. Techniques: Bioprospecting historical herbal texts by hunting for new leads in old tomes. Trends Pharmacol. Sci. 25 (9), 494–498.

Buenz, E.J., Bauer, B.A., Johnson, H.E., et al., 2006. Searching historical herbal texts for potential new drugs. BMJ 333 (7582), 1314–1315.

Directive 2004/24/EC of the European Parliament and of the Council. Official Journal of the European Union.L136/86 30th April 2004; Article 16 (a) 3 .

Dobre, D., van Veldhuisen, D.J., DeJongste, M.J., et al., 2007. The contribution of observational studies to the knowledge of drug effectiveness in heart failure. Br. J. Clin. Pharmacol. 64 (4), 406–414.

IMS/PhytoGold, 1998. Herbals in Europe. IMS SelfMedication International, London.

Kressman, S., Muller, W.E., Blume, H.H., 2002. Pharmaceutical quality of different *Ginkgo biloba* brands. J. Pharm. Pharmacol. 54 (5), 661–669.

McKee, M., Britton, A., Black, N., et al., 1999. Methods in health services research. Interpreting the evidence: choosing between randomised and non-randomised studies. BMJ 319, 312–315.

Moerman, D., 1998. Native American Ethnobotany. Timber Press, Portland Oregon.

Perry, L.R., 1980. Medicinal Plants of East and Southeast Asia. Massachusetts Institute of Technology Press, Cambridge, MA.

Radford, M.J., Foody, J.M., 2001. How do observational studies expand the evidence base for therapy? JAMA 286, 1228–1230.

The European Scientific Cooperative on Phytotherapy, 2003. The ESCOP monographs. Georg Thieme Verlag, Stuttgart, pp. 178–210, 257–281.

Williamson, E.M., 2001. Synergy and other interactions in phytomedicines. Phytomedicine 8 (5), 401–409.

Wolsko, P.M., Solondz, D.K., Phillips, R.S., et al., 2005. Lack of Herbal Supplement Characterization in Published Randomized Controlled Trials. Am. J. M. 118 (10), 1087–1093.

Scientific research in homeopathy

9

Peter Fisher • Robert T. Mathie
Harald Walach • Wayne B. Jonas

CHAPTER CONTENTS

INTRODUCTION

The authors of this chapter have been involved in research on various aspects of homeopathy for many years: two of us (PF, WBJ) are doctors who practise homeopathy. This chapter aims to describe homeopathy and the scientific issues it raises, to point out some paths that have been explored and abandoned as blind alleys and to highlight others that seem more promising. We do not attempt to cover all primary studies in depth. We believe we have referred to all systematic reviews and meta-analyses published, and some landmark studies, particularly those that have been replicated. The references to primary research are not comprehensive, but intended to give a flavour of the work. In view of the importance of a range of corroborative evidence, we will cover clinical research, biological models and basic research.

DOI: 10.1016/B978-0-443-06956-7.00009-4

HISTORY

Homeopathy (also spelt homoeopathy and homœopathy; Greek *homoios* = same or similar, *pathos* = suffering) is a system of medicine based on the idea of 'let like be cured by like', in Latin: *similia similibus curentur*. It was founded by the German physician Samuel Christian Hahnemann (1755–1843) in 1796 with his seminal 'Essay on a new principle for ascertaining the curative powers of drugs' with a few glances at those hitherto employed (Hahnemann 1796).

Coincidentally, this was the same year that Edward Jenner first vaccinated against smallpox. It also coincided with the period of so-called 'heroic medicine', which advocated treatments including bleeding and purging in 'heroic' doses – as large as the patient could tolerate and not infrequently larger, resulting in the death of the patient. Heroic medicine originated in the work of John Brown of Edinburgh (1735–1788), but had many influential advocates, including Benjamin Rush (1745–1813), a signatory of the American Declaration of Independence. It is notable that, although heroic medicine was briefly influential and widely accepted, it was rapidly abandoned, whereas homeopathy is still alive and well. Some historians of medicine attribute this to the fact that homeopathy was based on empirical observation, whereas heroic medicine was based on a purely theoretical model (Schwanitz 1983). A reaction against heroic medicine may, in part, explain the adoption by homeopaths of increasingly small doses.

Hahnemann delineated two main approaches to medical treatment: the homeopathic and the allopathic or enantiopathic method (based on '*contraria contrariis*': opposites oppose). It was Hahnemann who coined the words 'homeopathy' and 'allopathy'. The latter term is now sometimes, incorrectly, used to refer to all conventional medicine.

References to both these methods of treating disease can be found in the Hippocratic corpus, for instance:

> *Diseases are cured by opposites; for every disease there is something proper; so, for what is warm by nature, but sickened by cold, there is something to warm it up, and so on. This is another way: by similar (homoia) means a disease arises and by administering similar things health is restored from sickness; for instance the same which causes strangury that wasn't there before, when it is there, will make it stop. Likewise coughing arises, like strangury, and it stops by the same things.*
>
> (Hippocrates c 450BCE)

Homeopathy rapidly gained popularity in Europe in the first half of the 19th century. This seems to have been due to two main factors: its success in some high-profile cases and its success in epidemics (Jütte 1998). For instance, Radetzky, Field Marshal of the Austro-Hungarian Empire, declared 'the disease of my eye in 1841 was cured exclusively by the homoeopathic treatment of my staff physician, Dr Hartung', while famous violinist Paganini and the great naturalist Charles Darwin, among other prominent individuals, spoke highly of homeopathy. Darwin was initially very sceptical about high dilutions, but derived great benefit from treatment by Dr James Gully, a homeopath and hydrotherapist. Subsequently Darwin conducted experiments on the effects of highly dilute Ammonium phosphate on the carnivorous plant *Drosera* (Ullman 2009). (For an account of well-known users of homeopathy, see Ullman 2007).

The other factor in the rise of homeopathy was its success in the epidemics, particularly of cholera, which swept Europe during the 19th century. Homeopaths were much more successful in saving lives than their conventional counterparts. While in some conventional hospitals up to 74% of patients died, in homeopathic settings the figure was 4–11% (Glaz 1991). Homeopaths and the public usually attributed these successes to homeopathic treatment but historical analyses and modern data raise the question of whether the difference in outcomes (of which there is little doubt) was due to homeopaths curing their patients, or conventional physicians killing theirs! The mainstay of conventional treatment of cholera at that time was bloodletting which, as is now recognized, is just about the worst thing to do in a condition characterized by hypovolaemic shock. They also made frequent use of toxic medicines such as the mercury salt calomel but did not use rehydration (Leary 1994). A modern study of homeopathy in cholera showed no difference in death rates between homeopathy and placebo, because there were no deaths (Gaucher et al. 1994).

There are several distinct types of homeopathy. The main types are individualized or classical homeopathy, clinical homeopathy and isopathy. In individualized homeopathy typically a single homeopathic medicine is selected on the basis of the total 'symptom picture' displayed by a patient, including mental, general and constitutional features. In clinical homeopathy, one or more homeopathic medicines are administered for standard clinical situations or conventional diagnoses – sometimes several homeopathic medicines are combined in a fixed (complex) formulation. Isopathy is the use of homeopathic dilutions of allergens or causative infectious or toxic agents. Related medical systems which use homeopathic medicines include Homotoxicology, founded by HH Reckeweg and based on interpreting disease as an expression of the defensive effort of the organism against pathogenic toxins and detoxification with homeopathic medicines, and Anthroposophical Medicine, an approach founded by R Steiner and I Wegmann, integrating conventional medicine with the influence of soul and spirit.

Homeopathy is one of the most controversial forms of complementary and alternative medicine. Throughout its history of over 200 years it has been the focus of debate, often heated, with strong opinions expressed for and against. As long ago as 1846 John Forbes denounced homeopathy as 'ludicrously absurd' and an 'outrage to human reason' and any effect of homeopathy therefore impossible. More recently it has been claimed that 'Accepting that infinite dilutions work would subvert more than conventional medicine; it wrecks a whole edifice of chemistry and physics' (Vandenbroucke & de Craen 2001). Homeopathy has been described as 'implausible' and this has been used as a justification for scepticism concerning the claimed results of clinical trials of homeopathy (Kleijnen et al. 1991; Shang et al. 2005). Commentators have discussed homeopathy in terms of the 'growth of truth', including the relationship between bias, background knowledge and the concordance of clinical results with laboratory science findings, concluding that ultimately 'the proof of the pudding is in the eating': the ultimate proof of the validity of a scientific or medical idea is the extent to which it changes reality (Vandenbroucke 2005).

Others, more favourably disposed towards homeopathy, have examined the scepticism surrounding homeopathy in Bayesian terms, pointing to the importance of Bayesian 'prior beliefs' based in specific paradigms and the need for a range of sources of evidence to change deep-rooted assumptions (Rutten 2008). Still others have contended that requiring greater burden of proof for homeopathy than for other scientific hypotheses is itself unscientific: the same level of supporting evidence should be accepted for all scientific developments. If a lower level of proof is set for hypotheses that fit prior beliefs, science is biased in favour of such beliefs (Chaplin 2007). But such a stance describes an ideal; in reality, all humans, including scientists, are to some extent, Bayesians: they hold firm beliefs. Their perceptions are coloured and structured by what they see and deem possible. Hence the dispute about homeopathy is likely to be solved not only by data, but also by a convincing model that can alter such broader scientific belief systems. At present, no such universally accepted model exists.

Despite the controversies which have long surrounded it, homeopathy is popular in diverse regions of the world, including the Indian subcontinent, parts of Latin America and western Europe. In other regions it has experienced seemingly terminal declines, for instance in the USA during most of the 20th century and Eastern Europe and Russia during the communist period, only to rise again at the end of the 20th century. And its use is growing in regions as different as South Africa and Japan. It is clear that what has sustained homeopathy above all is not scientific evidence, but the fact that it was, and remains, popular with patients (Dinges 2002).

Central to the controversy surrounding homeopathy is the lack of a 'plausible' mechanism of action for the very high dilutions often used in homeopathy. Hahnemann initially used doses similar or somewhat smaller than those used in contemporary conventional medicine, but he gradually reduced the size of his doses to include 'ultramolecular dilutions' which are the focus of most of the argument. These dilutions are prepared by a process known as potentization, which involves repeated dilutions, usually in steps of 1:10 or 1:100, with succussion (vigorous shaking) between each dilution. Dilutions are denoted for instance 5x (in the Anglo-American convention) or 5dH (European convention) for the 5th decimal (i.e. 5 times 1:10 dilutions) or 30c/cH for the 30th centesimal (1:100 dilutions). 'H' denotes the Hahnemannian method, in which clean glassware (test tubes and pipettes) is used for each step of dilution (German Homoeopathic Pharmacopoeia 1993). This remains the most widely used dilution scale, but other dilutional scales are also used. In the Korsakovian method (denoted K), a single piece of glassware is used; this is emptied and refilled, the liquid adhering to the walls of the vessel in which it is diluted is equivalent to one part, to which 99 parts of new liquid is added. Otherwise it is similar to the method described above (British Homoeopathic Pharmacopoeia 1993). In the 50 millesimal or quinquagintamillesimal dilution method (denoted LM or Q), dilution is in steps of approximately 1:50 000; this is achieved by absorbing the dilution on to small lactose granules, which are then redissolved (German Homoeopathic Pharmacopoeia 1993).

The use of such dilutions creates a fundamental problem: the Italian aristocrat-scientist Count Amedeo Avogadro proposed in 1811 that the volume of a gas is proportional to the number of atoms or molecules regardless of the nature of the gas. The value of Avogadro's constant, the number of particles (atoms or molecules) in a mole of a pure substance was calculated by the Austrian scientist Johann Josef Loschmidt in 1865 as 6.022×10^{23}.

The inescapable implication is that dilutions above 23x/dH or 12c/cH (corresponding to dilutions of 10^{-23} and 10^{-24} respectively) are very unlikely to contain a molecule of the starting substance. Homeopathic medicines are used in both low dilutions, where the original substance is materially present, and in high dilutions, in which material quantities of the starting substance are much less likely to be present. In fact the 'molecular threshold' is usually crossed before this dilution, depending on factors including initial concentration and molecular weight. Classical pharmacological actions in vivo ('classical pharmacological action' is defined as interaction between pharmacologically active molecules and receptors) have been reported with dilutions as high as 10^{-22}mol/l and repeatedly with diilutions of 10^{-17}–10^{-18} (Eskinazi 1999). By definition dilutions beyond the 'molecular threshold' cannot. Many homeopathic medicines are of biological origin, and consist of complex mixtures of molecules often of unknown molecular weight and concentration, and in any case, even for pure substances of known molecular weight and concentration, the probability of a molecule of the initial substance being present can only be expressed in terms of probability. Homeopathic medicines in which a molecule of the starting substance is unlikely to be present are referred to as 'ultramolecular' or ultra-low dilutions (ULD), or beyond the reciprocal of Avogadro's number (BRAN).

It is important to remember that the first principle of homeopathy is that of similarity, and in this area there is substantial overlap with other areas of science, including hormesis (the stimulatory or beneficial effects of small doses of toxins) (Stebbing 1982; Calabrese & Blain 2005; Calabrese et al. 2006a, b), rebound effects, dose-dependent reverse effects and paradoxical pharmacology (Bond 2001; Teixeira 2006, 2007). The recent concept of 'postconditioning hormesis' refers to a small stimulus exerting a beneficial effect after a biological system has experienced a harmful stress of similar nature (Calabrese et al. 2007). These phenomena have in common that they are secondary, reverse or paradoxical effects of drugs and toxins in living organisms as a function of dose or time.

In order to understand the effects of drugs on healthy humans, Hahnemann conducted volunteer experiments, and homeopathy is the first form of medicine that aspired to base itself purely on empirical clinical trial evidence. As Hahnemann himself acknowledged, he was not the first to propose testing drugs on healthy volunteers – this had been proposed by the Swiss naturalist Albrecht von Haller (1708–1777) – but Hahnemann was the first to propose the systematic use of medicines on such data.

Hahnemann conducted a total of 99 *Prüfungen* (tests) of a wide range of substances on healthy individuals, and published these in his Materia Medica Pura and Chronic Diseases. *Prüfung* is traditionally translated into English as 'proving', but the more recent term 'homeopathic pathogenetic trial' (HPT) is more apt.

In the early 19th century homeopathy diffused widely around the world: it was introduced to the USA by German immigrants, most notably Dr Constantine Hering (1800–1880), who settled in Philadelphia, PA, USA, in 1833. Dr John Martin Honigberger (1795–1869), physician to Maharaja Ranjit Singhji of the Punjab, was the first to practise homeopathy in India, in 1839.

SCIENTIFIC QUESTIONS RAISED BY HOMEOPATHY

The scientific issues raised by homeopathy can be classified as follows:

1. Can substances diluted beyond the Avogadro limit have effects in living systems?
2. How might any such effects be mediated?
3. Do homeopathic medicines have beneficial effects in ill patients that are not attributable to placebo effects?
4. Do substances cure diseases or syndromes similar to those that they cause?
5. Do symptoms reported by healthy volunteers in homeopathic pathogenetic trials ('provings') reflect the therapeutic potential of substances?
6. Does homeopathy as a whole system of medicine provide benefit in terms of effectiveness and cost-effectiveness?
7. Is homeopathy safe?

These questions are ordered approximately from basic science to pragmatic. The fundamental claim of homeopathy is question 4, but the controversial aspects are questions 1–3. Most of the recent debate about homeopathy has revolved around question 3, the issue of placebo, and we will address this question first.

SYSTEMATIC REVIEWS AND META-ANALYSES OF CLINICAL TRIALS OF HOMEOPATHY

Systematic reviews and meta-analyses of randomized controlled trials (RCTs) are considered the strongest form of research evidence, sometimes referred to as type 1 evidence. A number of systematic reviews and meta-analyses of homeopathy as a whole or for specific conditions or of particular homeopathic medicines have been published.

SYSTEMATIC REVIEWS OF HOMEOPATHY AS A WHOLE

Most comprehensive systematic reviews and meta-analyses conclude that homeopathy differs from placebo. A meta-analysis published in *The Lancet* (Linde et al. 1997) included 186 placebo-controlled studies of homeopathy, from which data for analysis could be extracted from 89. The overall mean odds ratio for these 89 clinical trials was 2.45 (95% confidence interval, 2.05–2.93) in favour of homeopathy. This means that the chances that homeopathy would be of benefit were approximately 2–3 times greater than placebo. The main conclusion was that the results 'were not compatible with the hypothesis that the effects of homoeopathy are completely due to placebo'.

A subsequent analysis, by the same group, of the same data, looked at the effect of methodological quality on study outcome and found that studies with higher-quality scores tended to yield less positive results than those with lower-quality scores (Linde et al. 1999). These findings are comparable to those from similar analyses in conventional medicine (Moher et al. 1998). After discarding most of the lower-quality trials, homeopathic treatment remained statistically more effective than placebo – though less so than in their previous analysis. In both of Linde's systematic reviews, insufficient evidence was found to draw conclusions about the efficacy of homeopathy for any specific medical condition.

Linde's work prompted a review comparing the effectiveness of homeopathic treatments with that of conventional therapies (Ernst 1999a). Only six trials (each investigating a different medical condition) fulfilled the author's inclusion criteria, but all six were judged to be methodologically unsatisfactory. No clear trend emerged: results from two of the trials suggested homeopathic medicines were superior to conventional drug therapy, while two of the others suggested the opposite; the remaining two were judged inconclusive.

The Homeopathic Medicine Research Group, a joint group of researchers in conventional medicine and homeopathy, appointed by the Directorate General XII of the European Commission, produced an overview of clinical research in homeopathy and identified 184 clinical trials (Cucherat et al. 2000). They meta-analysed the highest-quality placebo-controlled RCTs, including a total of 2001 patients, and found strong evidence that homeopathy was more effective than placebo ($P < 0.001$), but concluded that 'the strength of this evidence is low because of the low methodological quality of the trials'.

In 2005, Shang et al. published a review comparing 110 placebo-controlled trials of homeopathy and 110 trials of conventional medicine. Homeopathy and conventional medicine showed a similar positive treatment effect overall. Twenty-one homeopathy trials and nine in conventional medicine were judged 'of higher quality'. From these, the results of 14 unspecified 'large trials of higher quality' (eight homeopathy, six conventional medicine) were analysed. The authors concluded that there was 'weak evidence for a specific effect of homoeopathic remedies, but strong evidence for specific effects of conventional interventions. This finding is compatible with the notion that the clinical effects of homoeopathy are placebo effects.'

However this last review gave no indication of which trials its conclusions were based on and was criticized for lack of transparency, absence of sensitivity analysis (for instance, not reporting the result of the analysis of the 21 homeopathy trials of higher quality) and failure to adhere to the Quality of Reporting of Meta-analyses (QUOROM) guidelines for reporting of systematic reviews (Moher et al. 1999). Subsequently a reconstruction of this review has found that the negative results were mainly due to a single trial on preventing muscle soreness in 400 long-distance runners, that its results were very sensitive to the definition of 'larger' sample sizes, and there was great heterogeneity between the trials. It concluded that the results were less definite than purported, although it did demonstrate that the quality of trials of homeopathy was generally higher than that of matched trials of conventional medicine (Lüdtke & Rutten 2008; Rutten & Stolper 2008).

SYSTEMATIC REVIEWS OF RANDOMIZED CLINICAL TRIALS IN SPECIFIC CLINICAL SITUATIONS

The following systematic reviews focused on particular clinical situations or homeopathic medicines have been published. Eleven of these 24 reviews included positive conclusions for homeopathy:

- adverse effects of cancer treatments (Kassab et al. 2009)
- allergies and upper respiratory tract infections, including otitis media (Bellavite et al. 2006; Bornhöft et al. 2006)

- childhood diarrhoea (Jacobs et al. 2003)
- influenza (Vickers & Smith 2006)
- postoperative ileus (Barnes et al. 1997)
- rheumatic diseases (Jonas et al. 2000)
- seasonal allergic rhinitis (hayfever) (Wiesenauer & Lüdtke 1996; Taylor et al. 2000; Bellavite et al. 2006)
- vertigo (Schneider et al. 2005).

Eight reviews were inconclusive (generally due to lack of high-quality evidence):

- anxiety (Pilkington et al. 2006)
- chronic asthma (McCarney et al. 2004a)
- dementia (McCarney et al. 2004b)
- depression (Pilkington et al. 2005)
- headache and migraine treatment (Owen & Green 2004)
- human immunodeficiency virus (HIV)/acquired immunodeficiency syndrome (AIDS) (Ullman 2003)
- induction of labour (Smith 2004)
- osteoarthritis (Long & Ernst 2001).

The remaining five reviews concluded there was little or no evidence for homeopathy:

- ailments of childhood and adolescence (Altunç et al. 2007)
- attention deficit hyperactivity disorder (Coulter & Dean 2007)
- cancer (Milazzo et al. 2006)
- delayed-onset muscle soreness (Ernst & Barnes 1998)
- headache and migraine prevention (Ernst 1999b).

Arnica has been the subject of two systematic reviews. Both found insufficient evidence overall to support the efficacy of this medicine (Ernst & Pittler 1998; Lüdtke & Hacke 2005).

RANDOMIZED CONTROLLED CLINICAL TRIALS OF HOMEOPATHY

A review of clinical trials in homeopathy reported from 1975 to 2002 found 93 studies comparing homeopathy with placebo or other treatment (Mathie 2003). Positive effects of homeopathy were found in 50. The evidence favoured a positive treatment effect of homeopathy in: allergic rhinitis, childhood diarrhoea, fibromyalgia, influenza, pain, side-effects of radio-/chemotherapy, sprains and upper respiratory tract infection. Reviewing 12 systematic reviews of homeopathy for specific medical conditions, Jonas et al. (2003) reached similar conclusions: homeopathy may be effective for allergies, childhood diarrhoea, influenza and postoperative ileus, but not for treatment of migraine, delayed-onset muscle soreness or prevention of influenza.

Single RCTs of homeopathy have been conducted in clinical areas, including asthma (White et al. 2003), life-threatening sepsis (Frass et al. 2005) and stomatitis induced by cancer chemotherapy (Oberbaum et al. 2001), chronic fatigue syndrome (Weatherley-Jones et al. 2004), premenstrual syndrome (Yakir et al. 2001), postpartum bleeding (Oberbaum et al. 2005) and Arnica for various clinical conditions (Tveiten et al. 1998; Stevinson et al. 2003). Most of these have yielded positive results.

In some clinical situations, both RCTs and clinical observational studies have been conducted, providing a fuller picture of the possible role of homeopathy. Such areas include upper respiratory tract and ear infections in children (de Lange et al. 1994; Frei & Thurneysen 2001a; Jacobs et al. 2001), attention deficit hyperactivity disorder (Frei & Thurneysen 2001b; Frei et al. 2005) and homeopathy for symptoms related to cancer treatment (Balzarini et al. 2000; Thompson & Reilly 2003; Jacobs et al. 2005a).

The group led by David Reilly has published an impressive series of trials of isopathy for respiratory allergies, including hayfever, perennial rhinitis and allergy, including a meta-analysis (Reilly & Taylor 1985; Reilly et al. 1986, 1994; Taylor et al. 2000). To date there has been no independent positive replication of these findings. Lewith et al. (2002) studied 242 patients with asthma who were sensitive to house dust mite; they were treated with three doses over 24 hours of house dust mite 30c and followed for 16 weeks. At the end of the study there was no statistically significant improvement in the treated group compared to placebo, though there was one clear difference between the groups: there was significantly more variation in the verum group than in the placebo group (Hyland & Lewith 2002). There were important differences between the design of Lewith et al.'s trial and those of the Reilly group. There were also differences in the objectives: the Reilly group's objective was to demonstrate efficacy compared to placebo, whereas Lewith's study was oriented to showing efficacy in asthma. Lewith's trial was multicentric, primary care-based, and of longer duration, with less rigorous diagnosis and entry criteria than the Reilly group's work. However, comparable studies in Norway with potentized birch pollen in subjects who were allergic to birch pollen did not demonstrate clear-cut effects (Aabel 2000, 2001).

Migraine is another area in which there have been replicated studies: a study on 60 patients by Brigo & Serpelloni (1991), using classical individualized homeopathy, was reported as showing a highly significant positive result. But attempted replications have been much less positive. The first, a close replication, showed weak effects approaching significance (Whitmarsh et al. 1997). In a subsequent study with individualized unrestricted homeopathy that included patients with all types of chronic headaches – not only migraine – no significant difference was found between homeopathy and placebo (Walach et al. 1997). Another study, conducted in Norway in 68 migraine patients, again used individualized homeopathy. Pain diaries showed no difference, but the neurologist rating was significantly in favour of homeopathy (Straumsheim et al 2000). However, an uncontrolled observational study reported major improvement in quality of life in patients undergoing homeopathic treatment for headache (Muscari-Tomaioli et al. 2001). Another observational study showed large effect sizes ($d = 2.44$) for improvement in headache days over the course of a year and in quality of life (Witt et al. 2009a).

Another model with independent replication is Arnica 30x to prevent delayed-onset muscle soreness. The results of two studies in the Oslo marathon have been pooled, and a small but significant effect on muscle soreness, but none on muscle enzymes, was shown (Tveiten & Bruset 2003). However, a larger-scale study replication, mostly on runners in the London marathon, was negative (Vickers et al. 1998). More recently the results of three linked studies of Arnica 30x in different types of knee surgery have yielded a positive result (Brinkaus et al. 2006). The models are so divergent, however, that no common quantitative measure can be derived.

Paralytic postoperative ileus has also been the subject of repeated studies: patients were treated with Opium and Raphanus C6; the time to resumption of intestinal transit was the outcome. Initial pilot studies were promising, but a large-scale multicentre study in France did not reproduce the initial results (GRECHO 1989). The initial results were so strong, however, that a pooled analysis still yielded significant results (Barnes et al. 1997).

Another area with mixed replications is rheumatology. An initial study of individualized homeopathy in rheumatoid arthritis was positive (Gibson et al. 1980), but independent studies failed to confirm these results (Andrade et al. 1991; Fisher & Scott 2001). A trial of a single homeopathic medicine (Rhus toxicodendron) in osteoarthritis with little or no individualization yielded a negative result (Shipley et al. 1983). However a replication, using the same homeopathic medicine but in a different rheumatological condition (fibromyalgia) and incorporating individualization, yielded a positive result (Fisher et al. 1989). Subsequently there have been two further positive results from RCTs of homeopathic treatment of fibromyalgia, but these have used different methods and outcomes: one looked at individualized homeopathy (Bell et al. 2004) and the other at the entire 'package' of homeopathic care, including consultation and medicine, compared to normal care (Relton et al. 2009).

In another area the apparently contradictory results of replications may be explicable by crucial methodological differences. Two placebo-controlled RCTs of homeopathy for attention disorder hyperactivity disorder were published at about the same time and were superficially similar: the patients recruited were similar and individualized homeopathy was used in both. However, closer scrutiny reveals that there were important differences in prescribing between the two studies: only one of the five most frequently prescribed homeopathic medicines was the same in the two studies (Frei et al. 2005; Jacobs et al. 2005b). But, importantly, one of these studies (Frei et al. 2005) was of unusual design: it was in fact a study of withdrawal of treatment. The optimum treatment was determined, then after improvement had occurred, randomly and blindly replaced with placebo for 6-week periods, then resumed. The patients deteriorated when on placebo. The crucial point is that it took a mean of three attempts to find the effective homeopathic medicine. It has been shown that if this study had randomized the patients at the time of the first homeopathic prescription, its results too would have been negative (Frei et al. 2007).

It has been contended that the lack of effect in some trials is due to confounding effects – toothpaste, coffee, diet and other factors believed to antidote homeopathy – or due to patients being unresponsive because of conventional drugs. An attempt was made to conduct a study of untreated patients only, but proved impractical largely because of recruitment problems (Siebenwirth et al. 2009). Another study, in depression, failed because of recruitment problems, reflecting strong patient preference issues related to homeopathy (Katz et al. 2005).

SUMMARY OF CLINICAL RESEARCH

Reviews of RCTs of homeopathy in the following conditions are broadly positive: childhood diarrhoea, influenza (treatment), postoperative ileus, seasonal allergic rhinitis, rheumatic diseases, upper respiratory tract diseases and vertigo. There is replicated RCT evidence that homeopathy may be effective in childhood diarrhoea, fibromyalgia, influenza (treatment), otitis media, seasonal allergic rhinitis, sinusitis and vertigo. There is also some evidence from individual RCTs that homeopathy may be effective in chronic fatigue syndrome, premenstrual syndrome, postpartum bleeding, sepsis and stomatitis.

For anxiety, childhood asthma, insect bites, menopausal symptoms in breast cancer, migraine, muscle soreness, prevention of upper respiratory tract infection, stroke and warts, the current RCT evidence is inconclusive or negative. For other medical conditions the current published evidence is fragmentary.

The evidence overall becomes less positive when filtered for internal trial validity and sample size. It can nevertheless be counterargued that many of these studies were of poor homeopathic quality, for instance lacking individualization or with unrealistic outcomes.

RESEARCH AND METHODOLOGICAL IMPLICATIONS

This debate also raises a fundamental methodological issue, concerning an assumption which underpins placebo-controlled studies: that specific and non-specific effects are separable and do not interact and that the total treatment effect is simply the sum of the two components. The effects of a treatment are traditionally divided into specific and non-specific: non-specific effects include explanation, reassurance, advice on diet, exercise and lifestyle. Placebo effects are a subset of non-specific effects: the psychological effects associated with an intervention, which include expectation of benefit, in part a response conditioned by previous experience of treatment, the patient's perception of the therapist and the setting, credibility of the therapy and others.

There is no a priori reason to suppose that specific and non-specific effects are separable and do not interact. Given the importance of this assumption, it is surprising how little it has been questioned or investigated. When it has been investigated the answer has usually been that this assumption is unsafe. The most comprehensive review of the topic concluded that 'specific and non-specific effects are sometimes synergistic, and at other times antagonistic, so the implicit model of the randomized clinical trial is too simple' (Kleinjen et al. 1994). For instance, a trial of analgesia for post dental surgery pain compared intravenous infusion given by a person at the bedside, by a person hidden in an adjacent room or by a preprogrammed syringe pump. The effect differed not only in scale but in sign: the patients who received the active drug given by a person, hidden or not, had more pain than the placebo group; the reverse was true when the drug was given by a pump (Levine & Gordon 1984).

An attempt to investigate interaction between specific and non-specific effects in homeopathy was confounded by differential recruitment between groups (Fisher et al. 2006). However, a subsequent RCT, also of double-dummy design but not placebo-controlled, demonstrated equivalence of individualized homeopathy to the antidepressant fluoxetine (Adler et al. 2009).

Clinical research in homeopathy provides a good example of why research in CAM needs to be multimodal, matched to specific utility benefits and not hierarchical, as described in Chapter 1. The impossibility of proving whether homeopathy in general works using heterogeneous studies was demonstrated statistically in a funnel plot-based sensitivity analysis by Linde et al. (2001). They demonstrated that over 1000 adequately powered placebo-controlled RCTs would be needed. The conclusion is that very meticulous basic research or whole-systems comparative trials should be the main focus of homeopathic research.

A strong case can be made that if the research question is, 'Do homeopathic medicines exert physiological effects?' then it is much better to use laboratory experiments. RCTs are a clumsy, expensive and difficult-to-reproduce way to answer the question. If the question is, 'Does homeopathy benefit patients?' or 'How much?' or 'At what cost?' or 'Is it safe?', then clinical studies are required. But they should be of pragmatic, not placebo-controlled, design.

COST-EFFECTIVENESS OF HOMEOPATHY

Cost-effectiveness studies in the public and insured primary care sectors in France and Germany suggest that integration of homeopathy is associated with better outcomes for equivalent costs. These studies were of 'quasiexperimental' design (i.e. different treatments were compared, but patients were not assigned randomly to the different treatments). A third, more recent, study was an RCT – the only one of its kind in homeopathy research to date.

Trichard et al. (2005; Trichard & Chaufferin 2004) compared two treatment approaches ('homeopathic strategy' versus 'antibiotic strategy') used in routine medical practice by allopathic and homeopathic GPs in the management of recurrent acute rhinopharyngitis in 499 children aged between 18 months and 4 years. The GPs using homeopathy had significantly better results in terms of clinical effectiveness, complications, parents' quality of life and time lost from work, for lower cost to social security. A study based in a public sector clinic in Italy and using data from the official Prescription Archive documented a large reduction in drug costs for patients receiving homeopathic treatment compared to patients who did not (Rossi et al. 2009a).

Witt and colleagues (2005a, b) compared homeopathic and conventional GPs' outcomes in chronic diagnoses commonly treated in general practice (adults – headache, low-back pain, depression, insomnia, sinusitis; children – atopic asthma, dermatitis, rhinitis). A total of 493 patients were treated by 101 homeopathic and 59 conventional GPs. The patients treated by the two groups of GPs were generally similar. The conclusion was that patients who sought homeopathic treatment had better outcomes for similar cost. Some of the same authors conducted a 12-month cohort study comparing homeopathic and conventional treatment of eczema in children. The two groups had similar improvements in perception of eczema symptoms (assessed by patients or parents) and disease-related quality of life (Keil et al. 2006). Also in the German context, the cost-effectiveness of the commercial homeopathic preparation Sinfrontal was assessed in a placebo-controlled RCT of adults with acute maxillary sinusitis (Kneis & Gandjour 2009). Sinfrontal led to average incremental savings of 275 euros per patient compared with placebo over

22 days; this was mainly due to reduced absenteeism from work (7.8 versus 12.9 workdays). In an indirect comparison, Sinfrontal had a higher cure rate than antibiotics, at similar or lower cost.

CLINICAL OBSERVATIONAL STUDIES

The clinical areas in which research on homeopathy has been done do not match well with those for which it is used in practice. For instance, homeopathy is commonly used to treat psychiatric problems, including anxiety and depression in France, Germany, the UK and USA (Davidson et al. 1998; Unutzer et al. 2000; Trichard et al. 2003; Becker-Witt et al. 2004), yet as mentioned above, clinical trial evidence is scant. Reasons for this include model simplicity (for instance, isopathic treatment of allergies has been relatively extensively investigated because it is a simple model), expediency and commercial motives. In practice homeopathy is frequently used for clinical problems, for instance dermatological or gastrointestinal conditions where there is little or no RCT evidence. But observational studies look at what happens to patients who receive homeopathic treatment. A comprehensive observational study at the Bristol Homoeopathic Hospital included over 6500 consecutive patients with over 23 000 attendances in a 6-year period (Spence et al. 2005). At follow-up, 70% of patients reported improved health, 50% major improvement. The best treatment responses were reported in childhood eczema or asthma, and in inflammatory bowel disease, irritable bowel syndrome, menopausal problems and migraine. A study at a public-sector clinic in Italy yielded similar results (Rossi et al. 2009b).

In a prospective, multicentre cohort study in Germany and Switzerland, 73% of 3709 patients with 8-year follow-up contributed data. The most frequent diagnoses were allergic rhinitis and headache in adults, and atopic dermatitis and multiple recurrent infections in children. Disease severity decreased significantly ($P < 0.001$) between baseline, 2 years and 8 years. Younger age, female gender and more severe disease at baseline correlated with better outcomes (Witt et al. 2008). An observational study by the same group followed 82 adults with psoriasis for 2 years. Mean disease duration was 15 years; 96% had had previous treatment. Their psoriasis improved with a large effect size and conventional treatment and health service use were reduced (Witt et al. 2009b).

A 500-patient survey at the Royal London Homoeopathic Hospital showed that many patients were able to reduce or stop conventional medication following homeopathic treatment (Sharples et al. 2003). The size of the effect varied between diagnoses: for skin complaints, for example, 72% of patients reported being able to stop or reduce their conventional medication; there was no reduction for cancer patients. In both these surveys, many of the patients were suffering from difficult-to-treat 'effectiveness gap' conditions. (Effectiveness gaps are clinical areas in which available treatments are not fully effective or satisfactory for any reason, including simple lack of effective treatment, adverse effects, acceptability to patients and cost: Fisher et al. 2004.)

Some observational studies have also addressed cost issues. For example, Frenkel & Hermoni (2002) reported that homeopathic intervention led to modest economic savings and modest reductions in the use of medications commonly used to treat allergic conditions and their complications. One homeopathic GP practice in London recorded costs of homeopathic medicines and calculated the costs of conventional drugs that would otherwise have been prescribed for 100 patients (Jain 2003). Average cost savings were £60 per patient. The majority of patients' health improved and most did not report any side-effects.

Although these observational studies showed significant and persistent outcomes, it is important to remember that the extent to which the observed effects are due to differential dropout, spontaneous improvement, regression to the mean, lifestyle changes, placebo or context effects is unknown and needs clarification in future explanatory studies.

SAFETY AND 'AGGRAVATION'

The available evidence suggests that patients' confidence in the safety of homeopathy is justified: the hazards from homeopathic products are modest in comparison with those of conventional medicine (Kirby 2002). A systematic review of the safety of homeopathy, including a search of the English-language literature between 1970 and 1995, came to the following conclusions: homeopathic medicines may provoke adverse effects, but these are generally mild and transient; adverse effects of homeopathy are underreported; there are cases of 'mistaken identity' where herbal medicines were described as homeopathic (Dantas & Rampes 2000). The main risks associated with homeopathy are indirect, relating to the prescriber rather than the medicine (Fisher et al. 2002). In two studies, adverse reactions were observed in approximately 2.7% of patients (Anelli et al. 2002; Endrizzi et al. 2005); in a third study, 7.8% of homeopathy patients had adverse reactions, compared to 22.3% in the corresponding group receiving conventional treatment (Riley et al. 2001). In addition, laboratory research has reported adverse effects in animals so some caution is needed in assuming all homeopathy is safe (Jonas & Ernst 1999).

A temporary deterioration on starting homeopathic treatment associated with a good long-term prognosis is widely described in the homeopathic literature – homeopathic 'aggravation' (or healing reaction) (Vithoulkas 1986; Kent 1990). A systematic review of double-blind randomized trials of homeopathy found no clear evidence of their occurrence (Grabia & Ernst 2003), but case series have reported rates of aggravation ranging from 2.68% to 24% (Thompson et al. 2004; Endrizzi et al. 2005).

HOMEOPATHIC PATHOGENETIC TRIALS

Eliciting symptoms with homeopathic reminders by giving them to healthy people and doing detailed analysis as the method called 'proving' was used by Hahnemann and others as a basis for seeing symptom pictures for certain remedies. They are now usually called 'human pathogenetic trials' or HPTs.

A systematic review of the modern literature identified 156 HPTs on 143 medicines, involving nearly 3000 volunteers, conducted worldwide between 1945 and 1995. The review concluded that there was a wide variation in methods and results, and that methodological quality was generally low (Dantas et al. 2007). Design flaws, particularly absence of proper randomization, blinding, placebo control and criteria for analysis of outcomes, were common. More symptoms were reported from HPTs of poor quality than from better ones. In addition considerable numbers of HPTs have been published outside the peer-reviewed literature, of substances as diverse as plutonium, chocolate, Coca-Cola and American bald eagle. These substances often seem to have been selected on symbolical or metaphorical grounds (Sankaran 1998; Sherr 1998, 2002). They often report large numbers of symptoms. The methodology is frequently not that of contemporary science, and we will not consider them further.

It has been objected that using RCT methods and excessive concern for statistical significance or the elimination of background noise risk 'throwing the baby out with the bathwater' (Sherr & Quirk 2007). And that modern provings unconsciously confound two different objectives: qualitative research and attributional clinical research. Qualitative research aims at maximizing variability to bring out the rich subtleties of the remedy administration and its experience, looking for striking, repeated (within individuals) and similar symptoms (between individuals). The validity of the symptom picture is later determined in clinical practice, not necessarily in other provers (Riley 2005). In attributional research the goal is to determine statistically if there are quantitatively different symptom counts between groups on the remedy and controls. A number of HPTs have been published subsequent to the cut-off date of the systematic review, with mixed results. Some of these have focused on the quality or 'typicality' of symptoms reported by volunteers, rather than their number, while preserving methodological rigour, and these do seem more likely to yield positive results (Signorini et al. 2005; Walach et al. 2008; Möllinger et al. 2009) than those which have focused only on symptom count (Walach et al. 2001; Brien et al. 2003; Teut et al. 2008).

BASIC SCIENCE

Although the basic idea of homeopathy is similarity, its most controversial claim concerns the properties of ultramolecular dilutions. Avogadro's constant, the number of particles (atoms or molecules) in a gram mole of a substance, is of the order of 10^{23}. In homeopathic terminology, 10^{23} corresponds to a 23X or 12C dilution. Homeopathic preparations in dilution less than those contain material traces of the original substance; those in high (ultramolecular) dilution are unlikely to do so. We will divide our discussion into biological models, physicochemical research and theoretical work on the basis of homeopathic and ultramolecular effects.

BIOLOGICAL MODELS

The largest body of research on biological models in homeopathy is based on experimental intoxication. A critical review and meta-analysis focused on 135 experiments published in 105 articles exploring the protective effect of homeopathic dilutions against toxins (Linde et al. 1994). The studies were extremely diverse and included many different experimental models: more than 70% of the high-quality studies reported positive effects. A more recent meta-analysis evaluated 67 in vitro biological experiments in 75 research publications and found high-potency effects were reported in nearly 75% of all replicated studies; however, no positive result was stable enough to be reproduced by all investigators. The most frequently used in vitro model was basophils, used in 42% of experiments (Witt et al. 2007).

A review of replicated basic studies in homeopathy identified 21 different models that have been repeated. The earliest experiments are those of Kolisko on the effect of homeopathically prepared silver nitrate on wheat seedlings, dating from 1923. This model has been the subject of four independent repetitions, three of them positive. The earliest in vitro model, first reported from the Soviet Union in 1932, on the effect of mercuric chloride on starch diastase, was not reproducible in the most recent repetition (Persson 1933; Boyd 1954; Witt et al. 2006).

Another relatively well-established plant model is the effect of the plant hormone gibberellic acid on plant growth. Again, repetitions have been mostly positive, although sometimes with qualitative differences between the results obtained by different groups. The problem of differing results between groups is mostly clearly seen with the wheat seedling/arsenic intoxication model (Brizzi et al. 2005). Multiple experiments, some of them with large datasets, have been conducted; most have shown statistically significant differences (Betti et al. 1997, 2005; Binder et al. 2005; Scherr et al. 2009). But these differences have been in different directions, and collaboration between the research teams has so far failed to elucidate the reason for this (Lahnstein et al. 2009).

The best-established and most repeated series of in vitro experiments in homeopathy is the model of the allergic response to antibody using the human basophil degranulation test. This exists in three main variants. All measure degranulation or activation (degranulation is a manifestation of activation) of human basophils in vitro, but the parameter measured has been variously: stimulation of degranulation by high dilutions of antiserum to IgE; or inhibition of such degranulation by high dilutions of *Apis mellifica;* or histamine. The latter model has now been the subject of 12 published positive reproductions. However this model got off to an inauspicious start: it was the source of the infamous 'Benveniste affair' of 1988, which followed the publication by a group led by Jacques Benveniste reporting inhibition of degranulation with ultramolecular dilutions of anti-IgE (Anonymous 1988a, b; Coles 1988; Davenas et al. 1988; Pool 1988). These experiments proved irreproducible (Ovelgönne et al. 1992; Hirst et al. 1993).

However, subsequent studies using ultramolecular dilutions of histamine to inhibit degranulation triggered by anti-IgE and other stimuli have shown positive results. Seventeen series of such experiments over 25 years have now been reported; these include multicentre and independent replications (Sainte-Laudy & Belon 1993; Belon et al. 2004; Chirumbolo et al. 2009). There has been steady refinement of the method, including automation by the use of flow cytometry. All but two repetitions have reported positive results. There is growing insight into possible mechanisms of action; for instance the response is highly specific to histamine. It is not induced by the structural analogue histidine, and it is blocked by histamine antagonist drugs. Experiments with series of dilutions show alternating peaks and troughs of effect at different dilutions. The reason for this is not understood, but there is a consistent peak of activity at 16c (histamine 10^{-32}M), well into the ultramolecular range.

These findings have been reproduced in several independent laboratories (Belon et al. 1999; Brown & Ennis 2001; Lorenz et al. 2003), as well as in a multicentre series of experiments. The effect is partly blocked by the H_2-receptor antagonists ranitidine and cimetidine (Belon et al. 2004).

Another relatively well-established model with multiple repetitions is the effect of aspirin in high dilution on platelet aggregation. In contrast to its effects in substantial dose, aspirin in high dilution promotes platelet aggregation (Doutemepuich et al. 1990; Eizayaga et al. 2005), something that might have important clinical relevance for postsurgery and injury (Jonas 1994). Again recent work casts light on possible pathways: work with 'knock-out' mice suggests it depends on the enzyme cyclooxygenase-2 (COX-2: Aguejouf et al. 2009). Several white blood cell-based models suggest that homeopathic medicines modulate cytokine expression (Fimiani et al. 2000; Ramachandran et al. 2007; de Oliveira et al. 2008; Smit et al. 2008).

Of the animal models, the best established is the effect of thyroxine on amphibians, particularly their rate of metamorphosis. Several independent studies have shown acceleration of the rate of metamorphosis (Endler et al. 1991; Zausner et al. 2002; Guedes et al. 2004); again, variations on this theme have been published (Endler et al. 1994). Several animal studies have focused on protection against toxins: models include the effects of homeopathically prepared arsenic and mercury on intoxication with the same substances and the protective effect of homeopathic phosphorus against carbon tetrachloride-induced hepatitis. Khuda-Bukhsh's group has reported remarkable results on the impact of homeopathic preparations on chemical carcinogens in rodents (Khuda-Buhksh 2007; Bhattacharjee et al. 2009). The effects of homeopathic medicines in rodent behavioural models have been the subject of a systematic review (Bellavite et al. 2009). There is relatively little reproduced work; one of the most promising models is the effect of Gelsemium on mouse exploratory behaviour. Another systematic review of conceptual aspects has drawn attention to inflammatory models (mostly using the rat paw oedema model), models examining host–parasite interaction and mathematical modelling of homeopathic effects. Some models suggest that intact animals respond more strongly than tissue cultures: for example, Thangapazham et al. (2006) showed anticancer effects from homeopathic intervention in whole animals but not in cell models of prostate cancer.

BIOLOGICAL MODELS OF SIMILITUDE

Given that the fundamental principle of homeopathy is that of similitude, it is surprising how little research has been done on this aspect. However the team led by Roel van Wijk and Fred Wiegant of the University of Utrecht in the Netherlands has conducted a scientific programme on similarity, rather than ultramolecular dilution effects. Their model is based on Reuber H35 rat hepatoma cells subjected to heat stress, followed by a stimulatory low dose. They have investigated both homologous treatment, where the initial harmful and the secondary stimulatory treatment are of the same nature, differing only in scale, equivalent to isopathy in clinical homeopathy; and heterologous experiments, where the two treatments differ in nature. They have used chemical toxins, including arsenite and cadmium. They have shown clear effects in terms of cell survival and production of stress proteins, and that the strength of the effect relates to the degree of similarity (as measured by the pattern of stress protein response), between the two stimuli (van Wijk & Wiedgant 1997; Wiegant et al. 1997, 1999). The HomBRex database provides a valuable resource, indexing over 1300 basic research experiments in homeopathy (Van Wijk & Albrecht 2007).

THE PHYSICAL BASIS OF ULTRAMOLECULAR EFFECTS

Despite the significant number of positive results, because a plausible mechanism of action of ultramolecular dilutions is lacking, many scientists have a low Bayesian 'prior' for homeopathy. The most widespread hypothesis to explain the mechanism of action of homeopathic dilutions refers to 'memory of water' effects: under appropriate circumstances, water retains information about substances with which it has previously been in contact and may then transmit that information to presensitized biosystems. In reviewing the possible mechanisms by which water might acquire a 'memory', Chaplin (2007) divides potential mechanisms into specific mechanisms, including remaining material and particle clusters, and imprinted silicates. In addition non-specific mechanisms include dissolved and particulate silicates, nanobubbles, redox molecules produced from water, natural and stabilized water clustering and ethanol solution complexity (Chaplin 2007). Some of these hypotheses have been further developed (Del Guidice et al. 1988; Anick & Ives 2007; Voeikov 2007).

On the experimental side, in a series of experiments, Elia's group used standard physicochemical techniques, including flux calorimetry, conductometry, pHmetry and galvanic cell electrode potential (Elia & Niccoli 1999; Elia et al. 2007), reporting large changes in physicochemical properties as a function of the history of dilutions, the solute previously dissolved and time. They report two surprising observations in homeopathic dilutions: an increase of the measured physicochemical parameters with sample age, and their dependence on the volume in which the dilution is prepared, with stronger effects observed with dilutions prepared in smaller volumes. Elia's group explain these observations in terms of dissipative structures. Thermoluminescence experiments suggest that the 'signature' of previous solutes is retained even after the solute has been diluted out, and that the atmosphere in which the dilutions are conducted is crucial – stronger effects are noted when dilutions are prepared in an oxygen atmosphere and weaker effects under reduced atmospheric pressure (Rey 2003, 2007).

Nuclear magnetic resonance (NMR) results have varied, depending on the parameters measured. Negative results have been reported (Aabel et al. 2001; Anick 2004), but when 20 MHz T1 and T2 water proton NMR relaxation rates are measured, homeopathic dilutions of histamine are distinguishable from solvents up to ultramolecular levels. The effect is attributed to stable supramolecular structures, involving nanobubbles of atmospheric gases and highly ordered water around them. It is deleted by heating (Demangeat et al. 2004; Demangeat 2008, 2009). Preliminary studies based on Raman and ultraviolet-visible spectroscopy (Rao et al. 2007; Roy et al. 2005) and other methods (Vybíral & Voráček 2007) are also reported as showing changes in the physicochemical properties of water as a function of its history. It remains to be proven whether such changes have the features to account for effects of homeopathic medicines in vivo (Chaplin 2007).[15]

The main competing hypotheses to the memory of water are those involving entanglement, known from quantum theory and postulated also as a systemic property for large systems by a 'weak quantum theory' (Atmanspacher et al. 2002). Such a model proposes that homeopathy involves coherence effects similar to those that occur between entangled subatomic particles and memorably described as 'spooky action at a distance' by Einstein (Walach 2003). Parts of an entangled system correlate instantaneously but acausally across infinite distances and time. This phenomenon has been repeatedly confirmed experimentally at the microscopic level, but never conclusively demonstrated at the macroscopic level. Entanglement hypotheses have been divided into: (1) one- way (entanglement between the starting substance and final medicine); (2) two-way (between patient and practitioner); and (3) three-way (between patient, practitioner and remedy) (Milgrom 2004). These hypotheses make a number of predictions, including 'smearing' of treatment effects across verum and placebo groups in randomized trials. Experimental evidence for this from a homeopathic pathogenetic trial has been claimed (Möllinger et al. 2004; Walach 2004), though this claim has been disputed (Lewith et al. 2005).

CONCLUSIONS

We have attempted to give a broad overview of the scientific aspects and issues around homeopathy, starting with the long-running debate over its use of ultramolecular dilutions, and covering its persistent popularity with patients and the public. We then moved on to the 'type 1' clinical evidence from meta-analyses and systemic reviews of RCTs. We looked at some example RCTs, focusing on those where there have been repetitions, or at least similar trials, or which illustrate particular points. We then briefly examined homeopathic pathogenetic trials (provings), biological models of ultramolecular responses and similitude. We concluded by considering the possible physicochemical basis of action, including some theoretical discussion.

Given its wide use, homeopathy is underresearched. Despite this a notable number of positive findings have been reported from RCTs and systematic reviews and meta-analyses of such trials for conditions, including: childhood diarrhoea, influenza, postoperative ileus, rheumatic diseases including fibromyalgia, seasonal allergic rhinitis, sinusitis and vertigo. There is some evidence that homeopathy may be effective in acute otitis media, chronic fatigue syndrome, premenstrual syndrome, postpartum bleeding, sepsis and certain symptoms related to cancer treatment.

Controlled but non-randomized, cost-effectiveness and observational studies show universally positive results, often in difficult-to-treat 'effectiveness gap' conditions. This might explain why homeopathy is favoured by patients despite the lack of a plausible theory or contested superiority over placebo. Even though the large effect sizes seen in observational studies might be due to the placebo effect, this is irrelevant from the patients' perspective. Homeopathy seems to be very safe.

The main barrier to scientific acceptance of homeopathy is its use of very high 'ultramolecular' dilutions. The leading hypothesis to explain the effects of such dilutions centres on the storage of information by aqueous solutions: there is some evidence from physical science of specific structural modifications in water, induced by the homeopathic preparation process, which might be capable of storing information. A number of biological models of high dilution effects and of similitude have been published, some of which have been reproduced in independent or multicentre experiments.

The evidence on homeopathy from the classical method of clinical research, the RCT, continues to be debated, as indeed is the cause of the disparate results of RCTs. Explanations for the lack of reproducibility range from poor trial quality, lack of true reproductions and variations in methodology, to those involving entanglement, which propose that the irreproducibility is inherent in the 'mechanism' of action (even the word 'mechanism' is inappropriate in this explanation). However the results of non-randomized studies using cohort and other designs are universally positive, suggesting that homeopathy has a useful role to play in health care, although taken alone, such data do not allow conclusions about effectiveness. This also points the way to the most promising strategy for clinical research. There is a lack of randomized pragmatic comparison studies that compare the system of homeopathy as a whole, and as normally practised, with conventional care. Such studies could be conceptualized as non-inferiority studies, with an emphasis on cost-effectiveness and side-effects.

The biggest changes in the homeopathic research scene since the first edition of this book was published a decade ago are at the level of basic research, both biological models and physicochemical. There are now a number of laboratory experiments that appear reproducible, including the human basophil degranulation/activation model which at one time appeared discredited. Although less advanced, there is also progress in the field of understanding the basic way in which homeopathic medicines might have effects. These developments have the potential to raise the very low Bayesian prior that currently exists in the minds of many members of the scientific community in respect of homeopathy.

Nevertheless, after 200 years of controversy, it would be an optimist who predicted the imminent resolution of scientific debate surrounding homeopathy! There is much research to be done, and a strong argument can be made, as was done by Linde et al. over a decade ago, that the agenda should divide into research exploring whether or not it provides a useful tool in health care (a question of great relevance to patients, health care providers and funders) and laboratory-based research exploring possible modes of action.

REFERENCES

Aabel, S., 2000. No beneficial effect of isopathic prophylactic treatment for birch pollen allergy during a low-pollen season: a double-blind, placebo-controlled clinical trial of homeopathic Betula 30c. British Homeopathic Journal 89, 169–173.

Aabel, S., 2001. Prophylactic and acute treatment with the homeopathic medicine Betula 30c for birch pollen allergy: a double-blind, randomized, placebo-controlled study of consistency of VAS responses. British Homeopathic Journal 90, 73–78.

Aabel, S., Fossheim, S., Rise, F., 2001. Nuclear magnetic resonance (NMR) studies of homeopathic solutions. British Homoeopathic Journal 90, 14–20.

Adler, U.C., Paiva, P.M., Cesar, A.T., et al., 2009. Homeopathic Individualized Q-potencies versus fluoxetine for moderate to severe depression: double-blind, randomized non-inferiority trial. Evidence-based Complementary and Alternative Medicine: eCAM doi:10.1093/ecam/nep114

Aguejouf, O., Eizayaga, F.X., Desplat, V., et al., 2009. Prothrombotic and hemorrhagic effects of aspirin. Clin. Appl. Thromb. Hemost. 15, 523–528.

Altunç, U., Pittler, M.H., Ernst, E., 2007. Homeopathy for childhood and adolescence ailments: systematic review of randomized clinical trials. Mayo Clin. Proc. 82, 69–75.

Andrade, L., Ferraz, M., Atra, E., et al., 1991. A randomized controlled trial to evaluate the effectiveness of homeopathy in rheumatoid arthritis. Scand. J. Rheumatol. 20, 204–208.

Anelli, M., Scheepers, L., Sermeus, G., et al., 2002. Homeopathy and health related Quality of Life: a survey in six European countries. Homeopathy 91, 18–21.

Anick, D.J., 2004. High sensitivity 1H-NMR spectroscopy of homeopathic remedies made in water. BMC Complement. Altern. Med. 4, 15.

Anick, D.J., Ives, J.A., 2007. The silica hypothesis for homeopathy: physical chemistry. Homeopathy 96, 189–195.

Anonymous, 1988a. Explanation of Benveniste. Nature 334 (6180), 285–286.

Anonymous, 1988b. When to publish pseudo-science. Nature 334 (6181), 367.

Atmanspacher, H., Römer, H., Walach, H., 2002. Weak quantum theory: complementarity and entanglement in physics and beyond. Found. Phys. 32, 379–406.

Balzarini, A., Felisi, E., Martini, A., et al., 2000. Efficacy of homeopathic treatment of skin reactions during radiotherapy for breast cancer: a randomized, double-blind clinical trial. British Homeopathic Journal 89, 8–12.

Barnes, J., Resch, K.L., Ernst, E., 1997. Homeopathy for postoperative ileus? A meta-analysis. J. Clin. Gastroenterol. 25, 628–633.

Becker-Witt, C., Ludtke, R., Weisshuhn, T.E.R., et al., 2004. Diagnoses and treatment in homeopathic medical practice. Forsch. Komplementärmed. Klass. Naturheilkd. 11, 98–103.

Bell, I.R., Lewis, D.A., Brooks, A.J., et al., 2004. Improved clinical status in fibromyalgia patients treated with individualized homeopathic remedies versus placebo. Rheumatology 43, 577–582.

Bellavite, P., Ortolani, R., Pontarollo, F., et al., 2006. Immunology and homeopathy. 4. Clinical studies – Part 1. Evidence-based Complementary and Alternative Medicine: eCAM 3, 293–301.

Bellavite, P., Ortolani, R., Pontarollo, F., et al., 2006. Immunology and homeopathy. 4. Clinical studies – Part 2. Evidence-based Complementary and Alternative Medicine: eCAM 3, 397–409.

Bellavite, P., Magnani, P., Marzotto, M., et al., 2009. Assays of homeopathic remedies in rodent behavioural and psychopathological models. Homeopathy 98, 208–227.

Belon, P., Cumps, J., Ennis, M., et al., 1999. Inhibition of human basophil degranulation by successive histamine dilutions: results of a European multi-centre trial. Inflamm. Res. 48 (Suppl. 1), S17–S18.

Belon, P., Cumps, J., Ennis, M., et al., 2004. Histamine dilutions modulate basophil activation. Inflamm. Res. 53, 181–188.

Betti, L., Brizzi, M., Nani, D., et al., 1997. Effect of high dilutions of *Arsenicum album* on wheat seedlings from seed poisoned with the same substance. British Homoeopathic Journal 86, 86–89.

Bhattacharjee, N., Pathak, S., Khuda-Bukhsh, A.R., 2009. Amelioration of carcinogen-induced toxicity in mice by administration of a potentized homeopathic drug, Natrum Sulphuricum 200. Evidence-based Complementary and Alternative Medicine. eCAM 6, 65–75.

Binder, M., Baumgartner, S., Thurneysen, A., 2005. The effects of a 45x potency of *Arsenicum album* on wheat seedling growth – a reproduction trial. Forsch. Komplementärmed. Klass. Naturheilkd. 12, 284–291.

Bond, R.A., 2001. Is paradoxical pharmacology a strategy worth pursuing? Trends Pharmacol. Sci. 22, 273–276.

Bornhöft, G., Wolf, U., Ammon, K., et al., 2006. Effectiveness, safety and cost-effectiveness of homeopathy in general practice – summarized health technology assessment. Forsch. Komplementärmed. 13 (Suppl. 2), 19–29.

Boyd, W.E., 1954. Biochemical and biological evidence of the activity of high potencies. British Homoeopathic Journal 44, 7–44.

Brien, S., Lewith, G., Bryant, T., 2003. Does ultramolecular homeopathy have any clinical effects? A randomised double blind placebo controlled pathogenetic trial of Belladonna 30c as a model. Br. J. Clin. Pharmacol. 56, 562–568.

Brigo, B., Serpelloni, G., 1991. Homoeopathic treatment of migraines – A randomized double-blind controlled study of sixty cases (homoeopathic remedy versus placebo). Berlin Journal of Research in Homeopathy 1, 98–106.

Brinkhaus, B., Wilkens, J.M., Lüdtke, R., et al., 2006. Homeopathic arnica therapy in patients receiving knee surgery: Results of three randomised double-blind trials. Complement. Ther. Med. 14, 237–246.

British Homoeopathic Pharmacopoeia. 1993. British Association of Homeopathic Manufacturers, London, p. 24.

Brizzi, M., Lazzarato, L., Nani, D., et al., 2005. Biostatistical insight into the As_2O_3 high dilution effects on the rate and variability of wheat seedling growth. Forsch. Komplementärmed. Klass. Naturheilkd. 12, 277–283.

Brown, V., Ennis, M., 2001. Flow-cytometric analysis of basophil activation: inhibition by histamine at conventional and homeopathic concentrations. Inflamm. Res. 50 (Suppl. 2), S47–S48.

Calabrese, E.J., Blain, R., 2005. The occurrence of hormetic dose responses in the toxicological literature, the hormesis database: An overview. Toxicol. Appl. Pharmacol. 202, 289–301.

Calabrese, E.J., Staudenmayer, J., Stanek, E.J., 2006a. Drug development and hormesis. Changing conceptual understanding of the dose response creates new challenges and opportunities for more effective drugs. Curr. Opin. Drug. Discov. Devel. 9, 117–123.

Calabrese, E.J., Staudenmayer, J.W., Stanek, E.J., et al., 2006b. Hormesis Outperforms Threshold Model in National Cancer Institute Antitumor Drug Screening Database. Toxicol. Sci. 94, 368–378.

Calabrese, E.J., Bachmann, K.A., Bailer, A.J., et al., 2007. Biological stress response terminology: Integrating the concepts of adaptive response and preconditioning stress within a hormetic dose–response framework. Toxicol. Appl. Pharmacol. 222, 122–128.

Chaplin, M.F., 2007. The memory of water: an overview. Homeopathy 96, 143–150.

Chirumbolo, S., Brizzi, M., Ortolani, R., et al., 2009. Inhibition of CD203c membrane upregulation in human basophils by high dilutions of histamine: a controlled replication study. Inflamm. Res. 58, 755–764.

Coles, P., 1988. Benveniste controversy rages on in the French press. Nature 334 (6181), 372.

Coulter, M.K., Dean, M.E., 2007. Homeopathy for attention deficit/hyperactivity disorder or hyperkinetic disorder *(Cochrane Review)*. In: The Cochrane Library. John Wiley, Chichester, UK, CD005648.

Cucherat, M., Haugh, M.C., Gooch, M., et al., 2000. Evidence of clinical efficacy of homeopathy – A meta-analysis of clinical trials. Eur. J. Clin. Pharmacol. 56, 27–33.

Dantas, F., Rampes, H., 2000. Do homeopathic medicines provoke adverse effects? A systematic review. British Homeopathic Journal 89, S35–S38.

Dantas, F., Fisher, P., Walach, H., et al., 2007. A systematic review of the quality of homeopathic pathogenetic trials published from 1945 to 1995. Homeopathy 96, 4–16.

Davenas, E., Beauvais, F., Amara, J., et al., 1988. Human basophil de-granulation triggered by very dilute antiserum against IgE. Nature 333, 816–818.

Davidson, J., Rampes, H., Eisen, M., et al., 1998. Psychiatric disorders in primary care patients receiving complementary medical treatments. Compr. Psychiatry. 39, 16–20.

de Lange de Klerk, E.S.M., Blommers, J., Kuik, D.J., et al., 1994. Effects of homoeopathic medicines on daily burden of symptoms in children with recurrent upper respiratory tract infections. Br. Med. J. 309, 1329–1332.

de Oliveira, C.C., de Oliveira, S.M., Goes, V.M., et al., 2008. Gene expression profiling of macrophages following mice treatment with an immunomodulator medication. J. Cell. Biochem. 104, 1364–1377.

Del Guidice, E., Preparata, G., Vitiello, G., 1988. Water as a free-electron dipole laser. Phys. Rev. Lett. 61, 1085–1088.

Demangeat, J.L., 2008. NMR water proton relaxation in unheated and heated ultrahigh aqueous dilutions of histamine: Evidence for an air-dependent supramolecular organization of water. Journal of Molecular Liquids 144, 32–39.

Demangeat, J.L., 2009. NMR water proton relaxation in unheated and heated ultrahigh aqueous dilutions of histamine: Evidence for an air-dependent supramolecular organization of water. Journal of Molecular Liquids 144, 32–39.

Demangeat, J.L., Gries, P., Poitevin, B., et al., 2004. Low-field NMR water proton longitudinal relaxation in ultrahighly diluted aqueous solutions of silica-lactose prepared in glass material for pharmaceutical use. Applied Magnetic Resonance 26, 465–481.

Dinges, M. (Ed.), 2002. Patients in the History of Homeopathy. European Association for the history of medicine and health publications. University of Sheffield, Sheffield.

Doutremepuich, C., de Seze, O., Le Roy, D., et al., 1990. Aspirin at very ultra low dosage in healthy volunteers: Effects on bleeding time, platelet aggregation and coagulation. Haemostasis 20, 99–105.

Eizayaga, F.X., Aguejouf, O., Belon, P., et al., 2005. Platelet aggregation in portal hypertension and its modification by ultra-low doses of aspirin. Pathophysiol. Haemost. Thromb. 34, 29–34.

Elia, V., Niccoli, M., 1999. Thermodynamics of extremely diluted aqueous solutions. Ann. N. Y. Acad. Sci. 879, 241–248.

Elia, V., Napoli, E., Germano, R., 2007. The 'memory of water': an almost deciphered enigma. Dissipative structures in extremely dilute aqueous solutions. Homeopathy 96, 163–169.

Endler, P.C., Pongratz, W., van Wijk, R., et al., 1991. effects of highly diluted successed thyroxin on metamorphosis of highland frogs. Berlin Journal of Research in Homeopathy 1, 151–160.

Endler, P.C., Pongratz, W., Kastberger, G., et al., 1994. The effect of highly diluted agitated thyroxin on the climbing activity of frogs. Vet. Hum. Toxicol. 36, 56–59.

Endrizzi, C., Rossi, E., Crudeli, L., et al., 2005. Harm in homeopathy: aggravations, adverse drug events or medication errors? Homeopathy 94, 233–240.

Ernst, E., 1999a. Classical homoeopathy versus conventional treatments: a systematic review. Perfusion (Nürnberg) 12, 13–15.

Ernst, E., 1999b. Homeopathic prophylaxis of headaches and migraine? A systematic review. J. Pain Symptom Manage. 18, 353–357.

Ernst, E., Barnes, J., 1998. Are homoeopathic remedies effective for delayed-onset muscle soreness? A systematic review of placebo-controlled trials. Perfusion (Nürnberg) 11, 4–8.

Ernst, E., Pittler, M.H., 1998. Efficacy of homeopathic arnica. A systematic review of placebo-controlled clinical trials. Arch. Surg. 133, 1187–1190.

Eskinazi, D., 1999. Homeopathy re-revisited – is homeopathy compatible with biomedical observations? Arch. Intern. Med. 159, 1981–1986.

Fimiani, V., Cavallaro, A., Ainis, O., et al., 2000. Immunomodulatory effect of the homoeopathic drug Engystol-N on some activities of isolated human leukocytes and in whole blood. Immunopharmacol. Immunotoxicol. 22, 103–115.

Fisher, P., Scott, D.L., 2001. A randomized controlled trial of homeopathy in rheumatoid arthritis. Rheumatology 4, 1052–1055.

Fisher, P., Greenwood, A., Huskisson, E.C., et al., 1989. Effect of homeopathic treatment on fibrositis (primary fibromyalgia). Br. Med. J. 299, 365–366.

Fisher, P., Dantas, F., Rampes, H., 2002. The safety of homeopathic products. J. R. Soc. Med. 95, 474–475.

Fisher, P., van Haselen, R., Hardy, K., et al., 2004. Effectiveness Gaps: A new concept for evaluating health service and research needs applied to complementary and alternative medicine. J. Altern. Complement. Med. 10, 627–632.

Fisher, P., McCarney, R., Hasford, C., et al., 2006. Evaluation of specific and non-specific effects in homeopathy: Feasibility study for a randomised trial. Homeopathy 95, 215–222.

Forbes, J., 1846. Homoeopathy, allopathy and 'young physic'. British and Foreign Medical Review 225–265. Available online at: www.jameslindlibrary.org/trial_records/19th_Century/forbes/forbes_kp_1.html (accessed 28 August 2009).

Frass, M., Linkesch, M., Banyai, S., et al., 2005. Adjunctive homeopathic treatment in patients with severe sepsis: a randomized, double-blind, placebo-controlled trial in an intensive care unit. Homeopathy 94, 75–80.

Frei, H., Thurneysen, A., 2001a. Homeopathy in acute otitis media in children: treatment effect or spontaneous resolution? Homeopathy 90, 180–182.

Frei, H., Thurneysen, A., 2001b. Treatment for hyperactive children: homeopathy and methylphenidate compared in a family setting. Homeopathy 90, 183–188.

Frei, H., Everts, R., von Ammon, K., et al., 2005. Homeopathic treatment of children with attention deficit hyperactivity disorder: a randomised, double blind, placebo controlled crossover trial. Eur. J. Pediatr. 164, 758–767.

Frei, H., Everts, R., von Ammon, K., 2007. Randomised controlled trials of homeopathy in hyperactive children: treatment procedure leads to an unconventional study design: Experience with open-label homeopathic treatment preceding the Swiss ADHD placebo controlled, randomised, double-blind, cross-over trial. Homeopathy 96, 35–41.

Frenkel, M., Hermoni, D., 2002. Effects of homeopathic intervention on medication consumption in atopic and allergic disorders. Altern. Ther. Health. Med. 8, 76–79.

Gaucher, C., Jeulin, D., Peycru, P., et al., 1994. A double blind randomized placebo controlled study of cholera treatment with highly diluted and succussed solutions. British Homoeopathic Journal 83, 132–134.

German Homoeopathic Pharmacopoeia (Homöopathische Arzneibuch), 5th supplement to 1978 Edition, English translation. 1993. British Homoeopathic Association, London, pp. 31–38 45–46.

Gibson, R.G., Gibson, S., MacNeill, A.D., et al., 1980. Homoeopathic therapy in rheumatoid arthritis; evaluation by double-blind clinical therapeutic trial. Br. J. Clin. Pharmacol. 9, 453–459.

Glaz, V.G., 1991. Hahnemann's theory in Russia. British Homoeopathic Journal 80, 231–233.

Grabia, S., Ernst, E., 2003. Homeopathic aggravations: a systematic review of randomised, placebo-controlled clinical trials. Homeopathy 92, 92–98.

GRECHO (Groupe de recherches et d'essais cliniques en homéopathie), 1989. Evaluation de deux produits homéopathiques sur la reprise du transit après chirurgie digestive – Un essai contrôlé multicentrique. [Evaluation of the effect of two homeopathic products on the restoration of intestinal peristalsis – A multicentre controlled trial.]. Presse Méd. 18, 59–62.

Guedes, J.R.P., Ferreira, C.M., Guimaraes, H.M.B., et al., 2004. Homeopathically prepared dilution of *Rana catesbeiana* thyroid glands modifies its rate of metamorphosis. Homeopathy 93, 132–137.

Hahnemann, S.C., 1796. Essay on a new principle for ascertaining the curative powers of drugs. In: Lesser Writings. 249–303, transl. Dudgeon. W Headland, London 1851.

Hippocrates. Des lieux dans l'homme. Oeuvres complètes d'Hippocrate, tr Littré E, Paris, 1839–1861 vol. 6. pp. 334–335.

Hirst, S.J., Hayes, N.A., Burridge, J., et al., 1993. Human basophil degranulation is not triggered by very dilute antiserum against human IgE. Nature 366, 525–527.

Hyland, M., Lewith, G., 2002. Oscillatory effects in a homeopathic clinical trial: an explanation using complexity theory, and implications for clinical practice. Homeopathy 91, 145–149.

Jacobs, J., Springer, D., Crothers, D., 2001. Homeopathic treatment of acute otitis media in children: a preliminary randomized placebo-controlled trial. Pediatr. Infect. Dis. J. 20, 177–183.

Jacobs, J., Jonas, W.B., Jimenez-Perez, M., et al., 2003. Homeopathy for childhood diarrhea: combined results and metaanalysis from three randomized, controlled clinical trials. Pediatr. Infect. Dis. J. 22, 229–234.

Jacobs, J., Herman, P., Heron, K., et al., 2005a. Homeopathy for menopausal symptoms in breast cancer survivors: a preliminary randomized controlled trial. J. Altern. Complement. Med. 11, 21–27.

Jacobs, J., Williams, A.L., Girard, C., et al., 2005b. Homeopathy for attention-deficit/hyperactivity disorder: a pilot randomized-controlled trial. J. Altern. Complement. Med. 11, 799–806.

Jain, A., 2003. Does homeopathy reduce the cost of conventional drug prescribing? A study of comparative prescribing costs in general practice. Homeopathy 92, 71–77.

Jonas, W.B., 1994. The effects of aspirin on gastric prostaglandins [letter]. Ann. Intern. Med. 121, 72.

Jonas, W.B., Ernst, E., 1999. The safety of homeopathy. In: Jonas, W.B., Levin, J.S. (Eds.), Essentials of Complementary and Alternative Medicine. Lippincott Williams & Wilkins, Philadelphia, pp. 167–171.

Jonas, W.B., Linde, K., Ramirez, G., 2000. Homeopathy and rheumatic disease. Rheumatic Disease Clinics of North America 26, 117–123.

Jonas, W.B., Kaptchuk, T.J., Linde, K., 2003. A critical overview of homeopathy. Ann. Intern. Med. 138, 393–399.

Jütte, R., 1998. The paradox of professionalisation: homeopathy and hydrotherapy as unorthodoxy in Germany in the 19th and 20th century. In: Jütte, R., Risse, G.B., Woodward, J. (Eds.), Culture, knowledge, and healing. European Association for the History of Medicine and Health Publications, Sheffield, pp. 65–88.

Kassab, S., Cummings, M., Berkovitz, S., et al., 2009. Homeopathic medicines for adverse effects of cancer treatments. Cochrane Database Syst. Rev. (2), CD004845. DOI: 10.1002/14651858.CD004845.pub2.

Katz, T., Fisher, P., Katz, A., et al., 2005. The feasibility of a randomised, placebo-controlled clinical trial of homeopathic treatment of depression in general practice. Homeopathy 94, 145–152.

Keil, T., Witt, C.M., Roll, S., et al., 2006. Homoeopathic versus conventional treatment of children with eczema: A comparative cohort study. Complement. Ther. Med. 16, 15–21.

Kent, J.T., 1990. Lectures in Homeopathic Philosophy, Lecture XXXV: Remedy Reactions. Homeopathic Book Service, Sittingbourne, UK.

Khuda-Bukhsh, A.R., 2007. An evidence-based evaluation of efficacy of homeopathic drugs in mice during induced hepatocarcinogenesis. Perspectives in Cytology and Genetics 13, 177–185.

Kirby, B.J., 2002. Safety of homeopathic products. J. R. Soc. Med. 95, 221–222.

Kleijnen, J., Knipschild, P., ter Riet, G., 1991. Clinical trials of homoeopathy. Br. Med. J. 302, 316–323.

Kleijnen, J., de Craen, A., Everdingen, J., et al., 1994. Placebo effects in double-blind clinical trials: a review of interactions with medications. Lancet 344, 1347–1349.

Kneis, K.C., Gandjour, A., 2009. Economic evaluation of Sinfrontal® in the treatment of acute maxillary sinusitis in adults. Appl. Health Econ. Health Policy 7, 181–191.

Kolisko, L., 1923. Physiologischer und Physikalischer Nachweis der Wirksamkeit kleinster Entitäten. [Physiological and physical proof of the efficacy of smallest entities.] Verlag "Der kommende Tag", Stuttgart.

Lahnstein, L., Binder, M., Thurneysen, A., et al., 2009. Isopathic treatment effects of *Arsenicum album* 45x on wheat seedling growth – further reproduction trials. Homeopathy 98, 198–207.

Leary, B., 1994. Cholera 1854: update. British Homoeopathic Journal 83, 117–121.

Levine, J., Gordon, N., 1984. Influence of the method of drug administration on analgesic response. Nature 312, 755–756.

Lewith, G.T., Watkins, A.D., Hyland, M.E., et al., 2002. Use of ultramolecular potencies of allergen to treat asthmatic people allergic to house dust mite: double blind randomised controlled clinical trial. Br. Med. J. 324, 520–523.

Lewith, G.T., Brien, S., Hyland, M.E., 2005. Presentiment or entanglement? An alternative explanation for apparent entanglement in provings. Homeopathy 94, 92–95.

Linde, K., Jonas, W.B., Melchart, D., et al., 1994. Critical review and meta-analysis of serial agitated dilutions in experimental toxicology. Hum. Exp. Toxicol. 13, 481–492.

Linde, K., Clausius, N., Ramirez, G., et al., 1997. Are the clinical effects of homoeopathy placebo effects? A meta-analysis of placebo-controlled trials. Lancet 350, 834–843.

Linde, K., Scholz, M., Ramirez, G., et al., 1999. Impact of study quality on outcome in placebo controlled trials of homeopathy. J. Clin. Epidemiol. 52, 631–636.

Linde, K., Jonas, W.B., Melchart, D., et al., 2001. The methodological quality of randomized controlled trials of homeopathy, herbal medicines and acupuncture. Int. J. Epidemiol. 30, 526–531.

Long, L., Ernst, E., 2001. Homeopathic remedies for the treatment of osteoarthritis: a systematic review. British Homeopathic Journal 90, 37–43.

Lorenz, I., Schneider, E.M., Stolz, P., et al., 2003. Sensitive flow cytometric method to test basophil activation influenced by homeopathic histamine dilution. Forsch. Komplementärmed. 10, 316–324.

Lüdtke, R., Hacke, D., 2005. On the effectiveness of the homeopathic remedy *Arnica montana*. Wien. Med. Wochenschr. 155, 482–490.

Lüdtke, R., Rutten, A.L.B., 2008. The conclusions on the effectiveness of homeopathy highly depend on the set of analysed trials. J. Clin. Epidemiol. 61, 1197–1204.

Mathie, R.T., 2003. The research evidence base for homeopathy: a fresh assessment of the literature. Homeopathy 92, 84–91.

McCarney, R.W., Linde, K., Lasserson, T.J., 2004a. Homeopathy for chronic asthma *(Cochrane Review)*. In: The Cochrane Library. John Wiley, Chichester, UK, CD000353.

McCarney, R., Warner, J., Fisher, P., et al., 2004b. Homeopathy for dementia *(Cochrane Review)*. In: The Cochrane Library. John Wiley, Chichester, UK, CD003803.

Milazzo, S., Russell, N., Ernst, E., 2006. Efficacy of homeopathic therapy in cancer treatment. Eur. J. Cancer. 42, 282–289.

Milgrom, L.R., 2004. Patient–practitioner–remedy (PPR) entanglement, part 4. Towards classification and unification of the different entanglement models for homeopathy. Homeopathy 93, 34–42.

Moher, D., Pham, B., Jones, A., et al., 1998. Does quality of reports of randomised trials affect estimates of intervention efficacy reported in meta-analyses? Lancet 352, 609–613.

Moher, D., Cook, D.J., Eastwood, S., et al., 1999. Improving the quality of reports of meta-analyses of randomised controlled trials: the QUOROM statement. Lancet 354, 1896–1900.

Möllinger, H., Schneider, R., Loeffel, M., et al., 2004. A double-blind, randomized, homeopathic pathogenetic trial with healthy persons: comparing two high potencies. Forsch. Komplementärmed. 11, 274–280.

Möllinger, H., Schneider, R., Walach, H., 2009. Homeopathic pathogenetic trials produce symptoms different from placebo. Forsch. Komplementärmed. 16, 105–110.

Muscari-Tomaioli, G., Allegri, F., Miali, E., et al., 2001. Observational study of quality of life in patients with headache, receiving homeopathic treatment. Homeopathy 90, 189–197.

Oberbaum, M., Yaniv, I., Ben-Gal, Y., et al., 2001. A randomized, controlled clinical trial of the homeopathic medication Traumeel S in the treatment of chemotherapy-induced stomatitis in children undergoing stem cell transplantation. Cancer 92, 684–690.

Oberbaum, M., Galoyan, N., Lerner-Geva, L., et al., 2005. The effect of the homeopathic remedies Arnica and *Bellis perennis* on mild postpartum bleeding – a randomized, double-blind, placebo-controlled study –preliminary results. Complement. Ther. Med. 13, 87–90.

Ovelgönne, J.H., Bol, A.W., Hop, W.C., et al., 1992. Mechanical agitation of very dilute antiserum against IgE has no effect on basophil staining properties. Experientia 48, 504–508.

Owen, J.M., Green, B.N., 2004. Homeopathic treatment of headaches: A systematic review of the literature. Journal of Chiropractic Medicine 3, 45–52.

Persson, W.M., 1933. Die Einwirkung von Mikrodosen saemtlicher Arzneimittel und Chemikalen auf fermente Urease, Diastase und Trypsin. Arch. Int. Pharmacodyn. Thér. 46, 249–267.

Pilkington, K., Kirkwood, G., Rampes, H., et al., 2005. Homeopathy for depression: a systematic review of the research evidence. Homeopathy 94, 153–163.

Pilkington, K., Kirkwood, G., Rampes, H., et al., 2006. Homeopathy for anxiety and anxiety disorders: A systematic review of the research. Homeopathy 95, 151–162.

Pool, R., 1988. Unbelievable results spark a controversy. Science 241 (4864), 407.

Ramachandran, C., Nair, P.K., Clèment, R.T., et al., 2007. Investigation of cytokine expression in human leukocyte cultures with two immune-modulatory homeopathic preparations. J. Altern. Complement. Med. 13, 403–407.

Rao, M.L., Roy, R., Bell, I.R., Hoover, R., 2007. The defining role of structure (including epitaxy) in the plausibility of homeopathy. Homeopathy 96, 175–182.

Reilly, D.T., Taylor, M.A., 1985. Potent placebo or potency? A proposed study model with initial findings using homoeopathically prepared pollens in hayfever. British Homeopathic Journal 74, 65–75.

Reilly, D.T., Taylor, M.A., McSharry, C., et al., 1986. Is homeopathy a placebo response? Controlled trial of homeopathic potency, with pollen in hayfever as model. Lancet ii, 881–885.

Reilly, D., Taylor, M.A., Beattie, N.G.M., et al., 1994. Is evidence for homeopathy reproducible? Lancet 344, 1601–1606.

Relton, C., Smith, C., Raw, J., et al., 2009. Healthcare provided by a homeopath as an adjunct to usual care for fibromyalgia (FMS): results of a pilot randomised controlled trial. Homeopathy 98, 77–82.

Rey, L., 2003. Thermoluminescence of ultra-high dilutions of lithium chloride and sodium chloride. Physica A 323, 67–74.

Rey, L., 2007. Can low temperature thermoluminescence cast light on

the nature of ultra-high dilutions? Homeopathy 96, 170–174.
Riley, D., Zagon, A., 2005. Clinical Homeopathic use of RNA: evidence from two provings. Homeopathy 94, 33–36.
Riley, D., Fisher, M., Sigh, B., et al., 2001. Homeopathy and conventional medicine: an outcomes study comparing effectiveness in a primary care setting. J. Altern. Complement. Med. 7, 149–159.
Rossi, E., Crudeli, L., Endrizzi, C., et al., 2009a. Cost–benefit evaluation of homeopathic versus conventional therapy in respiratory diseases. Homeopathy 98, 2–10.
Rossi, E., Endrizzi, C., Panozzo, M.A., et al., 2009b. Homeopathy in the public health system: a seven-year observational study at Lucca Hospital (Italy). Homeopathy 98, 142–148.
Roy, R., Tiller, W.A., Bell, I.R., Hoover, M.R., 2005. The structure of liquid water; novel insights from materials research; potential relevance to homeopathy. Materials Research Innovations 9, 577–608.
Rutten, A.L.B., 2008. How can we change beliefs? Homeopathy 97, 214–219.
Rutten, A.L.B., Stolper, C.F., 2008. The 2005 meta-analysis of homeopathy: the importance of post-publication data. Homeopathy 97, 169–177.
Sainte-Laudy, J., Belon, P., 1993. Inhibition of human basophil activation by high dilutions of histamine. Agents Actions 38, 525–527.
Sankaran, R., 1998. Provings. Homeopathic Medical Publishers, Mumbai.
Scherr, C., Simon, M., Spranger, J., et al., 2009. Effects of potentised substances on growth rate of the water plant *Lemna gibba* L. Complement. Ther. Med. 17, 63–70.
Schneider, B., Klein, P., Weiser, M., 2005. Treatment of vertigo with a homeopathic complex remedy compared with usual treatments: a meta-analysis of clinical trials. Arzneimittelforschung 55, 23–29.
Schwanitz, H.J., 1983. Homöopathie und Brownianismus 1795–1844. [Homoeopathy and Brownianism 1795–1844.] Gustav-Fischer-Verlag, Stuttgart.
Shang, A., Huwiler-Muntener, K., Nartey, L., et al., 2005. Are the clinical effects of homoeopathy placebo effects? Comparative study of placebo-controlled trials of homoeopathy and allopathy. Lancet 366, 726–732.
Sharples, F., Van Haselen, R., Fisher, P., 2003. NHS patients' perspective on complementary medicine. Complement. Ther. Med 11, 243–248.
Sherr, J.Y., 1998. Dynamic Provings, vol. 1. Dynamis Books, Malvern.
Sherr, J.Y., 2002. Dynamic Provings, vol. 2. Dynamis Books, Malvern.
Sherr, J., Quirk, T., 2007. Systematic review of homeopathic pathogenetic trials: an excess of rigour? Homeopathy 96, 273–278.
Shipley, M., Berry, H., Broster, G., et al., 1983. Controlled trial of homoeopathic treatment of osteoarthritis. Lancet i, 97–98.
Siebenwirth, J., Lüdtke, R., Remy, W., et al., 2009. Effectiveness of a classical homeopathic treatment in atopic eczema. A randomised placebo-controlled double-blind clinical trial. Forsch. Komplementärmed. 16, 315–323.
Signorini, A., Lubrano, A., Manuele, G., et al., 2005. Classical and new proving methodology: Provings of *Plumbum metallicum* and *Piper methysticum* and comparison with a classical proving of *Plumbum metallicum*. Homeopathy 94, 164–174.
Smit, E., Pretorius, E., Anderson, R., et al., 2008. Differentiation of human monocytes in vitro following exposure to Canova in the absence of cytokines. Ultrastruct. Pathol. 32, 147–152.
Smith, C.A., 2004. Homoeopathy for induction of labour *(Cochrane Review)*. In: The Cochrane Library. John Wiley, Chichester, UK CD003399.
Spence, D., Thompson, E.A., Barron, S.J., 2005. Homeopathic treatment for chronic disease: a 6-year university hospital based outpatient observational study. J. Altern. Complement. Med. 5, 793–798.
Stebbing, A.R.D., 1982. Hormesis – the stimulation of growth by low levels of inhibitors. Sci. Total Environ. 22, 213–234.
Stevinson, C., Devaraj, V.S., Fountain-Barber, A., et al., 2003. Homeopathic arnica for prevention of pain and bruising: randomized placebo-controlled trial in hand surgery. J. R. Soc. Med. 96, 60–65.
Straumsheim, P., Borchgrevink, C., Mowinckel, P., et al., 2000. Homeopathic treatment of migraine: A double blind, placebo controlled trial of 68 patients. British Homeopathic Journal 89, 4–7.
Taylor, M.A., Reilly, D., Llewellyn-Jones, R.H., et al., 2000. Randomised controlled trials of homoeopathy versus placebo in perennial allergic rhinitis with overview of four trial series. Br. Med. J. 321, 471–476.
Teixeira, M.Z., 2006. Evidence of the principle of similitude in modern fatal iatrogenic events. Homeopathy 95, 229–236.

Teixeira, M.Z., 2007. Bronchodilators, fatal asthma, rebound effect and similitude. Homeopathy 96, 135–137.

Teut, M., Dahler, J., Schnegg, C., 2008. A Homoeopathic Proving of *Galphimia glauca*. Forsch. Komplementärmed. 15, 211–217.

Thangapazham, R., Gaddipati, J., Rajeshkumar, N., et al., 2006. Homeopathic medicines do not alter growth and gene expression in prostate and breast cancer cells in vitro. Integr. Cancer Ther. 5, 356–361.

Thompson, E., Reilly, D., 2003. The homeopathic approach to the treatment of symptoms of oestrogen withdrawal in breast cancer patients. A prospective observational study. Homeopathy 92, 131–134.

Thompson, E., Barron, S., Spence, D., 2004. A preliminary audit investigating remedy reactions including adverse events in routine homeopathic practice. Homeopathy 93, 203–209.

Trichard, M., Chaufferin, G., 2004. Effectiveness, quality of life, and cost of caring for children in France with recurrent acute rhinopharyngitis managed by homeopathic or non-homeopathic General Practitioners. Disease Management and Health Outcomes 12, 419–427.

Trichard, M., Lamure, E., Chaufferin, G., 2003. Study of the practice of homeopathic general practitioners in France. Homeopathy 92, 135–139.

Trichard, M., Chaufferin, G., Nicoloyannis, N., 2005. Pharmacoeconomic comparison between homeopathic and antibiotic treatment strategies in recurrent acute rhinopharyngitis in children. Homeopathy 94, 3–9.

Tveiten, D., Bruset, S., 2003. Effect of Arnica D30 in marathon runners. Pooled results from two double-blind placebo controlled studies. Homeopathy 92, 187–189.

Tveiten, D., Bruseth, S., Borchgrevink, C.F., Norseth, J., 1998. Effects of the homoeopathic remedy Arnica D30 on marathon runners: a randomized, double-blind study during the 1995 Oslo Marathon. Complement. Ther. Med. 6, 71–74.

Ullman, D., 2003. Controlled clinical trials evaluating the homeopathic treatment of people with human immunodeficiency virus or acquired immune deficiency syndrome. J. Altern. Complement. Med. 9, 133–141.

Ullman, D., 2007. The Homeopathic Revolution: Famous People and Cultural Heroes who chose Homeopathy. North Atlantic Books, Berkeley, CA.

Ullman, D., 2009. The curious case of Charles Darwin. Evidence-based Complementary and Alternative Medicine: eCAM doi:10.1093/ecam/nep168.

Unutzer, J., Klap, R., Sturm, R., et al., 2000. Mental disorders and the use of the alternative medicine: results from a national survey. Am. J. Psychiatry 157, 1851–1857.

Van Wijk, R., Albrecht, H., 2007. Proving and therapeutic experiments in the HomBRex basic homeopathy research database. Homeopathy 97, 252–257.

van Wijk, R., Wiegant, F.A.C., 1997. The Similia Principle in Surviving Stress. Mammalian Cells in Homoeopathy Research. Utrecht University, Department of Molecular Cell Biology, Utrecht.

Vandenbroucke, J.P., 2005. Homeopathy and 'the growth of truth'. Lancet 366, 691–692.

Vandenbroucke, J.P., de Craen, J.M., 2001. Alternative medicine: a "mirror image" for scientific reasoning in conventional medicine. Ann. Intern. Med. 135, 507–513.

Vickers, A., Smith, C., 2006. Homoeopathic Oscillococcinum for preventing and treating influenza and influenza-like syndromes *(Cochrane review)*. In: The Cochrane Library. John Wiley, Chichester, UK, CD001957.

Vickers, A.J., Fisher, P., Wyllie, S.E., et al., 1998. Homeopathic *Arnica* 30X is ineffective for muscle soreness after long-distance running: a randomized, double-blind, placebo-controlled trial. Clin. J. Pain 14, 227–231.

Vithoulkas, G., 1986. The Science of Homeopathy. Thorsons, London.

Voeikov, V.L., 2007. The possible role of active oxygen in the Memory of Water. Homeopathy 96, 196–201.

Vybíral, B., Voráček, P., 2007. Long term structural effects in water: Autothixotropy of water and its hysteresis. Homeopathy 96, 183–188.

Walach, H., 2003. Entanglement model of homeopathy as an example of generalised entanglement predicted by Weak Quantum Theory. Forsch. Komplementärmed. 10, 192–200.

Walach, H., 2004. Homeopathic proving symptoms: result of a local, non-local or placebo process? Homeopathy 93, 179–185.

Walach, H., Häusler, W., Lowes, T., et al., 1997. Classical homeopathic treatment of chronic headaches. Cephalalgia 17, 119–126.
Walach, H., Köster, H., Hennig, T., et al., 2001. The effects of homeopathic belladonna 30CH in healthy volunteers – a randomized, double-blind experiment. J. Psychosom. Res. 50, 155–160.
Walach, H., Möllinger, H., Sherr, J., et al., 2008. Homeopathic pathogenetic trials produce more specific than non-specific symptoms: results from two double-blind placebo controlled trials. J. Psychopharmacol. 22, 543–552.
Weatherley-Jones, E., Nicholl, J.P., Thomas, K.J., et al., 2004. A randomized, controlled, triple-blind trial of the efficacy of homeopathic treatment for chronic fatigue syndrome. J. Psychosom. Res. 56, 189–197.
White, A., Slade, P., Hunt, C., et al., 2003. Individualised homeopathy as an adjunct in the treatment of childhood asthma: a randomised placebo controlled trial. Thorax 58, 317–321.
Whitmarsh, T.E., Coleston-Shields, D.M., Steiner, T.J., 1997. Double-blind randomized placebo-controlled study of homoeopathic prophylaxis of migraine. Cephalalgia 17, 600–604.
Wiegant, F.A.C., Van Rijn, J., Van Wijk, R., 1997. Enhancement of the stress response by minute amounts of cadmium in sensitized Reuber H35 hepatoma cells. Toxicology 116, 27–37.
Wiegant, F.A.C., Souren, J.E.M., Van Wijk, R., 1999. Stimulation of survival capacity in heat-shocked cells by subsequent exposure to minute amounts of chemical stressors: Role of similarity in hsp-inducing effects. Hum. Exp. Toxicol. 18, 460–470.
Wiesenauer, M., Lüdtke, R., 1996. A meta-analysis of the homeopathic treatment of pollinosis with *Galphimia glauca*. Forsch. Komplementärmed. Klass. Naturheilkd. 3, 230–236.
Witt, C., Keil, T., Selim, D., et al., 2005a. Outcome and costs of homeopathic and conventional treatment strategies: a comparative cohort study in patients with chronic disorders. Complement. Ther. Med. 13, 79–86.
Witt, C.M., Lüdtke, R., Baur, R., et al., 2005b. Homeopathic medical practice: long-term results of a cohort study with 3981 patients. BMC Public Health 5, 115.
Witt, C., Bluth, M., Hinderlich, S., et al., 2006. Does potentized $HgCl_2$ (mercurius corrosivus) affect the activity of diastase and alpha-amylase? J. Altern. Complement. Med. 12, 359–365.
Witt, C.M., Bluth, M., Albrecht, H., et al., 2007. The in vitro evidence for an effect of high homeopathic potencies – a systematic review of the literature. Complement. Ther. Med. 15, 128–138.
Witt, C., Lüdtke, R., Mengler, N., et al., 2008. How healthy are chronically ill patients after eight years of homeopathic treatment? Results from a long term observational study. BMC Public Health 8, 413.
Witt, C.M., Lüdtke, R., Willich, S.N., 2009a. Homeopathic treatment of chronic headache (ICD-9: 784.0) – a prospective observational study with 2 year follow-up. Forsch. Komplementärmed. 16, 227–235.
Witt, C., Lüdtke, R., Willich, S.N., 2009b. Homeopathic treatment of patients with psoriasis – a prospective observational study with 2 years follow-up. J. Eur. Acad. Dermatol. Venereol. 23, 538–543.
Yakir, M., Kreitler, S., Brzezinski, A., et al., 2001. Effects of homeopathic treatment in women with premenstrual syndrome: a pilot study. British Homeopathic Journal 90, 148–153.
Zausner, C., Lassnig, H., Endler, P.C., et al., 2002. Die Wirkung von 'homöopathisch' zubereitetem Thyroxin auf die Metamorphose von Hochlandamphibien – Ergebnisse einer multizentrischen Kontrollstudie. Perfusion (Nürnberg) 15, 268–276.

Massage therapy research methods

Tiffany Field

10

CHAPTER CONTENTS

AN EVOLVING RESEARCH PROCESS

HISTORICAL BACKGROUND

Massage therapy dates to prerecorded time and was epitomized by Hippocrates in 400 BC as 'medicine being the art of rubbing'. Research in the field of massage therapy also goes back many years. The first academic journal publications date back to the 1930s when massage therapy research on humans and animals was fairly popular. Many of those research projects focused on documenting the increased blood flow associated with massage therapy as well as reducing muscle atrophy. Although many of the questions then are the same questions

DOI: 10.1016/B978-0-443-06956-7.00010-0

now, the approach to research was limited by the measurement technology and the studies often featured either single cases or very small sample sizes, which were typically self-selected samples of clinical patients being treated for one condition. Measurement technology, for example, was limited to physiological measures such as heart rate, blood pressure and temperature and was basically a biomechanical model. The advent of biochemical assay technology has enabled more expansive models. Even in the last few years the ability to assay neurohormonal activity in non-invasive procedures has advanced the field significantly in terms of looking at underlying mechanisms.

Other methodological problems were that the control groups were non-treatment groups that did not control for attention from the therapist. Even more recently, massage therapy has been compared to other treatments such as relaxation therapy. However, these group comparisons were confounded by compliance problems as relaxation therapy is often viewed as requiring work and concentration. Thus we have been using a light pressure massage as a sham massage therapy group to control for touch/attention effects inasmuch as recent studies have documented the need for moderate pressure to achieve positive massage therapy effects (Diego et al. 2004).

THE RESEARCH QUESTION

Typically the research question for massage therapy studies is whether massage therapy is an effective and cost-effective treatment for a given condition. Much of research is 'me-search', the questions often derived from the investigator's personal interest, such as somebody close having experienced that condition or because that is a condition seen in one's practice or research setting or because the condition is a recent funding priority and the research is intended to provide pilot data for seeking funding in that area. Determining how effective the massage therapy is means finding meaningful variables such as the gold standard variables for that particular condition, designing the most effective massage therapy technique for that condition and selecting the most appropriate treatment comparison group and attention control group. To address these questions typically leads first to a literature search.

LITERATURE SEARCH

PubMed (accessed through Google) is the biggest source of current literature abstracts. Although it is fascinating to read the older literature, which often serves as a source of good ideas for replication studies using more sophisticated approaches to problems, the typical published paper features references from the last decade. Thus, literature searches are typically confined to the last decade. In searching through the abstracts yielded by the computer literature search, researchers look to see if the question has already been addressed, if the condition has been treated by massage therapy and if the literature suggests the next steps. Entering a term for the condition along with massage therapy is likely to yield the most specific information needed. However, starting with a more global approach using simply the terms 'treatment' or 'therapy' and the name of the condition would yield significantly more abstracts and more general information about:

- the condition
- the hypothesized underlying aetiology
- the gold standard and other measures that have been used in research on other treatments of the condition
- ideas for treatment comparisons that might serve as an attention control group.

The literature search can serve as the background for the first part of the paper, the introduction. To be sure one knows the problem being addressed and the methods used to study that problem, it is always a good idea to write the first half of the paper before starting the study. The literature search will provide background on the incidence of the problem, the symptoms, possibly the aetiology or hypothesized aetiology, previous treatments both allopathic and alternative medicine and the efficacy of those treatments. Once the background and methods sections are drafted, the paper can serve as a proposal that can go to potential collaborators who will facilitate the research.

SELECTION OF COLLABORATORS

Selecting a clinic or a hospital setting or a school setting for non-clinical problems is always advantageous given their provision of participants for the research. Another advantage is that clinical settings are often the places where potential collaborators work, such as allopathic or alternative physicians in osteopathic medicine. Having a medical collaborator is important in terms of being able to keep abreast of the most important clinical measures for the condition being studied, having a referral source and someone who can administer the clinical measures and having clinically relevant research that is considered credible by potential journals for publication and by potential reviewers for grant funding. Important scientific collaborators include a neuroscientist for assays of biochemical measures or for interpretation of physiological, e.g. electroencephalogram (EEG), data and a statistician or PhD researcher to assist with designing and conducting the statistical analyses for the project. Massage therapy collaborators are also needed, particularly if the researcher is not a massage therapist, for the design of the massage therapy procedure to be used and to help identify measures that can directly assess the effects of that procedure. Another important collaboration consideration is locating a source of volunteer massage therapists for the actual treatments or for demonstration of the treatments if parents or significant others are going to be the therapists.

SELECTING TREATMENT AND ATTENTION CONTROL COMPARISON GROUPS

Traditionally, the alternative treatment group has been compared to a standard treatment control group, for comparison assessments made on the first and last days of treatment. However, a potential placebo effect or an effect of the therapist simply providing attention to the subject has highlighted the need for using treatment comparison and/or attention control groups. In much of our early work we used relaxation therapy as a comparison treatment group because relaxation therapy has been shown to be effective particularly in alleviating stress and anxiety, which often exacerbate the medical conditions we are studying. Also, we considered it important to establish a greater efficacy of massage therapy (versus relaxation therapy) in order to justify the greater expense of massage therapy treatment. The problem we found was that it may be a biased comparison inasmuch as people view relaxation therapy as hard work, requiring significant concentration and self-discipline. Thus, we may be experiencing compliance problems when we use relaxation therapy as a control. In addition, because relaxation therapy requires a certain amount of cognitive sophistication along with a reasonable attention span, it may be too difficult for young children. Therefore, we have used attention controls such as rocking the child, holding the child or playing with toys and holding and reading to the child as comparison groups in massage therapy research with children.

More recently, since we discovered the critical importance of stimulating pressure receptors for the massage to be effective, we have elected to use a sham massage therapy procedure comparison group which receives exactly the same massage as the treatment group, but with light pressure. This also enables the subjects to be 'naïve' or 'blind' to expecting a unique effect of their particular treatment condition. The subjects or participants in each group would expect to receive some benefit from massage whether it was deep pressure (in the case of the real treatment group) or light pressure, as applied in the sham group. Double blinding is also possible insofar as the physicians who are providing the standard treatment and the massage therapists providing the experimental treatment do not necessarily have expectations that one or the other massage style is going to be more effective. This is the closest we can come to a double-blinded situation in massage therapy research. This way neither the participant nor the therapists are biased towards the treatment.

SELECTION OF SAMPLE PARAMETERS AND RANDOM ASSIGNMENT TO GROUPS

Demographic variables including age, gender, ethnicity and socioeconomic status are considered the most basic sampling parameters that need to be equivalent across groups. Generally, by virtue of the location and demographics of the clinical setting, the age, ethnicity and socioeconomic status of the participants are somewhat homogeneous. The ethnicity is often predominantly one ethnic group or another and the socioeconomic status is limited in range. This helps prevent the research design from being confounded by variability as a function of varying ethnicity or socioeconomic status and the random assignment to groups would be expected to result in a roughly equivalent distribution in each group. Clinics are also generally separated by paediatrics, adulthood and sometimes even by ageing, by function of the condition and by the specialty of the physician, so they are also typically homogeneous on age and condition.

Another critical background variable, particularly in medical research, is the severity of the condition. This variable is more likely to result in a heterogeneous grouping and therefore would need careful matching or stratification. Typically, participants are randomly assigned to groups by a table of random numbers or by flipping a coin and it is intended that the randomization would yield roughly equivalent groups on background variables. The most conservative way to ensure equivalent groups is to match subjects across groups. For example, in studies on premature babies, the subjects are frequently matched on birthweight and gestational age and then randomly assigned to treatment and control groups. The less conservative way is a random stratification procedure whereby cells would be made so that if there were two birthweight groups (low birthweight and very low birthweight) and two gestational age groups (short gestation and very short gestation), there would be four cells (a very short gestation and very low birthweight group, a very short gestation and low birthweight group, a short gestation and very low birthweight group, and a short gestation and low birthweight group). Subjects would then be randomly assigned to these cells and there would be a roughly equal number of subjects assigned to each cell in each group by the end of the study.

The selection of the sample size involves several considerations, including economic considerations. The typical first step for determining sample size is to conduct a power analysis to determine whether there will be enough statistical power for the data analysis given the sample size. Power can be determined by taking the difference of the two group means from a previous study and dividing that by the larger of the two standard deviations for the same means.

Despite the sample size determined by the power analysis, economic considerations constrain the sample size to a minimum. One way to remain economical is by conducting data analyses at intervals of 10 subjects per group to determine whether groups are significantly different on the key variables. If there is simply a trend for statistical significance for those variables, then the absence of significance may mean that the sample is still too small and more subjects are needed. This can be done at intervals of two subjects per group.

SELECTION OF VARIABLES

The most important variable is the gold standard clinical variable that is typically viewed as a criterion for clinical improvement in any condition. For example, in diabetes the gold standard variable is typically the glucose level and in asthma it is typically the peak air flow measure. The clinical gold standard measure can be designated by a collaborating physician or can be found in the literature. Often there is more than one clinical gold standard measure. If there are multiple variables that would be considered redundant, some selection needs to be made. For statistical analysis reasons, researchers try to keep in mind a five-subjects-to-one-variable ratio, attempting not to be variable-heavy.

The second important set of variables are stress variables as they are thought to exacerbate any clinical condition. Because of the subjective nature of stress, it is good to have not only self-report stress variables such as the State Anxiety Index and the Profile of Mood State measures (to be elaborated later) but also a converging physiological measure, e.g. vagal tone or a chemical measure, e.g. salivary cortisol, to provide validation of the subject's self-report on stress.

Typically, treatment research involves assessing the immediate effects of the therapy session and the longer-term effects at the end of the treatment period. Occasionally effects are also assessed after some interval of time after the end of therapy as a follow-up assessment. The immediate effects of the session are often measured by self-reports of how the subject feels, the anxiety level and the mood state, and saliva samples are taken for assaying stress hormone (cortisol). Sometimes a heart rate or a blood pressure measure would also be taken as a physiological index of stress. In the clinical condition of itching, as in burning during healing, some kind of temperature gauge of the itchiness immediately following the treatment would be made. Similarly, if the pain condition of juvenile rheumatoid arthritis was the subject of study, the immediate effects might be the response to a dolorimeter, which is a pressure gauge that determines the threshold beyond which the subject could no longer tolerate the pressure of the rod-like dolorimeter. Longer-term measures are, of course, the gold standard or criteria for the success of the therapy. Typically the longer-term measures include a clinical index such as the number of back pain-free days or number of migraine-free days, the glucose levels or the pulmonary measures taken in children with asthma. Those might also include a change in the level of depression and a change in the level of urinary stress hormones (noradrenaline (norepinephrine), adrenaline (epinephrine)).

The importance of having converging variables from several levels (behavioural, physiological and biochemical) cannot be overstated. Almost invariably, self-report measures are taken on pencil and paper forms. Recently, manual physiological assessments have been popular, such as heart rate and blood pressure. More sophisticated measures, such as vagal tone, which needs to be derived from the respiratory sinus arrhythmia of heart rate, are more difficult to collect because of the sophisticated equipment required and the data reduction that not only requires technical expertise but is also considered labour-intensive. Serious consideration needs to be given to biochemical assays and the significance of those to the research because assaying salivary and urinary cortisol levels requires expensive assay kits or neuroscientists in an expensively equipped laboratory. For example, a salivary cortisol assay costs $25. If you consider that at least two (one pre- and one posttherapy session) would need to be taken at each of the two assessment periods (first day, last day), the salivary cortisol protocol for each subject would cost approximately $100.

Other measures include sleep/wake behaviour observations which are typically valuable as they indicate how sleep and wake behaviour can be significantly affected across treatment and as the clinical condition changes. Because sleep and wake behaviour are the best index of the subject's functioning, these are important measures. They do, however, require training of observers either to conduct live observations by using time sample unit coding systems or laptop computers or to code videotapes of the behaviour if it has been videotaped. This then requires assessing interobserver reliability or the process whereby observers come to agree on the behaviours that they are observing and to code them similarly. The standard for interobserver reliability is 90%; that is, that the two observers agree on 90% of the time sample intervals on the behaviours being observed. This requires significant amounts of practice time on the part of the observers and interobserver reliability assessment time. Interobserver reliability needs to be calculated using what is called a kappa coefficient, a statistical calculation that corrects for chance disagreement.

Other important variables have already been mentioned, including the gold standard clinical measure that is typically performed by the physician. Sometimes when children are involved, it is important to tap measures of parental stress and mood state to determine whether their stress may be affecting the child's clinical course and whether the child's clinical course is, in turn, affecting them.

PROCEDURES

The treatment and research procedures need considerable attention and careful thought prior to the beginning of the study. In a sense, it is good to have completed the first half of the paper (the introduction and the methods) before starting the study so that they can be critiqued by colleagues and collaborators and so that every person in the treatment and research process is 'on the same page'.

One of the most important aspects of the research procedure is that the observers be blind to the hypotheses of the study and to the subject's group assignment. Otherwise their treatment of the subject and their observations would be biased by knowing the intent of the study and the subject's group assignment. Having multiple assessors and multiple observers often prevents this biasing process but training each of the individuals and then working to achieve interobserver reliability is a costly process.

Similarly, the treatment procedure requires careful thought. On the one hand, the procedures need to be extremely detailed and in most cases need to cover many muscle groups and different parts of the body to be effective. However, there are also cost considerations, like the length of the session, both for the cost of the study but also for the cost of transporting the treatment once it is determined to be effective. Most individuals are unable to afford more than one half-hour session of a professional massage therapist per week and even if their significant other is trained in the procedure, that person is not likely to conduct massages more than a couple of times a week at 20–30 minutes per session. Thus, these are important time and cost-effectiveness considerations. Volunteer massage therapists can often be found for research studies given that they appreciate the research experience, particularly when that involves children, whom they are rarely able to see otherwise. The research can end up being fairly inexpensive in that way. But, at the termination of the study, the subjects are less likely to continue their treatment if the procedure that has proven effective is too costly. Thus, in our studies we try to limit the therapy sessions to once or twice a week at approximately 20 minutes a session and have a built-in period for training a significant other to conduct the massage following the end of the study and we provide that individual with a video demonstration of the therapy procedure. In the case of children, parents are often the therapists for the massage studies and this becomes part of their ritual (typically bedtime ritual) that helps not only the children but themselves as well. We have documented that the therapist benefits from providing the massage in the same way that the recipient benefits (Field et al. 1998a). Massage therapy by parents, of course, is a very cost-effective procedure and one that not only helps the child's clinical condition but also helps make the parent feel empowered as part of the treatment process and helps the relationship between parent and child.

In the next section, special considerations are reviewed for specific research protocols, including growth and development prenatally and in early infancy, attention deficit disorders, psychiatric conditions and addictions, pain syndromes, autoimmune conditions including asthma, diabetes and dermatitis, and immune conditions including human immunodeficiency virus (HIV) and breast cancer.

SPECIFIC CONSIDERATIONS FOR SPECIFIC CONDITIONS

GROWTH AND DEVELOPMENT

Prenatal development

Elevated prenatal cortisol has been associated with several negative conditions, including excessive fetal activity, delayed fetal growth and development, prematurity and low birthweight (Wadwha 2005; Field et al. 2009). These data highlight the importance of conducting stress and depression-reducing interventions during pregnancy. In recent studies we have documented that pregnancy massage conducted twice a week over the last trimester of pregnancy reduced perinatal complications, the most important one being a reduction in prematurity (Field et al. 1999). In addition, the mothers' leg and back pains were reduced and, in turn, they were able to sleep better. In a more recent study we looked at the effects of pregnancy massage specifically on depressed mothers with the expectation that massage would not only reduce depression and anxiety but would also improve the newborn outcome, including a reduction in neonatal stress hormones and complications such as prematurity and an increase in birthweight (Field et al. 2004). Over the course of that study, the massage groups again experienced fewer symptoms and less prematurity. This study had the additional cost-effective advantage of showing that significant others could serve as the massage therapists. We later replicated this study using the women's partners and found similar results (Field et al. 2008a).

Labour massage

We also conducted a labour massage study using the significant others as the massage therapists (Field et al. 1998c). In that study we were able to reduce labour pain simply by the significant other being taught the labour massage and giving the massage for the first 15 minutes of every hour of labour. The labours were shorter, the need for labour medication was less and the mothers were hospitalized for a shorter period of time and experienced less postpartum depression.

Preterm growth and development

Unfortunately for some infants, preterm deliveries are unavoidable and those infants are hospitalized in neonatal intensive care units (NICUs) for sometimes 2–5 months. Prematurity-related stress is accompanied by the iatrogenic stresses of the nursery, including loud sounds and bright lights. At some point when the newborn is no longer in medical jeopardy, the only reason for the infant remaining in the intensive care unit is to gain sufficient weight to be discharged. At this time we conduct massage. Typically we have conducted the massages for three 15-minute periods a day for a 10-day period, although, in one study, we were able to establish a 47% weight gain (same weight gain achieved in the 10-day study) in a 5-day period (Dieter et al. 2001). Therefore, we have converted to using the more cost-effective 5-day treatment period. We are also trying to teach the parents to continue the massage following discharge.

In our early studies, the most important measure was weight gain. We also learned a significant amount about the infant's state by recording 45-minute sleep/wake sessions. We were able to document that indeterminate sleep (a sleep state that is very difficult to code because it is disorganized and does not look like deep sleep or active sleep) was a very important variable. In fact, the only neonatal variable that was noted to relate to childhood IQ was the amount of indeterminate sleep (which was negatively related). The other critical measures were the number of days in the hospital and the cost associated with that. We were able to document that we could save $4.7 billion in hospital costs if we were to provide 10 days of massage to the approximately 470,000 infants born prematurely in the US each year (saving $10,000 in hospital costs per infant). NICU costs have increased significantly since that time period, so the cost savings would now be even greater. One of the other important variables was conducting the Brazelton newborn assessments with these infants. If we had not known how much more responsive the baby was to social stimulation following the massage therapy, we would never have been able to hypothesize why these infants go on to have a weight and developmental advantage at 8 months postdischarge. Knowing that their newborn behaviour was more responsive, we argued that their interactions with their parents were better and thus, the infants were able to 'pull' better stimulation from their parents and eventually show better growth and development (Field et al. 1987).

In a more recent study we added growth hormone (insulin-like growth factor-1 or IGF-1) and insulin measurements (Field et al. 2008b). These variables are considered important for growth. In an earlier study we speculated that the underlying mechanism for the weight gain in the preterm babies following massage was that their vagal activity (activity of the 10th cranial nerve, the vagus) was increased and thereby gastric motility was increased, leading to more efficient food absorption (Diego et al. 2005). More hormones were being released for more efficient food absorption, since that is the function of the vegetative branch of the vagus nerve. Vagal activity was measured and shown to increase and plasma samples of insulin and IGF-1 increased (one of the more active growth hormones) (Field et al. 2008b). Having the additional measure of IGF-1 and insulin enabled us to determine further the underlying mechanism. Knowing underlying mechanisms is the most effective way to ensure that the massage gets put into practice in NICUs.

Attention and attention disorders

Two of the most reliable indicators of attention are vagal activity and EEG patterns. The stimulation of the 10th cranial nerve, the vagus, is critical for attention. Attention is accompanied by slower heart rate and increased vagal activity.

Vagal activity is the heart rate that accompanies sinus arrhythmia, so it can be easily transferred from heart rate recordings by a computer program. The very expensive $6000 vagal tone monitor is not necessary, although it more readily yields vagal activity than using the computer package. EEG also requires sophisticated equipment and technical expertise for reducing the data. EEG patterns that accompany attentiveness include decreased alpha, decreased beta and increased theta. In one study we have documented this pattern of heightened alertness/attentiveness following 15-minute chair massages in the subjects' offices (Field et al. 1997a). The heightened alertness/attentiveness EEG pattern was accompanied by improved performance on math computation tasks, including being able to perform them in less time with greater accuracy following the massage sessions. We have also documented enhanced performance by infants on habituation tasks (primitive learning tasks involving learning that a repeated stimulus like the sound of a bell, used in the Brazelton scale, becomes irrelevant because it does not signal anything else happening and is therefore no longer responded to) (Cigales et al. 1997). Finally, in a study on preschoolers we were able to show that following a brief massage the children were able to perform IQ tasks in less time and more accurately (Hart et al. 1998).

Children with attentional disorders

We have shown that children with autism (Field et al. 1997b; Escalona et al. 2001) and children with attention deficit hyperactivity disorder (ADHD) (Field et al. 1998b; Khilnani et al. 2004) are also able to perform better and stay on task for longer periods of time following massage therapy sessions. In the study on children with autism, we recorded their classroom behaviour, including how much time they were on task, how little attention they paid to irrelevant stimuli, how much stereotypic behaviour they showed and how much social relatedness was observed toward the teacher (Field et al. 1997b). Following massage therapy (two sessions per week by a massage therapist) these children were able to stay on task longer and relate more to their teachers. In a subsequent study we used parents as the therapists and we were able to show that the children not only spent more time being attentive and on task in the classroom but they also showed fewer sleep problems (Escalona et al. 2001). Since sleep problems are prevalent in children with autism, the sleep diaries recording the onset of sleep, duration of sleep and number of sleep wakings were a critical measure and one that surprisingly improved over this brief period of time.

Because parents of children with autism may be biased toward seeing any signs of improvement, it is particularly important to have converging measures. Since sleep behaviour is likely to affect classroom behaviour, classroom behaviour is worth observing. In addition, in some studies we have used time lapse video equipment to record nighttime sleep by simply turning on a nightlight and running the time lapse video camera. Subsequently, 8 hours of sleep can be coded in 1 hour. The movements on the tape look like Charlie Chaplin moving about, so they are very easy to record if you are interested in a gross rating of activity. Gross activity can differentiate deep sleep from active sleep and, of course, night wakings and moving out of the bed are easy to code from videotapes.

A measure somewhere between the use of videotaping, which can be somewhat intrusive and requires compliance of the subject, and the more subjective sleep diaries is a device called an actometer. The actometer is a Timex watch with the spring removed such that every time the subject moves his or her arm, the time hand on the watch moves so that the time elapsed from nighttime to daytime is a total amount of activity that has occurred during nighttime sleep. These are easy to use with all age groups.

Similar measures were used with ADHD children (Field et al. 1998b) and, in a subsequent study, with adolescents with ADHD (Khiilnani et al. 2004). Here again the most meaningful measures are those taken in the classroom where the children express and perhaps experience their worst problems. In these studies, we also used teacher and parent rating scales (the Conners Scale because it is shorter than the Child Behavior Checklist, which is another measure of the same type that is frequently used by parents and teachers).

PSYCHIATRIC CONDITIONS

Most psychiatric conditions are accompanied by depression or at least depressed mood state and anxiety. Thus, in all psychiatric conditions we have studied, we have used the following self-report scales:

- the Profile of Mood States (McNair et al. 1971) which taps depressed mood state, anxiety, anger and confusion.
- the Center for Epidemiological Studies Depression (CESD) scale (Radloff 1977) or the Beck Depression Inventory (Beck et al. 1961), both of which measure depressive symptoms. We have found that the CESD is more sensitive (detects more individuals with depressive symptoms) and is also more user-friendly or simpler, such that adolescents and less educated people are more able to complete this instrument.
- the State Trait Anxiety Inventory (Spielberger et al. 1970) (which also has a children's version called the STAIC) assesses state anxiety (current, short-term anxiety) and trait anxiety (closer to being a personality trait). The authors of these scales have now created two new instruments that measure depression and anger. These 20-item Likert-type scales are extremely easy to complete and have good psychometric properties, including good test–retest reliability.

In psychiatric conditions we also try to have a converging measure of behaviour, including the symptoms that are reported in the self-report scales such as depressed affect, behavioural agitation and angry behaviour. For behavioural observations we designed the Behavior Observation Scale. These behaviours, along with others, are rated on a five-point scale following a brief observation. Typically, like the mood scales which are completed by the subject before and after the therapy session, the behavioural observations are also made before the massage therapy session and after.

The third set of measures we have invariably collected in psychiatric conditions are saliva (for an assay of the stress hormone cortisol before and after the first and last massage therapy session) and urine (for assays of the stress neurotransmitters noradrenaline and adrenaline and the body's natural antidepressants, dopamine and serotonin). The salivary measure of cortisol is taken as an immediate index of the reduction of stress during the therapy session and the urinary assays are made to assess the longer-term effects of massage therapy over the course of the study.

We have recorded the above self-help, behavioural observation and biochemical samples in all of our studies on depressed children and adolescents (Field et al. 1991) and depressed mothers (Jones & Field 1999), as well as the studies we have conducted on anorexia (Hart et al. 2001) and bulimia (Field et al. 1998d) to assess the longer-term effects of the massage therapy treatment. While depression, eating disorders and addictions are considered to have an underlying depression base, which suggests the use of depression measures across studies, there are also, of course, measures that are unique to each of the conditions. Measures that were unique to the different studies include the following:

- Having time lapse videotaped sleep during the child and adolescent psychiatry study as well as a set of nurses' ratings of the children's and adolescents' behaviour on the psychiatric unit (Field et al. 1992).
- Additional measures for the eating disorder study included the Eating Disorders Inventory (Garner et al. 1983; Field et al. 1998d).
- For a smoking addiction study, the number of cravings and cigarettes smoked were recorded (Hernandez-Reif et al. 1999).
- For the depressed adult studies we have also recorded EEG. Depressed individuals typically have relative right frontal EEG during the expression or reception of emotional expressions. The right frontal area of the brain is an area for processing negative emotions. Activation of this area has been noted to shift to symmetry following massage therapy (Jones & Field 1999). Thus, in the depression studies we have employed the use of EEG (see Appendix D for an elaboration of these methods).
- For the posttraumatic stress disorder group of children (following Hurricane Andrew), we also employed the children's self-drawings using magic markers as an index of the children's change in depression (Field et al. 1996). The drawings are simply scored on seven points, including: (1) small self-figure on page; (2) use of dark colours; (3) missing facial features; (4) sad face; (5) distorted figure; (6) displaced body parts; and (7) agitated lines. Typically, depressed children have made drawings that feature very few facial features, distorted body parts and a small figure on the page. Self-drawings are a very reliable index of the children's mood state.

PAIN SYNDROMES

For pain alleviation, we have studied a number of pain syndromes, including migraine headaches, lower-back pain, premenstrual syndrome, pain from burns, fibromyalgia and juvenile rheumatoid arthritis. In these conditions we have used very similar self-report scales on pain, including the McGill Pain Questionnaire, the Pain Intensity Scale and a visual analogue scale which is generally in the form of a ruler with ratings along its scale or a thermometer with similar ratings or a series of sad to happy faces in the case of children's ratings of pain. In the case of adults these self-report scales are completed by the adults alone and, in the case of children, we often have parents rating the amount of pain existing as well as the physician making a rating. For each of the syndromes we have also used measures unique to that syndrome for assessing functioning of the individual. So, for example, for the burn subjects who we hoped would have higher pain thresholds following the massage therapy sessions, we assessed their affective reaction to debridement (skin brushing). For juvenile rheumatoid arthritis, we had a parent's assessment of the child's ability to continue activities of daily living (Field et al. 1997c). For lower-back pain we had functional assessments of range of motion and the ability to touch toes (Hernandez-Reif et al. 2001). For fibromyalgia we used a dolorimeter (a rod that exerts pressure until the patient winces, which represents the pain threshold) (Sunshine et al. 1996) and, for migraine headaches, we had a measure of headache-free days (Hernandez-Reif et al. 1998).

Because anxiety exacerbates pain syndromes, we also used anxiety scales (State Trait Anxiety Inventory) to assess the pre–post massage therapy session anxiety levels. In addition, we used salivary cortisol as the secondary index of anxiety/stress levels before and after massage therapy sessions. In addition, because sleep is considered disturbed in most pain syndromes, either because of the pain or because the sleep syndrome is contributing to the pain (the direction of effects is not certain here), we have used sleep recordings (typically sleep diaries). More recently, because we have come to notice that in all of the pain syndrome studies sleep improved following massage therapy and pain in turn was reduced, we are now trying to get better measures of sleep, including actometer readings during sleep. One current theory about the origins of pain syndromes is that there is insufficient quiet or restorative sleep and when that happens, there are increased levels of substance P which causes pain. Because substance P can be measured in salivary samples, we are assaying substance P at the beginning and end of the massage therapy treatment periods.

AUTOIMMUNE DISORDERS

Once again, because stress and particularly stress hormones such as cortisol are known to interact and affect autoimmune and immune conditions, we measure cortisol in saliva before and after the massage therapy sessions and in urine at the beginning and end of the study period. In all of the autoimmune diseases we have studied to date (asthma, diabetes and dermatitis) we have studied children and used the parents as the massage therapists. We know that the parents are also likely to benefit from the therapy because grandparent volunteer massage therapists who massaged infants became less depressed and had lower cortisol levels (Field et al. 1998a).

For asthma, the gold standard clinical measure is the peak air flow monitor value recorded by the child and parent (Field et al. 1998e). Typically these are done on a daily basis and a diary-like recording is made. The pulmonologist also has standard pulmonary measures that are recorded at the beginning and the end of the study.

In the case of diabetes, a self-report measure was completed by the parents, in this case on the child's glucose regulation, insulin and food regulation and exercise (Field et al. 1997d). In addition, glucose levels were measured by the children and their parents using a calibrated glucometer which we provided. Here it was important for the readings to be taken at the same time of day by the parents.

IMMUNE DISORDERS

One of the immune measures that seems to be invariably improved following massage therapy across all of our immune studies, including HIV in adults (Ironson et al. 1996), HIV in adolescents (Diego et al. 2001) and breast cancer (Hernandez-Reif et al. 2004, 2005), is the increased production of natural killer cells. Natural killer cells are considered the front line of the immune system and they ward off viral and cancer cells. In more immune-compromised conditions such as the study on HIV men, the CD4 cell number was so low that it was not possible to reverse those numbers, whereas in the less immune-compromised adolescent HIV study, we were able not only to increase natural killer cells but also reverse the CD4 cell number and improve the CD4:CD8 ratio (the HIV disease marker).

STATISTICAL ANALYSES

The statistical analyses should be left to a statistician or a PhD trained researcher on the project. While the actual use of the statistical analysis software is like following a recipe, it is important to know the appropriate statistics to use and how to interpret the results. A brief description of the basics will be given here.

In any group treatment comparison research, the scores or values of the variables are averaged across the group to obtain a mean score/rating/value. The distribution of the individuals around the mean performance is called variability and a typical distribution would have a mean in the middle of a line with most of the individuals falling in a hill around the mean but as individuals depart from the group value, they become farther out on 'downward slopes of the hill' either to the left or to the right of the peak of the hill. To give an example, the mean IQ score for the population at large is 100. However, there are many individuals who perform higher and many who perform lower. One standard deviation from the mean would be 16 points higher, or a score of 116, or 16 points lower, or a score of 84. Two standard deviations would be twice 16 or 132 or 100 minus 32, and very few people would be out beyond the two standard deviations. The standard deviation is the term for variability.

A simple statistical comparison between groups can be made by a *t*-test where the group means and the group standard deviations are taken into consideration to arrive at a *t*-value which is then indicated as being significant if this value could only happen five times out of 100 times or significantly more often than chance (which would be five in 100 times) (at the $P \geq 0.05$ level). Typically *t*-values greater than 2.00 are significant. After performing a *t*-test by hand on the calculator or computer, the *t*-values can be looked for in a table of *t*-values and the *P*-value or significance level also checked. The significance level only indicates whether the test result was statistically significant, suggesting that the groups were significantly different on that value.

Another group comparison test is called the *F*-test, which is basically the same as a *t*-test but is performed when there are more than two groups being compared. The test for yielding an *F*-value is called the analysis of variance (ANOVA). Once again, an *F*-test would be checked in a statistics table to determine the *P*-level (significance level). Typically *F*-values greater than

4.00 are significant. More complex ANOVAs can be performed when there are more than two groups and more than three variables. These are called MANOVAs, which is an abbreviation for multivariate analyses of variance. Whenever there are multiple variables and multiple groups, a MANOVA is performed on the group of variables followed by post hoc ANOVAs on each of the variables. The MANOVA indicates whether the groups are significantly different on the group of variables as a whole. Subsequently, the ANOVAs are conducted to determine whether the groups are different on each of the individual variables. If there is more than one independent measure describing the group, for example age and gender, and the MANOVAs and ANOVAs yield significant differences, it is then necessary to conduct post hoc *t*-tests to test all the possible comparisons.

Another way of looking at the data is to determine the relationships between the variables. For example, does gender relate to anxiety scores such that higher anxiety scores are noted for males versus females? The entire group of variables can be entered into a correlation analysis and the relationships between variables can be determined. The computer program prints out a matrix of correlation coefficients that range from 0 to 0.99. If gender and anxiety are correlated 0.83, this is an extremely high correlation or a strong relationship. If anxiety levels run from low to high with higher values reflecting higher anxiety and males are classified as a 1 and females as a 2, then the relationship between gender and anxiety would be a negative 0.83 (−0.83) relationship, with males having higher anxiety. If females had higher anxiety, the correlation coefficient would be a positive 0.83. Again, the table of numbers is checked for the *P*-level (if the computer output does not provide that).

Further analyses can be conducted, for example stepwise regression analyses. In this analysis it is possible to determine the relative importance of the predictor variables or the independent variables. Again, if we are discussing gender and anxiety we would enter into the stepwise regression analysis the anxiety score as the dependent measure (or the outcome measure) and gender along with age would be entered as the predictor variables. If gender has a high correlation (0.83), as was already noted, the computer program will enter gender as a predictor variable into the equation. This would be interpreted as explaining 64% of the outcome variance or variability. If you multiply 0.83 (which is the *R* or the correlation coefficient by itself to get the *R* square or variance), this would tell you how much the variable gender is contributing to the outcome variable anxiety (64%). If then age came into the equation at the second step and the correlation coefficient was 0.91 with an *R* square of 0.81 or 81%, that would have added 17% to the variance (64% plus 17% equalling 81%).

These, then, are some of the simplest analyses performed in treatment research. Many things are considered in selecting the types of data analysis, including whether the data are normally distributed or skewed, for example. It may be necessary to use non-parametric statistics (instead of the parametric statistics just described) because the database fails to meet the required assumptions to perform the parametric analyses. These considerations are complex and understanding them as well as using them appropriately requires considerable coursework in statistics.

ACKNOWLEDGEMENTS

We would like to thank the subjects who participated in our research and the researchers who collected and analyzed data. This research was supported by a National Institute of Mental Health (NIMH) Senior Research Scientist Award (MH#00331) and a National Center for Complementary and Alternative Medicine Senior Research Scientist Award (AT#001585) and by a merit award from NIMH to Tiffany Field (MH#46586) and by funding from Johnson & Johnson Pediatric Institute.

REFERENCES

Beck, A., Ward, C., Mendelson, M., et al., 1961. An inventory for measuring depression. Arch. Gen. Psychiatry 4, 561–571.

Cigales, M., Field, T., Lundy, B., et al., 1997. Massage enhances recovery from habituation in normal infants. Infant Behav. Dev. 20, 29–34.

Diego, M.A., Hernandez-Reif, M., Field, T., 2001. Massage therapy effects on immune function in adolescents with HIV. Int. J. Neurosci. 106, 35–45.

Diego, M.A., Field, T., Sanders, C., et al., 2004. Massage therapy of moderate and light pressure and vibrator effects on EEG and heart rate. Int. J. Neurosci. 114, 31–35.

Diego, M.A., Field, T., Hernandez-Reif, M., 2005. Vagal activity, gastric motility, and weight gain in massaged preterm neonates. J. Pediatr. 147, 50–55.

Dieter, J., Field, T., Hernandez-Reif, M., et al., 2001. Maternal depression and increased fetal activity. J. Obstet. Gynaecol. 21, 468–473.

Escalona, A., Field, T., Singer-Strunk, R., et al., 2001. Brief report: Improvements in the behavior of children with autism following massage therapy. J. Autism Dev. Disord. 31, 513–516.

Field, T., Scafidi, F., Schanberg, S., 1987. Massage of preterm newborns to improve growth and development. Pediatr. Nurs. 13 (6), 385–387.

Field, T., Morrow, C., Valdeon, C., et al., 1992. Massage reduces anxiety in child and adolescent psychiatric patients. J. Am. Acad. Child Adolesc. Psychiatry 31, 125–131.

Field, T., Seligman, S., Scafidi, F., et al., 1996. Alleviating posttraumatic stress in children following Hurricane Andrew. J. Appl. Dev. Psychol. 17, 37–50.

Field, T., Quintino, O., Henteleff, T., et al., 1997a. Job stress reduction therapies. Altern. Ther. 3, 54–56.

Field, T., Lasko, D., Mundy, P., et al., 1997b. Brief report: autistic children's attentiveness and responsivity improved after touch therapy. J. Autism Dev. Disord. 27 (3), 333–338.

Field, T., Hernandez-Reif, M., Seligman, S., et al., 1997c. Juvenile rheumatoid arthritis: Benefits from massage therapy. J. Pediatr. Psychol. 22, 607–617.

Field, T., Hernandez-Reif, M., Lacoreca, A., et al., 1997d. Massage therapy lowers blood glucose levels in children with diabetes mellitus. Diabetes Spectrum 10, 237–239.

Field, T., Hernandez-Reif, M., Quintino, O., et al., 1998a. Elder retired volunteers benefit from giving massage therapy to infants. J. Appl. Gerontol. 17, 229–239.

Field, T., Quintino, O., Hernandez-Reif, M., et al., 1998b. Adolescents with attention deficit hyperactivity disorder benefit from massage therapy. Adolescence 33, 103–108.

Field, T., Hernandez-Reif, M., Taylor, S., et al., 1998c. Labor pain is reduced by massage therapy. J. Psychosom. Obstet. Gynecol. 18, 286–291.

Field, T., Schanberg, S., Kuhn, C., et al., 1998d. Bulimic adolescents benefit from massage therapy. Adolescence 33, 555–563.

Field, T., Henteleff, T., Hernandez-Reif, M., et al., 1998e. Children with asthma have improved pulmonary function after massage therapy. Journal of Pediatrics 132, 854–858.

Field, T., Hernandez-Reif, M., Hart, S., et al., 1999. Pregnant women benefit from massage therapy. J. Psychosom. Obstet. Gynecol. 20, 31–38.

Field, T., Diego, M.A., Hernandez-Reif, M., Schanberg, S., Kuhn, C., 2004. Massage therapy effects on depressed pregnant women. J. Psychosom. Obstet. Gynecol. 25, 115–122.

Field, T., Figueiredo, B., Hernandez-Reif, M., et al., 2008a. Massage therapy reduces pain in pregnant women, alleviates prenatal depression in both parents and improves their relationships. J Bodyw Mov Ther 12, 146–150.

Field, T., Diego, M., Hernandez-Reif, M., et al., 2008b. Insulin and Insulin-Like Growth Factor I (IGF-1) Increase in Preterm Infants Following Massage Therapy. J. Dev. Behav. Pediatr. 29, 463–466.

Field, T., Diego, M., Hernandez-Reif, M., et al., 2009. Pregnancy massage Reduces Prematurity, Low Birthweight and Postpartum Depression. Infant Behav. Dev. 32, 454–460.

Garner, D.M., Olmstead, M.P., Polivy, J., 1983. The Eating Disorders Inventory: a measure of cognitive behavioral dimensions of anorexia nervosa and bulimia. In: Darby, P.L., Garfinkel, P.R., Garner, D.M., et al. (Eds.), Anorexia nervosa: recent developments in research. Alan R Liss, New York, pp. 173–184.

Hart, S., Field, T., Hernandez-Reif, M., et al., 1998. Preschoolers' cognitive performance improves following massage. Early Child Dev Care 143, 59–64.

Hart, S., Field, T., Hernandez-Reif, M., et al., 2001. Anorexia nervosa symptoms are reduced by massage therapy. Eat. Disord. 9, 289–299.

Hernandez-Reif, M., Dieter, J., Field, T., et al., 1998. Migraine headaches are reduced by massage therapy. Int. J. Neurosci. 96, 1–11.

Hernandez-Reif, M., Field, T., Hart, S., 1999. Smoking cravings are reduced by self-massage. Prev. Med. 28, 28–32.

Hernandez-Reif, M., Ironson, G., Field, T., et al., 2005. Immunological responses of breast cancer patients to massage therapy. Int. J. Neurosci. 115, 495–510.

Hernandez-Reif, M., Field, T., Krasnegor, J., et al., 2001. Lower back pain is reduced and range of motion increased after massage therapy. Int. J. Neurosci. 106, 131–145.

Hernandez-Reif, M., Ironson, G., Field, T., et al., 2004. Breast cancer patients have improved immune and neuroendocrine functions following massage therapy. J. Psychosom. Res. 1, 1–8.

Ironson, G., Field, T., Scafidi, F., et al., 1996. Massage therapy is associated with enhancement of the immune system's cytotoxic capacity. Int. J. Neurosci. 84, 205–218.

Jones, N.A., Field, T., 1999. Massage and music therapies attenuate frontal EEG asymmetry in depressed adolescents. Adolescence 34, 529–534.

Khilnani, S., Field, T., Hernandez-Reif, M., et al., 2004. Massage therapy improves mood and behavior of students with attention deficit/hyperactivity disorder. Adolescence 152, 623–638.

McNair, D.M., Lorr, M., Droppleman, L.F., 1971. POMS – profile of mood states. Educational and Industrial Testing Services, San Diego, CA.

Radloff, L., 1977. The CES-D Scale: a self-report depression scale for research in the general population. Applied Psychological Measures 1, 385–401.

Spielberger, C.D., Gorusch, T.C., Lushene, R.E., 1970. The State Trait Anxiety Inventory. Consulting Psychologists Press, Palo Alto, CA.

Sunshine, W., Field, T., Schanberg, S., et al., 1996. Massage therapy and transcutaneous electrical stimulation effects on fibromyalgia. J. Clin. Rheumatol. 2, 18–22.

Wadwha, P.D., 2005. Psychoneuroendocrine processes in human pregnancy influence fetal development and health. Psychoneuroendocrinology 30 (8), 724–743.

Acupuncture

Adrian White • Claudia M. Witt

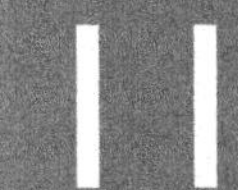

CHAPTER CONTENTS

This chapter should not be read in isolation, but in the context of both Chapter 1, which discusses the place for, interpretation of, and problems in complementary and alternative medicine (CAM) research, and Chapter 5, which discusses the fundamental principles of research, particularly the randomized controlled trial (RCT). Both these chapters illustrate several points with examples from acupuncture research, which will not be repeated here. This chapter will discuss the particular applications of these general principles to acupuncture research.

INTRODUCTION

At the time of writing, the recent history of acupuncture research has been dominated by the Modellvorhaben Akupunktur, a programme of trials funded by German health insurance companies using various designs to investigate

DOI: 10.1016/B978-0-443-06956-7.00011-2

the effectiveness, efficacy, safety and cost-effectiveness of acupuncture treatment for common conditions (headache, migraine, neck pain, back pain, osteoarthritis of hip and knee, allergic rhinitis and dysmenorrhoea) (Linde et al. 2006; Witt et al. 2006a). Anyone planning an RCT of acupuncture would be well advised to study the published protocols and reports of these research projects in detail, as they were exemplary in many ways.

The results of the programme with regard to the effectiveness of acupuncture can be briefly summarized as follows: for musculoskeletal conditions, acupuncture was much more effective than usual care, or standardized care; so was sham acupuncture (shallow needling of wrong points, sometimes called 'placebo', as discussed below); there was a small trend for acupuncture to be superior to sham acupuncture, but the difference was significant in only one study (Witt et al. 2005). Similarly for tension headache, acupuncture was better than waiting list (Melchart et al. 2005) and not superior to sham (Endres et al. 2007). In the case of migraine, acupuncture's effect was no different from the effect of standard prophylactic medication (beta-blockers, flunarizine or valproic acid) (Diener et al. 2006).

The programme was designed specifically to provide evidence for the decision on whether to reimburse treatment with acupuncture, and on the basis of the results it was decided to refund acupuncture treatment for:

- knee pain, where acupuncture was clearly effective and in one of two trials superior to sham acupuncture
- back pain, where acupuncture was clearly more effective than existing guideline-based care, though not superior to sham acupuncture

However, only doctors who have advanced diplomas in psychological medicine and in pain qualify for reimbursement.

The results of these trials have not been as conclusive as acupuncturists had hoped – particularly the lack of clear, consistent superiority of acupuncture over placebo. Various aspects of the studies have generated debate, such as what is 'adequate' acupuncture, how important is choice of point location and what is a satisfactory 'placebo' for acupuncture. For some commentators, acupuncture remains 'on trial' but others dismiss it as no more than a placebo. The history of acupuncture research is full of studies with negative results which could, in retrospect, have been anticipated from features of the design – such as inappropriate conditions or patients, suboptimal treatment regimes, poorly chosen control groups or insensitive measures. In order to end up with a representative and truthful evaluation of acupuncture, study design is crucial: studies must have the best chance of showing an effect as well as high methodological quality. This chapter will discuss important aspects of study design.

APPROACH

Acupuncture treatment can be seen as having two components, each of them complex: (1) the insertion and stimulation of the needle – which is largely mechanical and reproducible; and (2) the other aspects of the therapeutic interaction, such as the belief and expectations of the practitioner and the patient, the demeanour of the practitioner, the formulation of a diagnosis – which are essentially subjective and difficult to reproduce and measure. This chapter mainly deals with the mechanical aspects of needling, not because this is necessarily more important but because it is what acupuncturists spend much time and effort in learning. The process of needling is also what is understood by the world at large as the principle component of acupuncture. And it seems important to demonstrate somehow that the correct form of acupuncture needling is superior to placebo (even though, in practice, the effect of acupuncture is considerably enhanced by the other aspects of treatment), since health regulators have come to regard this as essential precondition for integration and reimbursement.

This chapter assumes that needles act principally by stimulating the nervous system. It will adopt the PICO (participants, intervention, control, outcomes) sequence, then will offer some comments on study design and economic evaluation.

PARTICIPANTS

It is still not known why some patients respond better than others (i.e. what are the predictor variables of an acupuncture response), apart from the general statement that less severe cases are more likely to respond than severe ones. It would be an ideal arrangement if controlled trials of acupuncture could include only known responders, as happens in many studies of non-steroidal anti-inflammatories: patients are recruited only if they are already taking the drug, and they are asked to stop (Bjordal et al. 2004). Then they are randomized only if they show a significant worsening of symptoms, i.e. they are responders. However, with acupuncture, patients who have received treatment are likely to identify if they are subsequently given placebo/sham acupuncture. In addition, selecting only the responders would decrease the external validity of the results.

It is also important to choose participants with a clinical condition that is known to respond. Acupuncture has gained a reputation as a panacea for all kinds of condition, but it is still most commonly used for musculoskeletal conditions, and this is where it seems to hold most promise according to systematic reviews. The effects of acupuncture on other forms of chronic pain, such as cancer pain or fibromyalgia, are less clear. The balance of evidence shows an effect in nausea and vomiting, though some well-run studies have also had negative results, and other promising areas include postoperative pain and allergic rhinitis.

It is probably most difficult to measure an effect of acupuncture when this is likely to be rather small in relation to the 'placebo response' of patients. Some conditions, such as menopausal hot flushes and irritable bowel syndrome, are known to have relatively large psychological responses to any treatment, so studies in these conditions are likely to have to use large sample sizes.

THE ACUPUNCTURE INTERVENTION

Acupuncture can be standardized (formula acupuncture); semi-standardized, for example allowing variation in prespecified ways in response to certain symptoms; or individualized, given as in daily practice. There is no evidence published so far that one type of acupuncture is more effective than any other, though individualized acupuncture is certainly more satisfying for the practitioner.

ADEQUATE ACUPUNCTURE

This section reproduces in part an article on dose of acupuncture to which many authors contributed in a consensus process (White et al. 2008).

Acupuncture's development over 2000 years has taken place in different centres in China, Japan, Korea and other parts of the world, and understandably many different styles of practice now exist. Currently, there is considerable disagreement among acupuncturists, particularly those trained in different schools, about what constitutes the best treatment for different conditions and for different patients. A treatment protocol (i.e. a precise description of the procedures and the schedule for a course of treatment) that is one practitioner's favourite may be dismissed by another.

It is inconceivable that any pharmaceutical company would spend resources on clinical trials of a new drug until they know the characteristics of the dosage and the patients likely to respond. Yet, because acupuncture research has, for the most part, skipped some of the necessary earlier phases of research in which the dose–response relationship is carefully examined (Campbell et al. 2000), there is a dearth of data upon which to base decisions about optimal acupuncture protocols.

A definition of the 'dose' of acupuncture has been suggested (Box 11.1). Clearly, the effect of needling will vary at different sites in the body, but for simplicity we shall not consider the location of needling in these general comments. The dose required to treat different health conditions will vary depending on the intended mechanism of the effect, e.g. whether local, segmental, extrasegmental or central. Some conditions, e.g. migraine or fibromyalgia, probably require several mechanisms to be activated if treatment is to be effective (Filshie & White 1998). And some conditions, again including fibromyalgia, may require wide variations in dose according to the degree to which the nervous system is sensitized in a particular patient (Lundeberg & Lund 2007).

Please note that the patient's response is also part of the dose. This looks odd at first, because a response is usually what is elicited by the dose. However, the dose of acupuncture consists of more than just the mechanical stimulation: patients come to acupuncture with beliefs and expectations already formed, and these may subsequently be altered by the experience of the treatment. These cognitive factors are known to influence the effects of acupuncture, so they should be regarded as part of the total dose, and measured if we are to know fully what treatment the patient has received. Unfortunately, measurement of these factors is not easy or reliable.

The components that make up the purely mechanical aspects of acupuncture are set out in the Standards for Reporting Interventions in Controlled Trials of Acupuncture (STRICTA) guidelines (MacPherson et al. 2002), which are discussed below.

BOX 11.1 Dose of acupuncture needling

The physical procedures applied in each session, using one or more needles, and the patient's resulting perception, sensory as well as affective and cognitive

Different doses will be required for different conditions and for different states of the nervous system

DECIDING ON AN ADEQUATE DOSE OF ACUPUNCTURE

There are several approaches for deciding what is 'adequate' for any condition, and the original references should be consulted for full descriptions:

1. Clinical opinion. What clinicians think is the best treatment can be determined in several ways. Firstly, by observing different practitioners (Napadow et al. 2004). Secondly, by establishing some kind of clinical consensus, either using methods such as the Delphi method (Webster-Harrison et al. 2002), consensus surveys or conference-type processes (Foster et al. 1999; Witt et al. 2005; Molsberger et al. 2006a, b; MacPherson & Schroer 2007) or by using a stepwise procedure to develop protocols in a 'treatment manualization' process (Schnyer & Allen 2002). Thirdly, by examining the traditional acupuncture texts (Birch 1997), though the value of this approach may be limited by difficulties of translation.
2. Clinical trials. The most reliable method of determining an adequate acupuncture protocol would be by directly comparing different protocols in patients in a tightly controlled, explanatory trial, ideally in conditions in which one form of acupuncture has already been shown to be effective. The protocols would need to be established first, using various combinations of clinical consensus and basic research. The choice of protocol for testing would vary between different 'schools'. One group of researchers used this approach for fibromyalgia, and found that relief of symptoms depended neither on the point location nor the manner of stimulation of the needles – though it did depend on how frequently the treatment was given (Harris et al. 2005). Studies in other conditions may have very different results. The major problem with direct comparisons is that studies need to be large to demonstrate the small differences that are likely to exist between protocols.
3. Basic research. Laboratory studies have mostly explored the effect of different treatment parameters on an outcome such as pain threshold in healthy human volunteers (Marcus 1994; Barlas et al. 2000; Zaslawski et al. 2003). Results suggest that stimulation intensity is the single most important determinant of analgesia, and that there is interindividual variation as to how people respond to this type of stimulation. However, it may not be appropriate to apply the findings of experiments in healthy volunteers to patients with clinical conditions since our knowledge of the mechanisms of symptoms such as chronic pain, joint stiffness, depression, hot flushes and so on is incomplete.
4. Reviews. Systematic reviews of RCTs offer the opportunity to compare the effects of different treatment regimens. In one well-known example, Ezzo and colleagues (2000) demonstrated that trials using six or more sessions of acupuncture for osteoarthritis of the knee were more likely to be positive than those using fewer than six.
5. Individual patient data. The different treatment effects in individual patients could be revealed by the use of individual patient data, as in the Acupuncture Trialists' Collaboration. Individual patient data from many trials will be combined into a single database and analysed to determine whether characteristics of acupuncture such as the number of treatment sessions, treatment style or practitioner qualifications affect outcome.

A combination of clinical opinion and some published evidence was used in one systematic review to set a threshold for 'adequate' acupuncture for treating knee osteoarthritis: 'at least six treatments, at least one per week, with at least four points needled for each painful knee for at least 20 minutes, and either needle sensation (deqi) achieved in manual acupuncture, or electrical stimulation of sufficient intensity to produce more than minimal sensation' (White et al. 2007).

REPORTING ACUPUNCTURE TREATMENT – STRICTA GUIDELINES

Acupuncture is a procedure that has many variable components. In order to encourage researchers to report it in a way that can be reproduced and interpreted, a group of researchers formed a consensus on what criteria need to be reported. These are known as the STRICTA criteria – standing for Standards for Reporting Interventions in Clinical Trials of Acupuncture (MacPherson et al. 2002). They cover:

- rationale behind the particular use of acupuncture in the study
- details of needling
- regimen of treatment over time
- other components of treatment
- practitioner background
- control or comparison groups, where relevant.

Descriptions of the criteria can be presented either in the text or in a table. The criteria should be applied flexibly according to the context, as it will not be necessary to provide all details in all circumstances – for example, not all studies use co-interventions or control groups.

These guidelines are currently (2010) under revision and readers should search for the latest version. STRICTA should be used in addition to the general Consolidated Standards of Reporting Trials (CONSORT) guidelines for reporting trials and may come to be regarded as an extension to CONSORT.

CO-INTERVENTIONS

Most studies test acupuncture as a sole intervention, for the obvious reason that this is the only way to be sure that any changes are due to the acupuncture itself. At most, the only other intervention available to patients is rescue analgesia.

However, in practice acupuncture is often used together with massage, manipulation, exercise and so on, and a few studies have investigated such combinations. In one of the German studies of acupuncture for knee pain, all patients received physiotherapy involving strengthening and aerobic exercises, the acupuncture group received additional acupuncture whereas the control group received additional sham acupuncture (Scharf et al. 2006). Interestingly, a review found that the effect of acupuncture in this study was much smaller than in studies in which acupuncture patients received rescue medication only (White et al. 2007).

Further, in a UK study also in patients with knee osteoarthritis, acupuncture (or sham acupuncture) was given in addition to individualized strengthening and aerobic exercises. This study also found that acupuncture had no additional effect (Foster et al. 2007). It seems possible that appropriate exercise can have a 'ceiling' effect in osteoarthritis, so that acupuncture is unable to show any additional effect. The size of the effect of exercise in this study was rather similar to the average size of the effect of acupuncture in the review (White et al. 2007). If this ceiling effect of exercise is supported by other evidence, the implication for practice is that the choice between exercise and acupuncture could depend on their cost-effectiveness, or on patient preference.

CONTROL INTERVENTIONS

Two of the fundamental research questions for acupuncture – does it have a useful effect for patients? does it have a biological effect? – require different control groups: standard care and 'placebo' control.

STANDARD CARE

There is now good evidence that acupuncture is a good alternative to conventional treatment for a number of conditions. Two of the German studies used standard care based on guidelines as the control. For back pain, for example, acupuncture was compared with standardized, multimodal care according to German, evidence-based guidelines (Haake et al. 2007). Participants received 10 consultations with the physician, exercise therapy and analgesics (paracetamol or non-steroidal anti-inflammatory drugs) during painful periods. The response rate in the acupuncture group was 47.6%, compared with 27.4% in the standardized care group ($P<0.001$). Interestingly, the response rate in the sham acupuncture group was 44.2%, also statistically superior to standardized care ($P<0.001$), and not significantly different from acupuncture.

Although acupuncture appears to have had an impressive effect in this study, we should bear in mind that these patients had experienced pain for at least 6 months, were recruited for a trial of acupuncture through media advertisements, and might expect or at least hope to receive acupuncture. Those who were randomized to continue with the same treatment would be disappointed, possibly leading to some negative bias in scoring the effect of treatment, though it might be unreasonable to argue that bias could account for the whole of the difference between groups. Therefore the results are open to interpretation: detractors of acupuncture will dismiss the results as due entirely to the placebo effect.

SHAM ('PLACEBO') ACUPUNCTURE

When it comes to demonstrating the biological activity of acupuncture, the questions resolve into several issues, the main ones being: What are the active components of needle stimulation? Does needle stimulation have an effect at acupuncture points, according to classical theory? Does needle stimulation have an effect anywhere that it stimulates a nerve (i.e. including outside acupuncture points), according to neurophysiological theory? The existence of a true acupuncture placebo would greatly help in resolving these issues.

Terminology for sham acupuncture

Any realistic control intervention for acupuncture must press or at least touch the patient's skin, and so stimulate nerve endings. Therefore it will not be completely inactive and cannot be called a 'placebo' control. Other terms have been suggested, though are not used consistently. 'Sham' acupuncture has been used to mean needling wrong points (Lewith et al. 1983; Hammerschlag 1998; Lewith & Vincent 1998); 'minimal' acupuncture has been used for superficial needling. Some authors have argued that the term 'sham' should be used for all methods as it places emphasis on the psychological impact on the subject (Park et al. 1999), so the procedure should always be described in full.

Here, we shall use the term 'sham' for any procedure that pretends to be acupuncture. The sham may be either 'penetrating' or 'non-penetrating'. This concept is somewhat similar to the recommend use of the terms 'invasive needle control' and 'dummy needling control' (White et al. 2006).

The essential features of the ideal acupuncture sham are: (1) that it should match what the subject (or at least, the acupuncture-naïve subject) expects to see and experience with needling; but (2) that it should not produce the specific needle sensation, deqi. Margolin et al. (1998) suggest an additional test, that it should have the same likelihood of adverse events leading to dropout as the real intervention, but this applies only to its appearance and acceptability, and not to its physiological effects.

Sham procedures

Several sham acupuncture procedures have been devised, including both penetrating and non-penetrating types:

1. Standard needles inserted into inappropriate sites and/or superficially. This is by far the most common form of sham acupuncture.
2. Standard needles used in an abnormal way, either pressing with the handle (Hesse et al. 1994) or just pricking the surface of the skin and immediately being removed (Moore & Berk 1976).
3. Other devices used to touch or press the skin, such as the fingernail (Junnila 1982), an empty guide tube (Lao et al. 1994) or a cocktail stick (White et al. 1996). Ingeniously, Lao et al. (1995) attached leads from inactive electrostimulation apparatus to both groups in order to reduce the perceived differences between the procedures.
4. Sham forms of other treatments, such as inactivated transcutaneous electrical nerve stimulation or laser apparatus (Macdonald et al. 1983; Dowson et al. 1985). These are less than ideal, because the placebo effects of inactivated electrical devices are likely to be different from those of needles. Therefore, any differences in the outcomes of the two groups cannot be attributed solely to the specific effect of acupuncture.

5. Non-penetrating, blunted needles. A major advance was the development by Streitberger & Kleinhenz (1998) of a sham needle that is blunt and in which the shaft of the needle is free to move inside the handle. When pressed on the skin, the needle appears to penetrate but the handle simply telescopes over the shaft. The needle is supported vertically on the skin by an adhesive dressing applied over an O-ring around the point. In a validation study, 22% of volunteers could feel 'a dull sensation' with the sham needle, compared with 57% with a real needle. This 'dull sensation' was called deqi by the authors, though it may not accurately reflect true needle sensation. This sham needle needs to be tested in a variety of locations, with different methods of manual stimulation and with variation in direction of needle insertion (Kaptchuk 1998). An RCT using the sham needle showed a significant difference in treatment effect between real needle and sham needle in treatment of rotator cuff lesions in sportsmen (Kleinhenz et al. 1999). The credibility of the intervention was not different between the groups.

A different method of supporting the needle was developed by Park et al. (1999), consisting of an oversize guide tube with a silicon flange which adheres to the skin by means of double-sided tape. The standard guide tube makes a sliding fit within the Park tube.

Another sham needling set comprising genuine and sham needles has recently been developed, using a guide tube with adhesive base like the Park tube (Takakura & Yajima 2007). The needle handle has a stopper to determine depth of insertion. While the real needle penetrates skin and muscle, the sham needle penetrates a stopper at the base of the guide tube, designed to reproduce the feel of natural tissue. Evidence from the group that developed the new placebo suggests that it is successful at blinding both patient and practitioner, but more experience is required from other centres before it can be adopted with confidence.

Selection of sham points

Although the non-penetrating sham needle may prove a satisfactory control for use at genuine points, it may still have physiological activity. Until this is established, it is better to use it on sham points. Choice of sham points involves several considerations. A sufficient number and variety of sham points should be defined before the study to give the user some choice (Zaslawski et al. 1997). The practical process of locating them (for example, measuring from landmarks) should be comparable to using real points, and practitioners must become as familiar with using them as with real points. It is not known how close sham points should be to the site of the complaint in order to be credible. Some studies have placed needles in the knee (Jobst et al. 1986; Williamson et al. 1996; Waite & Clough 1998), but the credibility was not tested. The points should not be in the affected anatomical segment: a meta-analysis of 90 sham-controlled studies found that real acupuncture was much more likely to be superior when controls were not in the relevant segment than when they were close to it (Araujo 1998). Finally, sham points should be properly validated, as exemplified by Margolin and colleagues (1998) in preparation for a definitive study of auricular acupuncture for cocaine dependence.

Activity of sham acupuncture

Evidence is accumulating that whatever procedure is undertaken as a sham for acupuncture, it will have a physiological effect if given in a therapeutic setting. The clearest evidence for this showed that a blunt needle, described as an active treatment, produced responses in the limbic system (part of the brain related to pain control), whereas a shallow penetration described as a placebo did not. In the same study, deep penetration with deqi also stimulated the insula, which is particularly important for analgesia (Pariente et al. 2005).

The arguments that support the activity of sham acupuncture have been set out by Lundeberg and colleagues (2008), and the original article should be consulted for detailed references. The physiological findings include the following:

- Light touch on the skin, such as is obtained during sham acupuncture, results in activity in the insular region of the brain.
- Mechanical, non-penetrating, sham acupuncture as well as low-frequency electro-acupuncture evokes brain responses localized to the contralateral primary somatosensory cortex in healthy subjects.
- Superficial and deep acupuncture needle stimulation elicits similar blood oxygen level-dependent (BOLD) responses in the central nervous system of healthy subjects.
- Sham acupuncture and traditional Chinese acupuncture reduced both clinical and experimental pain in patients suffering from fibromyalgia. Both modalities resulted in neural activity in the brain, as assessed with functional magnetic resonance imaging, though traditional acupuncture generally had a more pronounced effect.
- Reduction of serum cortisol concentration and anxiety level were observed following both verum (real) and sham (placebo) acupuncture, although there were no significant differences in the changes between the two groups. These changes could not be attributed to rest.
- Acupuncture and sham acupuncture may activate the reward system and modulate the functional connectivity, including the default mode.

Evidence that sham acupuncture is not inert is also provided by some clinical trials:

- Superficial needling as sham acupuncture is superior to a placebo pill, demonstrating that superficial and sham acupuncture is not inert.
- Superficial needling has been advocated as a treatment technique in its own right.
- Sham acupuncture has been proven to be as effective as verum acupuncture and dedicated analgesics in headache and migraine.
- Sham acupuncture and verum acupuncture have been shown to be more effective than conventional therapeutic interventions in low-back pain.
- Sham (placebo) acupuncture was associated with a significantly higher overall pregnancy rate when compared with real acupuncture in in vitro fertilization treatment.

Testing the success of blinding

The success of blinding should be tested, either indirectly by comparing the credibility of real and sham interventions, to show that they have the same psychological impact, or directly by asking subjects which intervention they believe they received. Neither method is entirely straightforward.

The common indirect approach (Vincent & Lewith 1995) to credibility testing involves four questions:

1. How confident do you feel that this treatment can alleviate your complaint?
2. How confident would you be in recommending this treatment to a friend who suffered from similar complaints?
3. How logical does this treatment seem to you?
4. How successful do you think this treatment would be in alleviating other complaints?

The responses can be on a six-point scale or visual analogue scale (Petrie & Hazleman 1985). The original questionnaire was developed as an exercise to rate the credibility of novel therapies and control procedures that had just been described to (though not experienced by) a class of healthy psychology students (Borkovec & Nau 1972). Although the original context was very different from a clinical trial, the questionnaire was shown to have test–retest validity and internal consistency in the context of a clinical trial (Vincent 1990) and has been used in several subsequent studies (White et al. 1996; Wood & Lewith 1998; Kleinhenz et al. 1999; Linde et al. 2005). However, the subjects' response could vary according to information they received on recruitment, for example whether they were told 'You will receive one of two forms of acupuncture' or 'You will receive either acupuncture or a placebo'. The subjects must be judging the intervention they have actually experienced, and not just giving answers about acupuncture in general. For example, Kleinhenz et al. report that, even after treatment had failed, 'acupuncture was continued to be judged as effective'. The questionnaire wording must be both precise and fully understood.

Other investigators have used a direct question, such as: 'You were told you would receive either acupuncture or another treatment very similar to it. Which do you believe you have received?' (Moore & Berk 1976; White et al. 1996; Zaslawski et al. 1997; Berman et al. 2004). This method may be less than ideal: subjects may try to give the answer which they think the researcher wants (interviewer bias), and the question focuses their attention on the details of therapy, which may cause doubt and confound the outcome. Also, we observed that it is quite stressful for subjects who do not want to 'lose face' by not recognizing the fact that they had false treatment. Zaslawski et al. (1997) analysed the responses in some detail and found that the subjects' decision depended on four factors: (1) layout of the needles; (2) needle sensation; (3) general responses such as drowsiness; and (4) alteration of symptoms.

In order to provide some method of evaluating the success of blinding, two forms of a Blinding Index have been developed which test whether patients guess according to chance (Park et al. 2008). In view of the unknown factors (such as timing of the question, or how to deal with don't know responses), it is probably premature to draw conclusions from these index calculations but hopefully with further development it will become meaningful.

It seems, then, that there is no entirely satisfactory method of testing subject blinding, and it is provisionally recommended to use the credibility questions as they are less stressful for subjects, taking great care in setting the correct context.

Practitioner blinding

The influence of the therapist can be powerful, possibly more powerful than many interventions (Balint 1957), and is best minimized by masking (blinding) the practitioner. However, it is difficult or impossible to mask an acupuncturist and still offer technically optimal treatment. In one attempt, a doctor with no special knowledge of acupuncture was trained specifically for the study, learning two sets of points without knowing which were the correct ones (Lagrue et al. 1977). In another attempt, the practitioner was given either the true or false diagnosis made by another physician (Godfrey & Morgan 1978). This method has been adapted for rigorous, truly 'double-blind' studies of individualized acupuncture (Allen et al. 1998): the diagnosing practitioner (or, preferably, team) would write down both appropriate and inappropriate selections of points, place them in different envelopes marked A and B, and leave the room. An independent practitioner would then enter, select one envelope according to a code and treat the subject. This way, all acupuncture practitioners would remain blinded as well as the subject, so it only remains to arrange a blinded assessor. This method is, however, still not acceptable by practitioners who use immediate feedback from the patient, e.g. by feeling the pulse, as a guide for further treatment.

One substitute for practitioner blinding is standardized, minimal interaction (Hansen & Hansen 1985), in which the acupuncturist must avoid discussing the therapy or the response with the patient. A modification involves answering questions about acupuncture using prepared responses (Kleinhenz et al. 1999). Social discussion should also be forbidden, even though this creates a rather stilted atmosphere. Care must be taken that the actual performance of the intervention is identical in both groups. If subjects might see different practitioners on subsequent attendances, the approaches must be standardized. In a study in the UK, it was found that interventions were more credible when they were given by a male practitioner than a female, and working in a holistic manner rather than symptomatically (Choi & Tweed 1996).

The recent development of a placebo needle that mimics insertion (described above) appears to offer the chance of double-blinding, though more experience with its use is required before it is generally adopted.

OUTCOMES

For measuring the main outcome, there is no reason why acupuncture studies should choose a different measure than conventional trials of the same condition. Triallists can add secondary measures for particular outcomes that are of interest, often quality of life. For cost-effectiveness analysis based on quality-adjusted life years (QALYs) it is is essential to use generic quality-of-life measurement instruments such as the SF-36 or the EuroQol (EQ-5D).

EXPECTATION

As discussed in detail elsewhere (Chapter 5), the patient's expectation for the treatment outcome can have a relevant effect on the outcome. This applies to acupuncture as well. In a pooled analysis of the data of four German studies (Linde et al. 2007), the authors found that a higher expectation could predict a better treatment outcome. It appears wise to account for patient expectations by measuring them at baseline and to analyse the main outcomes data by taking them into account.

ECONOMIC ANALYSIS IN ACUPUNCTURE STUDIES

Patients want to know how effective a treatment is. Purchasers want to know in addition how much this will cost. Therefore national institutes such as the National Institute for Health and Clinical Excellence (NICE) in the UK introduced arbitrary cost limits for the reimbursement of new treatments. Yet for most established conventional treatments such information about cost-effectiveness is still missing. In this situation, several cost-effectiveness analyses for acupuncture have been published in recent years. Most of them are part of a large German research initiative after the first from the UK (Wonderling et al. 2004) had found acupuncture to be more cost-effective than conventional routine care.

Unfortunately, the results of cost-effectiveness analyses are mainly valid only for the country where the study was performed. They are based on the respective national health system, the local costs of the treatments, the assumptions on which the analysis is based (e.g. societal or third-party payer perspective), and thus vary between countries. This makes the field of economic analysis more complicated than other areas of medical research. All cost-effectiveness studies have shown that acupuncture is associated with better outcome than usual care, but at additional costs. The above German studies, taking a societal approach, calculated total and diagnosis specific costs. The total costs per QALY varied according to the diagnosis between € 3000 for dysmenorrhoea (Witt et al. 2008a) and €18 000 for osteoarthritis of the knee or the hip (Reinhold et al. 2008). The costs per QALY for low-back pain (Witt et al. 2006b), neck pain (Willich et al. 2006) and headache (Witt et al. 2008b) were ranked somewhere in between. It would be interesting to see whether acupuncture might help to save costs in the long term. The German cost-effectiveness studies lack such an analysis, whereas the study on low-back pain from the UK (Ratcliffe et al. 2006) stretched over a period of 2 years. Here, the costs for the additional acupuncture treatment were not compensated by other savings after 2 years. Based on the available data we can currently assume that additional acupuncture treatment is associated with a higher benefit for the patients but also with higher costs for the purchasers. Because economic aspects are important, future studies should include them whenever possible.

COMMENT ON STUDY DESIGN (EXPLANATORY AND PRAGMATIC STUDIES)

The single-blinded studies in the Modellvorhaben Akupunktur series in Germany were three-arm trials, comparing acupuncture, sham acupuncture (shallow needling to non-classical sites) and no acupuncture – this last group was on a waiting list for acupuncture, or received usual care or standardized care. Superficially this is an efficient design, since it answers two questions (Does acupuncture have a biological effect? Is acupuncture clinically useful?) in one study.

However, when the differences between explanatory and pragmatic approaches (Chapter 5) are considered, it soon becomes clear that design features that suit the first question may not be ideal for the second. The 'biological effect' question has the best chance of a truthful answer if it recruits patients who are likely to respond (they have no other medical conditions, and are not receiving any other treatments); in contrast, the 'useful' question should include a sample representing potential patients who might receive this treatment in usual care, with other conditions and existing treatments. Studies of the 'biological effect' question should apply acupuncture and sham acupuncture to a high technical standard, which is best achieved by using experienced practitioners who receive extra training for the study purpose; in contrast, the 'useful' question requires practitioners trained to the standard commonly available in the health service. Finally, the 'biological effect' question can be answered at any appropriate time point, and usually the end of treatment is chosen as that is when the effect will be the greatest; in contrast, the 'useful' question should have a long follow-up of at least 6 months, since this is the information that is relevant to patients.

In one study, 340 practitioners recruited an average of three patients each: the effect was measured at 6 months (Haake et al. 2007). This study design is good for addressing the pragmatic question of the effectiveness of acupuncture in normal practice, but may not provide the most accurate information on the biological effect of acupuncture: there may be doubts about the technical standards of the acupuncture and sham procedures, and any effect at the end of treatment might have dissipated by 6 months. These limitations could reduce the internal validity of the study in addressing the explanatory (biological effect) question.

At the present time, a blunt, non-penetrating needle control applied away from acupuncture points seems the best approximation to placebo (inert) acupuncture, but does require considerable expertise. Placebo-controlled studies require careful control of all variables, which needs considerable resources for multicentre studies so may be best conducted in single centres.

The German study had large sample sizes, and were thought to be sufficient to detect even relatively small biological effect of acupuncture. However, with the exception of one study in knee pain (Witt et al. 2005) they found no significant differences between acupuncture and sham acupuncture and provoked an international discussion on the benefits and pitfalls of sham acupuncture procedures in clinical studies. Thus they have not produced the hoped-for 'definitive answers' to whether acupuncture has biological effects.

The main lessons from this experience are that explanatory (sham-controlled) studies that address the placebo question should:

- have a small number of well-trained centres
- preferably use non-penetrating needles as the control

CONCLUSION

The design of acupuncture studies is far from straightforward, but there is now considerable international expertise, and collaboration with experts is essential in designing studies. It is important to consider in detail the types of patient to be included, the type and dose of acupuncture to be used, the control group and the measurement of outcome. Different study designs are required to address different research questions. Pragmatic randomized studies evaluating acupuncture as an add-on or comparing it to standard treatment are helpful for decision-making. Studies that address the placebo question should carefully consider the limitations of the sham controls for acupuncture that are currently available, some of which may have activity of their own, as well as methods for testing the success of blinding. Cognitive factors in patients, particularly their expectations of acupuncture, should always be assessed as these influence the outcome in individuals.

REFERENCES

Allen, J.J.B., Schnyer, R.N., Hitt, S.K., 1998. The efficacy of acupuncture in the treatment of major depression in women. Psychol. Sci. 9, 397–401.

Araujo, M.S., 1998. Does the choice of placebo determine the results of clinical studies on acupuncture? Forsch. Komplementärmed. 5 (Suppl), 8–11.

Balint, M., 1957. The doctor, the patient and the illness. Pitman Medical.

Barlas, P., Lowe, A.S., Walsh, D.M., et al., 2000. Effect of acupuncture upon experimentally induced ischemic pain: a sham- controlled single-blind study. Clin. J. Pain 16 (3), 255–264.

Berman, B.M., Lao, L., Langenberg, P., et al., 2004. Effectiveness of acupuncture as adjunctive therapy in osteoarthritis of the knee: a randomized, controlled trial. Ann. Intern. Med. 141 (12), 901–910.

Birch, S., 1997. Issues to consider in determining an adequate treatment in a clinical trial of acupuncture. Complement. Ther. Med. 5, 8–12.

Bjordal, J.M., Ljunggren, A.E., Klovning, A., et al., 2004. Non-steroidal anti-inflammatory drugs, including cyclo-oxygenase-2 inhibitors, in osteoarthritic knee pain: meta-analysis of randomised placebo controlled trials. BMJ 329 (7478), 1317.

Borkovec, T.D., Nau, S.D., 1972. Credibility of analogue therapy rationales. Journal of Behavioural and Experimental Psychiatry 3, 257–260.

Campbell, M., Fitzpatrick, R., Haines, A., et al., 2000. Framework for design and evaluation of complex interventions to improve health. BMJ 321 (7262), 694–696.

Choi, P.Y.L., Tweed, A., 1996. The holistic approach in acupuncture treatment: implications for clinical trials. J. Psychosom. Res. 41, 349–356.

Diener, H.C., Kronfeld, K., Boewing, G., et al., 2006. Efficacy of acupuncture for the prophylaxis of migraine: a multicentre randomised controlled clinical trial. Lancet Neurol. 5 (4), 310–316.

Dowson, D.I., Lewith, G., Machin, D., 1985. The effects of acupuncture versus placebo in the treatment of headache. Pain 21, 35.

Endres, H.G., Bowing, G., Diener, H.C., et al., 2007. Acupuncture for tension-type headache: a multicentre, sham-controlled, patient-and observer-blinded, randomised trial. J. Headache Pain 8, 306–314.

Ezzo, J., Berman, B., Hadhazy, V., et al., 2000. Is acupuncture effective for the treatment of chronic pain? A systematic review. Pain 86 (3), 217–225.

Filshie, J., White, A.R., 1998. Medical Acupuncture: a Western scientific approach. Churchill Livingstone, Edinburgh.

Foster, N., Barlas, P., Daniels, J., et al., 1999. Use of acupuncture by physiotherapists in the treatment of osteoarthritis of the knee: current trends inform a clinical trial. Proceedings of the Chartered Society of Physiotherapists Congress, Birmingham, UK, p. 27.

Foster, N.E., Thomas, E., Barlas, P., et al., 2007. Acupuncture as an adjunct to exercise based physiotherapy for osteoarthritis of the knee: randomised controlled trial. BMJ 335 (7617), 436.

Godfrey, C.M., Morgan, P., 1978. A controlled trial of the theory of acupuncture in musculoskeletal pain. J. Rheumatol. 5 (2), 121–124.

Haake, M., Muller, H.H., Schade-Brittinger, C., et al., 2007. German Acupuncture Trials (GERAC) for chronic low back pain: randomized, multicenter, blinded, parallel-group trial with 3 groups. Arch. Intern. Med. 167 (17), 1892–1898.

Hammerschlag, R., 1998. Methodological and ethical issues in clinical trials of acupuncture. J. Altern. Complement. Med. 4, 159–171.

Hansen, P.E., Hansen, J.H., 1985. Acupuncture treatment of chronic tension headache – a controlled cross-over trial. Cephalalgia 5, 137–142.

Harris, R.E., Tian, X., Williams, D.A., et al., 2005. Treatment of fibromyalgia with formula acupuncture: investigation of needle placement, needle stimulation, and treatment frequency. J. Altern. Complement. Med. 11 (4), 663–671.

Hesse, J., Mogelvang, B., Simonsen, H., 1994. Acupuncture versus metoprolol in migraine prophylaxis: a randomised trial of trigger point inactivation. J. Intern. Med. 235, 451–456.

Jobst, K., Chen, J.H., McPherson, K., et al., 1986. Controlled trial of acupuncture for disabling breathlessness. Lancet 328, 1416–1418.

Junnila, S.Y.T., 1982. Acupuncture therapy for chronic pain. Am. J. Acupunct. 10, 259–262.

Kaptchuk, T., 1998. Placebo needle for acupuncture. Lancet 352, 992.

Kleinhenz, J., Streitberger, K., Windeler, J., et al., 1999. Randomised clinical trial comparing the effects of acupuncture and a newly designed placebo needle in rotator cuff tendinitis. Pain 83 (2), 235–241.

Lagrue, G., Poupy, J.L., Grillot, A., et al., 1977. Acupuncture anti-tabagique. La Nouvelle Presse Médicale 9, 966.

Lao, L., Bergman, S., Anderson, R., et al., 1994. The effect of acupuncture on post-operative pain. Acupunct. Med. 12, 13–17.

Lao, L., Bergman, S., Langenberg, P., et al., 1995. Efficacy of Chinese acupuncture on postoperative oral surgery pain. Oral Surg. Oral Med. Oral Pathol. Oral Radiol. Endod. 79, 423–428.

Lewith, G.T., Vincent, C.A., 1998. The clinical evaluation of acupuncture. In: Filshie, J., White, A. (Eds.), Medical Acupuncture: a Western Scientific Approach. Churchill Livingstone, Edinburgh, pp. 205–224.

Lewith, G., Field, J., Machin, D., 1983. Acupuncture compared with placebo in post-herpetic pain. Pain 17, 361–368.

Linde, K., Streng, A., Jurgens, S., et al., 2005. Acupuncture for patients with migraine: a randomized controlled trial. JAMA 293 (17), 2118–2125.

Linde, K., Streng, A., Hoppe, A., et al., 2006. The programme for the evaluation of patient care with acupuncture (PEP-Ac) – a project sponsored by ten German social health insurance funds. Acupunct. Med. 24 (Suppl), 25–32.

Linde, K., Witt, C.M., Streng, A., et al., 2007. The impact of patient expectations on outcomes in four randomized controlled trials of acupuncture in patients with chronic pain. Pain 128 (3), 264–271.

Lundeberg, T., Lund, I., 2007. Did 'The Princess on the Pea' suffer from fibromyalgia syndrome? The influence on sleep and the effects of acupuncture. Acupunct. Med. 25 (4), 184–197.

Lundeberg, T., Lund, I., Naslund, J., et al., 2008. The Emperors sham – wrong assumption that sham needling is sham. Acupunct. Med. 26 (4), 239–242.

Macdonald, A.J.R., Macrae, K.D., Master, B.R., et al., 1983. Superficial acupuncture in the relief of chronic low back pain. Ann. R. Coll. Surg. Engl. 65, 44–46.

MacPherson, H., Schroer, S., 2007. Acupuncture as a complex intervention for depression: A consensus method to develop a standardised treatment protocol for a randomised controlled trial. Complement. Ther. Med. 15 (2), 92–100.

MacPherson, H., White, A., Cummings, M., et al., 2002. Standards for reporting interventions in controlled trials of acupuncture: The STRICTA recommendations.STandards for Reporting Interventions in Controlled Trails of Acupuncture. Acupunct. Med. 20 (1), 22–25.

Marcus, P., 1994. Towards a dose of acupuncture. Acupunct. Med. 12 (2), 78–82.

Margolin, A., Avants, K., Kleber, H., 1998. Investigating alternative medicine therapies in randomized controlled trials. JAMA 280, 1626–1627.

Melchart, D., Streng, A., Hoppe, A., et al., 2005. Acupuncture in patients with tension-type headache: randomised controlled trial. BMJ 331 (7513), 376–382.

Molsberger, A.F., Boewing, G., Diener, H.C., et al., 2006a. Designing an acupuncture study: the nationwide, randomized, controlled, German acupuncture trials on migraine and tension-type headache. J. Altern. Complement. Med. 12 (3), 237–245.

Molsberger, A.F., Streitberger, K., Kraemer, J., et al., 2006b. Designing an acupuncture study: II. The nationwide, randomized, controlled German acupuncture trials on low-back pain and gonarthrosis. J. Altern. Complement. Med. 12 (8), 733–742.

Moore, M.E., Berk, S.N., 1976. Acupuncture for chronic shoulder pain. Ann. Intern. Med. 84 (4), 381–384.

Napadow, V., Liu, J., Kaptchuk, T.J., 2004. A systematic study of acupuncture practice: acupoint usage in an outpatient setting in Beijing, China. Complement. Ther. Med. 12 (4), 209–216.

Pariente, J., White, P., Frackowiak, R.S., et al., 2005. Expectancy and belief modulate the neuronal substrates of pain treated by acupuncture. Neuroimage 25 (4), 1161–1167.

Park, J., Bang, H., Canette, I., 2008. Blinding in clinical trials, time to do it better. Complement. Ther. Med. 16 (3), 121–123.

Park, J., White, A.R., Lee, H., et al., 1999. Development of a new sham needle. Acupunct. Med. 17, 110–112.

Petrie, J.P., Hazleman, B.L., 1985. Credibility of placebo transcutaneous nerve stimulation and acupuncture. Clin. Exp. Rheumatol. 3, 151–153.

Ratcliffe, J., Thomas, K.J., MacPherson, H., et al., 2006. A randomised controlled trial of acupuncture care for persistent low back pain: cost effectiveness analysis. BMJ 333 (7569), 626–628A.

Reinhold, T., Witt, C.M., Jena, S., et al., 2008. Quality of life and cost-effectiveness of acupuncture treatment in patients with osteoarthritis pain. Eur. J. Health Econ. 9 (3), 209–219.

Scharf, H.P., Mansmann, U., Streitberger, K., et al., 2006. Acupuncture and knee osteoarthritis – a three-armed randomized trial. Ann. Intern. Med. 145 (1), 12–20.

Schnyer, R.N., Allen, J.J., 2002. Bridging the gap in complementary and alternative medicine research: manualization as a means of promoting standardization and flexibility of treatment in clinical trials of acupuncture. J. Altern. Complement. Med. 8 (5), 623–634.

Streitberger, K., Kleinhenz, J., 1998. Introducing a placebo needle into acupuncture research. Lancet 352, 364–365.

Takakura, N., Yajima, H., 2007. A double-blind placebo needle for acupuncture research. BMC Complement. Altern. Med. 7, 31.

Vincent, C., 1990. Credibility assessments in trials of acupuncture. Complementary Medical Research 4, 8–11.

Vincent, C., Lewith, G., 1995. Placebo controls for acupuncture studies. J. R. Soc. Med. 88, 199–202.

Waite, N.R., Clough, J.B., 1998. A single-blind, placebo-controlled trial of a simple acupuncture treatment in the cessation of smoking. Br. J. Gen. Pract. 48 (433), 1487–1490.

Webster-Harrison, P., White, A., Rae, J., 2002. Acupuncture for tennis elbow: an E-mail consensus study to define a standardised treatment in a GPs' surgery. Acupunct. Med. 20 (4), 181–185.

White, A.R., Eddleston, C., Hardie, R., et al., 1996. A pilot study of acupuncture for tension headache, using a novel placebo. Acupunct. Med. 14 (1), 11–15.

White, P., Golianu, B., Zaslawski, C., et al., 2006. Standardization of nomenclature in acupuncture research (SONAR). *eCAM* 4 (2), 267–270.

White, A., Foster, N.E., Cummings, M., et al., 2007. Acupuncture treatment for chronic knee pain: a systematic review. Rheumatology (Oxford) 46 (3), 384–390.

White, A., Cummings, M., Barlas, P., et al., 2008. Defining an adequate dose of acupuncture using a neurophysiological approach – a narrative review of the literature. Acupunct. Med. 26 (2), 111–120.

Williamson, L., Yudkin, P., Livingstone, R., et al., 1996. Hay fever treatment in general practice: a randomised controlled trial comparing standardised Western acupuncture with sham acupuncture. Acupunct. Med. 14 (1), 6–10.

Willich, S.N., Reinhold, T., Selim, D., et al., 2006. Cost-effectiveness of acupuncture treatment in patients with chronic neck pain. Pain 125 (1–2), 107–113.

Witt, C., Brinkhaus, B., Jena, S., et al., 2005. Acupuncture in patients with osteoarthritis of the knee: a randomised trial. Lancet 366 (9480), 136–143.

Witt, C.M., Brinkhaus, B., Reinhold, T., et al., 2006a. Efficacy, effectiveness, safety and costs of acupuncture for chronic pain – results of a large research initiative. Acupunct. Med. 24 (Suppl), S33–S39.

Witt, C.M., Jena, S., Selim, D., et al., 2006b. Pragmatic randomized trial evaluating the clinical and economic effectiveness of acupuncture for chronic low back pain. Am. J. Epidemiol. 164 (5), 487–496.

Witt, C.M., Reinhold, T., Brinkhaus, B., et al., 2008a. Acupuncture in patients with dysmenorrhea: a randomized study on clinical effectiveness and cost-effectiveness in usual care. Am. J. Obstet. Gynecol. 198 (2), 166–168.

Witt, C.M., Reinhold, T., Jena, S., et al., 2008b. Cost-effectiveness of acupuncture treatment in patients with headache. Cephalalgia 28 (4), 334–345.

Wonderling, D., Vickers, A.J., Grieve, R., et al., 2004. Cost effectiveness analysis of a randomised trial of acupuncture for chronic headache in primary care. BMJ 328 (7442), 747–749.

Wood, R., Lewith, G., 1998. The credibility of placebo controls in acupuncture studies. Complement. Ther. Med. 6, 79.

Zaslawski, C., Rogers, C., Garvey, M., et al., 1997. Strategies to maintain the credibility of sham acupuncture used as a control treatment in clinical trials. J. Altern. Complement. Med. 3, 257–266.

Zaslawski, C.J., Cobbin, D., Lidums, E., et al., 2003. The impact of site specificity and needle manipulation on changes to pain pressure threshold following manual acupuncture: a controlled study. Complement. Ther. Med. 11 (1), 11–21.

FURTHER READING

Altman, D.G., 1991. Practical Statistics for Medical Research. Chapman & Hall, London.

MacPherson, H., Hammerschlag, R., Lewith, G., et al., (Eds.), Acupuncture Research: Strategies for Building an Evidence Base. Elsevier, Edinburgh.

White, A., Cummings, M., Filshie, J., 2008. An Introduction to Western Medical Acupuncture. Churchill Livingstone Elsevier, Edinburgh.

Research methodology for studies of prayer and distant healing

Elisabeth Targ* • Harald Walach

12

CHAPTER CONTENTS

*This chapter is dedicated to the memory of Elisabeth Targ, the author of the chapter in the last edition. She has passed away since the original chapter was written. I have kept the original text as much as was feasible and adapted it slightly to fit with the new edition and its overall plan. I have also provided an updated reference list and have put the text in context. Harald Walach.

DOI: 10.1016/B978-0-443-06956-7.00012-4

INTRODUCTION

The topic of distant healing or healing intentionality brings some of the most controversial and central questions to the area of complementary medicine. Within the scientific community, the usual explanation for any beneficial effects of prayer, energy, spiritual or 'psychic' healing efforts is that hope, expectation or the relationship with the healer mobilizes a psychogenic improvement in the patient's health. Such psychogenic effects have been well described in the psychophysiology and psychoimmunology literature and are now being researched under the heading 'placebo effects'. They are discussed in Chapter 16. Here we consider research approaches for assessing whether the intentions of one person can benefit the health of another independently of or in addition to any psychological factors. The term 'distant' when applied to healing intentionality is used to emphasize the removal of ordinary channels of communication between healer and patient, but certainly the modality of healing intention could be present when a healer and patient are in proximity. More than 80% of Americans believe that their 'thoughts can cause healing for another person at a distance', and most of the complementary and alternative medicine (CAM) practices said to be used by Americans refer to prayer (Barnes et al. 2002). Anecdotal reports of healing in a wide variety of conditions have stimulated more than 150 controlled studies dealing with human and/or biological systems. Of these, two-thirds found a statistically significant effect (for review, see Benor 1992, 2001; Dossey 1993; Targ 1997). The US National Center for Complementary and Alternative Medicine (NCCAM) now even has a category entitled 'energy medicine' that comprises the concept of distant healing. This implies a type of consciousness-mediated causality that has never been accepted within the medical sciences.

Few fields of research routinely raise such heartfelt opposition as research in distant healing; as one National Institutes of Health (NIH) reviewer wrote to this author, 'healing is intrinsically a matter of faith, and therefore cannot be studied by science'. Such remarks illustrate a popular belief among the scientific community. Some healers have voiced the concern that research cannot test or study the subtle effects of their treatments. Religionists have objected that research in distant healing may dissuade people from prayer for the purpose of strengthening faith and mistakenly focus them on a causal interaction between prayers and physical outcomes (Thomson 1996). Typical concerns are that testing healing is 'testing God' and therefore blasphemous, if not impossible (Dossey 1997).

These concerns, when removed from the debate, do reflect important issues in studying distant healing. Clearly we must consider the limits of our studies. As we interpret results, we must remember that:

- finding that a change occurs in a biological system in the context of a directed prayer or healing intention neither proves nor disproves the tenets of anyone's religion

- the spiritual, cultural and psychological contexts in which healing efforts are embedded are complex and may have many benefits (or detriments) apart from their efficacy in affecting clinical change through intention alone
- use of the double-blind randomized clinical trial has multiple inherent constraints that preclude testing of distant healing exactly as it is practised in the community.

Researchers interested in pursuing studies in this area will take heart from a list of basic research tenets published by the NIH Panel Report on CAM Research Methodology. This report states the underlying assumptions that:

- research is always feasible – and essential, regardless of the therapy under consideration
- research rarely provides unequivocal answers
- good research aims to minimize the effects of bias, chance variation and confounding
- our priority is research that investigates whether treatments do more good than harm (Vickers et al. 1997).

The methodological questions in research in distant healing necessarily rest on defining a specific intervention and evaluating its impact on a target system. This will be the main focus of this chapter. Questions of mechanisms depend on the successful negotiation of these first tasks, on theoretical and paradigmatic assumptions, and will be discussed more briefly at the end.

DEFINING THE INTERVENTION

There are no established protocols or practice standards for distant healing practitioners as a group. Healer inclusion criteria in published studies have ranged from novice volunteers in many studies (Braud 1989; O'Laoire 1997) to 'people who believe in God' (Harris et al. 1999), to healers of international renown (Grad 1965; Rauscher & Rubik 1983) or with many years of professional experience (Snel & Hol 1983; Sicher et al. 1998; Astin et al. 2006; Walach et al. 2008). Each experimenter must carefully choose and document the approach and experience level of healers in a study. The choice may have a theoretical basis, e.g. an attempt to compare one approach to another or to manipulate healing parameters. Or it may be based on a practical issue, e.g. an experimenter may wish to evaluate a method being used in a particular clinic. Documentation of healer approach or experience does not require that healers be identical on all descriptors. For example, one approach might be to require 5 years of experience or a certain score on a test of concentration but not to discriminate on the basis of philosophical approach.

Because the efficacy of distant healing as a modality has not been established, there is no test by which to choose an effective healer. In addition, unlike a pharmacological agent or a technical device, distant healing depends specifically on the consciousness of a human being. This raises the important issue that, in addition to possible differing efficacy of various approaches, there may be differing skill levels of practitioners of a particular approach or even of an individual practitioner on a day-to-day basis. In a large study, one runs the risk that certain patients might be treated by an effective healer and others by healers of no ability. One novel approach used by us (Sicher et al. 1998;

Astin et al. 2006) has been to have healers that meet certain inclusion criteria work on different patients on a rotating schedule, so that if some of the healers were effective and others not, all patients would have contact with a range of practitioners, or have several healers working on the same patient in parallel (Walach et al. 2008). Because a healer might not always be performing at his or her maximum ability, it may also be appropriate to plan several intervention periods, rather than using a one-healer, one-session approach. Another way to think about this is that in studying intentionality as a healing modality, one has to ensure that the intentionality effort is really present and maximize the potential effects.

Many terms have been used to describe interventions which may fall into the category of distant healing. These include: intercessory prayer, non-directed prayer, energy healing, shamanic healing, non-contact therapeutic touch, spiritual healing. Each of these describes a particular theoretical, cultural and pragmatic approach to attempts to mediate a healing or biological change through mental intentions. The following are some operational definitions of modalities which include elements of distant healing.

- Intercessory prayer. Any form of requesting a transcendent reality or God to bring about a specific desired outcome (O'Laoire 1997).
- Non-directed prayer. Intercessory prayer in which the person praying wishes only that God's will be done in the life of the subject (O'Laoire 1997). This prayer may typically be worded 'Thy will be done' (Dossey 1997).
- Energy healing. This large category describes attempts by a practitioner to send or direct atypical or 'subtle energy' flows either to or within the subject. Examples include attempts to interact with the Asian concept of chi, ki or prana (or life energy) through chi gong, jin shin jyutsu or reiki or chakra (human energy centres) energetic manipulations as taught in schools influenced by Ayurvedic teaching (Brennan 1987).
- Shamanic healing. This approach is typical of Native American and other indigenous cultures (Halifax 1979). These complex practices involve the healer entering a profound altered state of consciousness in which he or she experiences moving into different 'realms' and interacting with spirits whose aid may be enlisted in healing the patient.
- Therapeutic touch. A technique developed by nurse Dolores Krieger (1975) in which the healer uses meditative practice to induce a calm and focused state and moves his or her hands over the patient (without touching) while holding a mental intention for the patient's healing.
- Spiritual healing. This very general term has been used to refer to a wide range of techniques including spiritist healing seances (Krippner & Villoldo 1979), as well as meditations focused on visualizing the patient connected with God, a universal force of love or the Absolute. Such healing efforts may be performed in a religious or a non-denominational context.

In a qualitative analysis of what he termed 'transpersonal healers', Cooperstein (1992) found that, whatever the cultural or religious orientation of the healer, most typically begin with a period of relaxation, followed by enhanced concentration, culminating in visualization. Types of healing can be distinguished according to whether they employ a rather technical metaphor ('energy') or more a spiritual one ('divine light') for the imagery, and according to the degree of altered states of consciousness induced.

Most healing efforts in the community occur within a cultural context either of interaction between the healer and the patient or expectation by the patient that healing is being performed on his or her behalf. This may or may not be the case in a study of distant healing.

WHAT IS THE HEALER DOING?

Healer strategy should be documented before any trial via interview of the healer and in extended studies healers should be asked to write daily logs describing their healing efforts. Healer selection might also involve questions as to level of experience and professional training or other issues of relevance to the study such as healer ability at concentration. Since it has not yet been established whether healer experience and training are significant for outcome, this will be an important variable to explore.

FOR HOW LONG IS HEALING ATTEMPTED?

Periods of time for healing interventions in the literature range from a few seconds in experiments attempting to arouse anaesthetized mice (Watkins & Watkins 1971) to 60 hours (Sicher et al. 1998). A majority of studies have required healers to perform their healing efforts serially on a daily or weekly basis for a series of treatments. Few, however, have indicated how much time the healer should spend on the healing efforts. For example, in three major intercessory prayer studies (Byrd 1988; Walker et al. 1997; Harris et al. 1999) no indication is given if prayers are prayed for a few seconds at bedtime or concentrated for minutes or hours. This problem can be addressed by requiring a set amount of time for the healing effort (Sicher et al. 1998) and providing healers with a log to document the extent of their compliance (Walach et al. 2008). In addition, it may be important to stay in communication with and actively encourage healers during extended studies, for the purpose of motivating their performance and ensuring that healing efforts will in fact be performed.

INDIVIDUAL VERSUS GROUP EFFORTS

Most distant healing interventions have been organized such that one subject is treated by one healer. A variation of this approach described above involves sequential treatment of each subject by a series of different healers, or a simultaneous treatment of one patient by several healers operating independently. Another variation is seen in the Harris study: the name of each patient was given simultaneously to a 'team of intercessors' (Harris et al. 1999). Thus each patient was receiving pooled prayer efforts from a group of people working individually. In the study by Byrd (1988), prayer was performed as a group effort, by pre-existing Christian prayer groups. At this point there is no evidence to suggest that individual or group healing efforts are more successful. A logistical concern is the risk that, in a group setting, group members may distract one another from the task of focusing on the subject. In addition, studies using healing groups and pooled efforts have tended to use less experienced healers than those studying individual efforts. In order to comment meaningfully on the relative roles of experience versus number of interveners, it will be important that investigators considering one or another of these approaches document the experience and practice level of the healers.

EXTRANEOUS PRAYER

Dossey (1997) has pointed out that, in clinical healing studies, especially ones in which the patient is very ill, it is quite likely that patients may be receiving prayer or healing efforts from friends and family members or may be praying for him- or herself. In fact, on a daily basis, hundreds of thousands of people worldwide offer prayers 'for all the sick'. Although one of the first studies of such a type of prayer by Galton (1872) did not reveal any benefit of such generic prayers, there is concern that such additional prayer might 'interfere with' or 'dilute' experimental effects of prayer. Although this might be true, it could be expected to be a typical random variable that is controlled for by random allocation (see below).

DEFINING THE HEALING INTENTION

The investigator has the responsibility to define parameters of the healing intervention engaged. This may or may not involve defining the specific mental techniques used by the healers. It does, however, require carefully defining the intentions of the treatment. Intentions may be very specifically prescribed, such as having healers hold intention for 'lower blood pressure', 'reduced tumour size', 'decreased anxiety' or even 'increased emotional and physical well-being' if the investigator plans to use a broad range of measurement tools. It is not appropriate for healers to pray for 'religious conversion' for patients and some studies have specifically directed healers not to do this.

It is also not useful for healers to focus their intentions for change in an area which the investigator cannot measure, e.g. 'change in the etheric field' or 'balancing the heart chakra'. If within a healer's theoretical orientation such an action is believed also to be associated with changes in the target system as defined by the experimenter, this type of focus may be acceptable as part of the healer's working style but a measurable outcome intention should be defined and specified by the investigator.

WORKING WITH HEALERS

Most healers have not worked in a laboratory or experimental setting and many are not comfortable with or sympathetic to the constraints put on their activity in the research setting. This represents a limitation of distant healing as it is performed in the community. It has been our experience that there is a great range of healing practitioners and some are eager to participate, very flexible and appreciative of research efforts. Others have been very angry about not being allowed to, for example, touch experimental Petri dishes or have felt investigators were discourteous because they were questioning the ability of the healers. As with all social and working situations, it is important that the healer–investigator team work toward mutual understanding, respect and consideration. Because of the history of scientists doubting healers, it is especially important to examine unconscious tendencies in the team to be dismissive toward healers. In addition, it is important to respect and understand cultural differences which may be present, such as whether it is important or insulting for a healer to be paid. Likewise, healers who participate in research studies should be fully appraised of the limitations they will experience and should be assessed for their motivation to participate in the study.

TARGET SYSTEMS

Distant healing studies have historically shown significant effects in trials of influence not only on human medical problems but also human physiology in the laboratory, on animals (Grad 1965; Snel & Van Der Sijde 1995; Bengston & Krinsley 2000; Chen et al. 2002; Bengston 2004; Bengston & Moga 2007), bacteria (Rauscher & Rubik 1983) and cells in vitro (Baumann et al. 1986; Braud 1989; Yount et al. 1997, 2004; Radin et al. 2004; Taft et al. 2005). Animal and in vitro targets are often chosen for reasons including lower cost, less complexity in running a trial and ease of isolating a particular outcome measure. In addition, in animals and certainly in in vitro systems, it is much easier to eliminate psychological and placebo effects.

POPULATION COMPARABILITY

The same general rules for choosing target populations in any study apply to distant healing, with special emphasis on population homogeneity and the need for thorough baseline assessments of factors which may influence outcome, such as social support, levels of depression and anxiety, meditation practice and spiritual beliefs. In smaller samples it may be appropriate to stratify or use pair-matching to ensure balance between comparison groups on these and other relevant medical factors.

HEALER ATTITUDE

Studies of distant healing, as with many psychosocial interventions, are studies of consciousness either directly or indirectly interacting with another living system. For this reason, it is important to consider issues pertaining to the relationship between the healer and the healing target. At the same time, we must consider the possibility of a target system contribution to the healing effect. Specifically, it may be important for the healing task to be motivating and relevant to the healer. For example, in developing studies in our own laboratory, we interview many healers who state that their preference would be to attempt to heal someone who was very ill, rather than to try and influence a minor problem. Despite staff concerns that healing someone very ill might be too hard, the healers insisted that this would bring forth their better efforts.

Another example of the importance of healer attitude toward the task and the target is a situation in which a chi gong master acting as a healer in our laboratory was asked to attempt to 'kill cancer cells in vitro'. He vehemently objected that, as a healer, he was prohibited from killing anything. The situation was resolved when he agreed to 'emit harmonizing chi energy' toward the cells, holding an intention equivalent to 'Thy will be done' with regard to the cells. The cells died significantly faster than controls (Yount et al. 1997). Similarly, in studies at Lawrence Berkeley Laboratories, CA, USA, healer Olga Worrel was not willing to attempt to kill *Salmonella* bacteria in vitro but she was willing (and able) to protect the *Salmonella* from the harmful effects of antibiotics (Rauscher & Rubik 1983).

SUBJECT BELIEFS

Questions have often been raised as to the relevance of subject beliefs about healing, religious orientation and desire for healing. Studies from the literature in parapsychology, for example, have repeatedly found that subjects who believe in clairvoyance or telepathy show higher scores on tests of psychic functioning than do non-believers (Schmeidler 1998). Very few studies have examined the contribution of belief specifically to healing. In our distant healing study EUHEALS patients blind to the intervention who believed that they had received healing had large and clinically relevant improvements, irrespective of the actual treatment (Walach et al. 2008).

SUBJECT COMFORT WITH HEALING

In addition to differences in belief in distant healing, there may also be differences among patients in their comfort level with being the target of distant healing efforts. For example, in the Byrd study, which used 393 subjects, an additional 57 patients who were invited to participate refused. Byrd (1988) states that some of these refusals were based on religious convictions – a point of view reiterated by a commentator in the *Wall Street Journal* who stated that if any doctor tried to pray for him, 'I would sue him'. We do not know if such opposition would modify the efficacy of distant healing efforts but it emphasizes the importance of documenting patients' attitude as well as obtaining informed consent.

SUBJECT DESIRE FOR HEALING

A potential confounder in healing experiments became clear with the publication of a study by Walker et al. (1997), in which it was found that alcoholic patients did worse if they believed family or friends were praying for them. This emphasizes the complexity of prayer in a social context. Patients might have relied on prayer, instead of on their own decision to come clean. In designing a healing study, it would therefore be reasonable to ask subjects to indicate their own level of desire for recovery, as well as their comfort with the possibility of others praying for them.

SUBJECT PARTICIPATION IN HEALING

There has been debate among researchers doing studies in distant healing as to whether it is important for subjects to know they are receiving healing efforts. The primary objection to such trials is that telling subjects they are receiving healing eliminates the blinding and introduces possible placebo or expectation effects. This can be achieved by three- or four-armed trials in which some patients are informed about being prayed for and some are not (Benson et al. 2006; Walach et al. 2008). The recent Study of the Therapeutic Effects of Intercessory Prayer (STEP) study (Benson et al. 2006) showed worse outcome for patients who knew that they were prayed for, pointing to a potential nocebo effect: it is difficult to predict what conclusions patients draw from the information they are given (see Chapter 16).

OUTCOME MEASURES

The choice of a measurable, definable, non-confounded outcome measure is crucial to the development of a meaningful study of distant healing. Ideally, study endpoints should include those that are objective, have adequate variability in the study population and are not modified by the measurement process or study participation. The outcome measurement tools should have been validated in work separate from the study. Some guidance can be found in Chapter 18.

RICH VERSUS SIMPLE MEASUREMENT

Also with healing studies there are different stages in research. Typically, early research, where not much is known, will want to describe a wide variety of potential outcomes to find out which ones might be sensitive measures, or in which areas effects can be detected. Such a broad array of outcomes is useful, but it is fraught with some statistical complications (see Chapter 17). This is the reason why researchers, especially at a later stage, tend to narrow down their outcome measures to a few, even to only one. This allows for very simple statistical tests and clear decisions. Normally, such an approach presupposes a very clear theory about the potential effect of the intervention, and some prior background knowledge. Neither is normally abundant in healing research. Hence a good alternative is a reasonable varied amount of outcome measures that are then tested in a multivariate approach. Here, single outcome measures are combined into one variate, a vector of all outcomes. Such a method produces one statistic and makes use of the intercorrelations of the measures. In further steps, one can then analyse which domains contribute to an effect, if there is any at all.

ESTABLISHING CAUSALITY

The biggest question in the field of distant healing is: Do distant healing efforts modify biological systems? Trials exploring this question will be successful only if they avoid the two central research errors: false-positive and false-negative conclusions. Avoidance of the false-positive result has been the chief focus of researchers and critics of distant healing research; however, to the extent that we are trying to sort one type of consciousness effect (distant healing) from another (hope and expectation), the false negative also presents a significant pitfall.

AVOIDING THE FALSE-POSITIVE RESULT

Hope and expectation are the chief confounders in studies of distant healing. While it is likely that hope and expectation effects would be synergistic with any true non-local healing effects, the focus of distant healing experiments is exploration of the role of healer intentionality in modifying subject outcomes, independent of subject or experimenter intentionality. The classical way of finding out is a clinical experiment (see Chapter 5). This consists of three elements that are not necessarily interlinked, but are often used conjointly: randomization, blinding and sham control.

Randomization means that out of a population of individuals the allocation of an individual to the treatment group is purely random. This distributes potential, and more importantly, unknown, confounding variables evenly in the population and so the only difference between the group is the experimental intervention. Blinding means that patients, researchers, nurses or doctors dealing with patients and taking measurements and study personnel in general do not know which group a patient belongs to.

Different types of studies answer different questions. While the common knowledge still is that double-blind, placebo-controlled randomized trials are preferable, because they are most rigorous, the view adopted in this book is that each type of study answers different questions and they should all be used when indicated, and no single study type preferred. For instance, if one wants to know whether spiritual healing is more effective than doing nothing in wound recovery, a simple large randomized open study might tell us. If we want to know whether the healing effect is specific and different from the expectation of patients to receive healing, we will have to blind some of the patients to the treatment they receive. The benefit of distant healing studies is that sham control can be avoided, as the healing happens or does not happen at a distance and patients and personnel have no way of telling. It has to be borne in mind, though, that extraordinary claims require extraordinary proofs. So only rigorous studies will be able to settle the dispute.

Double-blind randomized controlled trials (RCTs)

The purpose of blinding in the RCT is to minimize any elements of hope, expectation or belief that might mediate a differential outcome.

Blinding protocols. Adequate blinding is essential. For a definitive test of efficacy of a distant healing modality, it is required that:

- patients do not know their group assignment
- no research staff member may know of subject group assignment
- no outside treating personnel may know of group assignment.

The only person who may know a subject's group assignment is the healer. Ideally, the healer and patient never meet and the healer has insufficient information about the patient to describe or contact him or her (e.g. first name or photo only). An elaborate example of how blinding can be achieved in an organizationally complex study can be found in the study by Walach et al. (2002).

Use of sham control conditions. Under some conditions, for example when the healing treatment requires that the healer be present in the room with the patient, alternative blinding schemes can be used. In studies of non-contact therapeutic touch, Quinn (1989) used a sham condition in which the healer was present for control patients, made hand passes over the patient's body but did not 'hold a healing intention'. Instead she performed mental arithmetic. This protocol has the advantage of preserving the integrity of the intervention as it is performed in the community but raises concerns either that the healer may not be able to 'turn off' her healing ability (leading to a false negative) or that the patient might perceive in the healer's affect whether or not healing is being performed (false positive). Another example involves stage actors mimicking the actions of healers without further healing intentions (Abbot et al. 2001). However, as long as we do not know what might be the underlying mechanism, it is difficult to tell whether the lack of difference seen in the Abbot study is due to the strong placebo effect induced by the actors in the sham condition, or whether actors mimicking healers might in fact be healers unbeknown to themselves.

In studies in which the principal outcome measure is believed to be objectively stable, e.g. stroke-related paralysis that has been documented stable for years, tests of in-person healing can be done if subject condition is documented over an initial waiting period of 1 or 2 months, then an intervention or sham intervention is performed and an investigator blind to the condition makes a second assessment. Both these types of protocol allow testing of hands-on healing or healing in which the healer believes he or she must be in the room.

It is not recommended that investigators use a control condition that does not mimic the healing condition, as the expectation effect for prayer and distant healing may be presumed in certain individuals to be the guiding principle of their lives.

In vitro trials. In in vitro trials it is also important to create sham treatment conditions for control samples. Any control sample should travel to the same room on the same schedule as treatment samples, be handled in the same way, and position in test tube racks or incubators should be the same as for treatment samples. To assess mechanical and environmental factors further, in laboratory comparison studies, it is also useful to use systematic negative controls as introduced by Walleczek (2000) and used by Yount (Radin et al. 2004; Yount et al. 2004; Taft et al. 2005). In this methodology, some trials compare a treated sample with a sham-treated sample whereas others compare sham treatment with sham treatment. This allows assessment of baseline variability in the treatment system. Many investigators have also used thermistor devices to ensure that healer hand temperatures do not affect treatment samples.

AVOIDING THE FALSE-NEGATIVE RESULT

While most of the attention in distant healing studies is on eliminating the false-positive or type I error, there are a number of ways in which a positive result could be ignored or washed out by the experimental protocol. This mostly applies to situations where subject self-report of symptoms is a primary outcome or where outcomes are known to be modified by a subject's emotional state. This type of potential confounder has been seen in studies of distant healing in blood pressure (Beutler 1988), asthma (Attevelt 1988) and depression (Greyson 1996), in which patients were required to make regular clinic visits for interviews or attend sessions of relaxing in an empty room while blind to a treatment condition, or where baseline medication introduced a ceiling effect on top of which healing could not add much.

Subject study-related activity should be minimized, e.g. it is preferable that subjects do not come to the lab or clinic for regular study-related activities, that they do not keep a study-related journal, that they are not instructed to meditate once a day to make them 'more receptive' and that they are not telephoned by staff members to 'see how they are doing'. Any such activity has the potential to alter (usually reduce) symptoms. This symptom reduction will be equally present in both the treatment and control groups and may wash out a possibly more subtle treatment effect. Unless the healing intervention is thought to require the immediate presence of the healer, it is best that, once enrolled in the study, subjects have little or no contact with study personnel and that outcome measurement activities be kept to a minimum.

Effects of social pressure and expectation are well known in the social sciences (e.g. Hawthorn effect: see Chapters 16 and 18). If subjects in double-blind experiments are overly encouraged to think an effect may occur, if they feel they have to 'please' the experimenter by showing improvement or if they interact with other study subjects who may be receiving the treatments, the effects of psychological pressure may lead to patients either psychophysically self-generating improved symptoms or simply inflating improvement scores on assessment tools. This 'pleasing' or 'peer pressure' effect is an equal risk among control or treatment subjects. These factors could wash out a potential distant healing effect, too. For this reason it is recommended that subjects do not interact with each other and that, at study enrolment, investigators limit their enthusiasm for the treatment.

EXPERIMENTER EFFECTS

Experimenter effects have been widely documented and discussed in the literature (Rosenthal 1976, 1984). They can lead to either false-positive or false-negative results. We should be aware of the following paradox: if we are using experimental methodology to prove distant intentionality true, we are in fact violating the very principle on which experimentation rests, or rather, we assume that it is not valid. Experimental methodology relies on the assumption that the experimental system is isolated against any outside effects, especially non-material intentionality effects. If we use that methodology to study such intentionality effects, we are in fact tacitly assuming that we can somehow confine inentionality effects within the experimental system which we create. This might, or might not, be the case. There is no reason to assume, if intentionality effects at a distance can occur in patients, why the experimenter should not have the same potential influence over his or her system, i.e. the whole experiment. Thus, research in distant healing presents a special case in which the assumptions underlying the RCT are challenged.

In fact, this issue was raised in the context of studies of the ability of research volunteers to influence the electrodermal activity of subjects in the next room (Braud & Schlitz 1983, 1991; Schlitz & Braud 1997; Schmidt et al. 2004). This double-blind randomized study was replicated in numerous laboratories in the USA but failed in the laboratory of a sceptical investigator, Richard Wiseman, in England. After repeated failures of the protocol in his laboratory, Wiseman invited a successful experimenter (Marilyn Schlitz) to replicate the experiment in his laboratory. In alternating trials, when Schlitz functioned as chief investigator, the positive results were found; when Wiseman was chief investigator the experiment failed (Wiseman & Schlitz 1997). We also found that experimenters may have distinctive influences unknown to them (Walach & Schmidt 1997), and in fact the parapsychology literature is full of similar examples (Kennedy & Taddonio 1976). Such studies highlight the point that when investigating effects of consciousness over distance, all sources of influence must be considered. It does not preclude the possibility of meaningful double-blind RCTs; if an investigator's non-local influence on an experimental population is minimal, neutral or equal then it is possible to determine whether or not the experimental treatment is effective. These observations suggest, first, the importance of the experimenter's interaction with subjects, especially with regard to whether he or she appears encouraging or discouraging. Second, it may be important in the future to conduct trials comparing outcomes by investigators with different levels of belief.

INTERPRETATION OF DATA

Because the implications of experimental claims for the efficacy of distant healing are so profound, the experimenter is obliged to hold his or her studies up to the most rigorous statistical scrutiny and maintain the highest methodological standards. In addition to keeping internal validity as high as possible, the researcher should also focus on adequate model validity, for instance by using expert healers' advice and opinion in design planning.

EVALUATION OF BASELINE FACTORS

It is especially important when analysing data from distant healing trials to discover whether there are interactions among relevant baseline variables and outcome measures. Unless these baseline–outcome correlations are measured and understood, the study will be open to criticism. It is therefore important to run correlation analyses between all baseline differences and all outcome measures, and control for such correlations by general linear models that include such variables (analysis of covariance). Specific baseline and independent variables which should be examined include: baseline psychological status, comorbidity, anxiety or depression, status of the disease, other sources of distant healing, beliefs about distant healing and the subject's guess as to whether he or she was in the treatment group or the control group, to name but the most important potential predictor variables.

STATISTICAL POWER

There has been a recent trend in meta-analyses to report data not only in terms of *P*-value but also to calculate an effect size. The reason for this is that in a trial with small numbers of subjects the power to detect treatment effects may be small, even if an effect is present. The use of effect size measurement in addition to standard analysis may assist in evaluation of pilot studies and may allow comparisons between degree of efficacy in treatments that have not yet been evaluated in direct comparison trials.

INTERPRETING RESULTS: QUALITATIVE AND MIXED-METHODS APPROACHES

Although the double-blind RCT is conventionally held to be the gold standard for establishing causality in clinical trials, qualitative studies are important to understand trial outcomes, especially if they have been equivocal. Hence, an increasing number of clinical researchers start to embark on qualitative studies embedded within or parallel to clinical trials. Such studies probe patients' experiences and document what they have understood of the information given to them, or what conclusions they have drawn from the complex ritual of a clinical study they have been exposed to. Such information might yield decisive insights into shortcomings of trial planning or other psychological processes triggered in patients through a study that might have been instrumental to changes, but not captured by outcome measures.

ETHICAL ISSUES

Research in distant healing raises the usual ethical issues involved in testing a treatment with unknown effects. One could argue that scientists have an ethical obligation to study distant healing as it is a modality for which important claims have been made, it is widely available and some people are choosing it over conventional therapies. Others argue that such research is not ethical because of a potential negative impact on subject belief systems as well as concerns as to possible negative uses of information from trials.

INFORMED CONSENT

As for all trials of an untested intervention, it is required that informed consent be obtained under the guidance of a certified human subjects safety review committee. Some investigators (Harris et al. 1999) have argued that, because there has not been definitive evidence of harm to patients in distant healing trials, informed consent is not required. We disagree. There is considerable evidence already in the published literature for the modification of biological states via the mechanism of distant healing (Benor 1992). Some of these data include the possibility of negative effects (Dossey 2002). As with all studies, potential loss of confidentiality should be considered a risk. As evidenced by the 14% refusal rate in the Byrd (1988) study, not all subjects are keen to receive healing. As evidenced by the negative outcome for alcoholics who knew they were prayed for by relatives in the study by Walker et al. (1997), there is clearly at least some psychological risk. An additional risk includes the possibility of anger and disappointment in subjects after they learn they have been in the control group, as occurred in one of our studies. Lastly, in psychiatric populations there may be an additional risk of paranoia or delusions associated with the idea of an unknown person at a distance attempting to influence one's body.

For the protection of the subjects, as well as of the investigators, informed consent should be obtained. Subjects should be told the probability of their being assigned to a treatment or a control group and that it is not known whether the treatment will be beneficial, neutral or harmful. They should be offered psychological or medical consultation if distress occurs as a result of participation in the trial.

MECHANISM OF EFFECT

This chapter has focused on methodology for establishing whether or not an effect is occurring, rather than exploring possible mechanisms of action. One reason for this is that one cannot investigate mechanisms before the effect is known to occur. Nevertheless, investigators who feel they have established replicable protocols may wish to pursue studies of mechanism. These trials can proceed in many ways, probably principally by identifying limits on efficacy, such as studying whether certain techniques or individuals show a more reliable effect, or examining potential shielding of targets or looking at a cellular or molecular level to understand what systems are being affected at a microscopic or chemical level.

Basically, there are two generic and quite contradictory ways of looking at such effects. The first one operates on the assumption that the effect is due to a subtle causal influence, for want of a good concept termed 'subtle energies'. This is conceptualized along the lines of a physical field, causative and stable, which can be isolated by good research (Rubik 1995). The prediction from such a conceptual framework would be that once a good experimental model has been identified and replicated, we will distil out an effect. The latest news is not good for such a concept. The initially positive results of the Byrd prayer study (Byrd 1988), that was the template for three replications, could not be replicated in full. While the first follow-up study was still positive (Harris et al. 1999), a subsequent trial reported a considerably smaller, non-significant effect (Aviles et al. 2001). The most recent one was quite puzzling: those who knew that they had been prayed for had significantly worse outcome (Benson et al. 2006).

The same pattern can be observed with an initially very positive outcome in a study of distant healing in acquired immunodeficiency syndrome (AIDS) (Sicher et al. 1998) that could not be replicated in a larger study (Astin et al. 2006). The Monitoring and Actualization of Noetic Training (MANTRA) study that explored prayer-augmented visual imagery in angioscopy had a very promising start as a pilot (Krucoff et al. 2001) but could not be replicated (Krucoff et al. 2005). Our own study did not show any indication of a specific healing effect either (Walach et al. 2008). Experimental models that have been sufficiently replicated tended not to replicate initially positive results (Taft et al. 1997, 2005; Radin et al. 2004; Yount et al. 2004; Zachariae et al. 2005). Hence, the general assumption about the purported 'subtle' causal effect rests on shaky ground at the moment. These findings fit well with the current focus on the importance of expectancy and belief for self-healing (see Chapter 16). While most people now draw the conclusion that healing is likely to be just a placebo or expectancy effect, this is not the only option.

The second way of looking at these results is to question the underlying assumptions and proceed on the hypothesis that the effects are not due to causal influences but due to non-local correlations that are not causal, but nevertheless meaningful (Walach 2005). Such a model could explain both the fact that in uncontrolled practice healing is potentially useful, but not replicable in experimental research. It would in fact predict just that (Lucadou et al. 2007). If this model is true, then no matter how much we experiment, we will not find the effect. Such an approach would call for a more naturalistic study that does not interfere with the system to be studied too much. It would predict that healing might be researchable in difficult situations, single case studies, and wherever no manipulation is carried out. Hence observational or open randomized studies would be the designs of choice here.

BARRIERS TO RESEARCH

Until these conceptual questions are not answered well there will be a paradigmatic barrier between the mainstream research paradigm and the one possibly required by healing research. But only research will be able to tell us how these questions are to be answered.

An additional barrier to research is caused by the existence of a social and academic stigma toward researchers who engage in studies of what many consider to be an implausible or laughable treatment. The only place in the medical literature where paranormal abilities are currently indexed, for example, is within psychiatry under the definitions for psychosis and schizophrenia. It is therefore not surprising that many experimenters feel uncomfortable about expressing an interest in pursuing studies in the area of conscious influence at a distance.

Another, somewhat surprising source of resistance has been religious communities. Some religious people have understandably objected to scientists equating 'intentionality' with prayer. This has led to the concern that testing distant healing is a form of 'testing God' and therefore interfering with the sacred and highly personal relationship of faith.

WHY DO DISTANT HEALING RESEARCH?

Prayer and distant healing have been part of nearly every culture since the dawn of civilization. If research determines that it has a measurable effect, under double-blind conditions, on any group of physical or psychological findings, this might encourage health care practitioners of all descriptions to include distant healing modalities as part of their treatment plans. If no effects are measured, research should focus on understanding the ways in which the culture around prayer or healing activities serves to lift the spirits and enrich the lives of patients.

Without evidence from rigorous trials, it is not appropriate for physicians either to recommend or discourage distant healing; with such evidence, they will be in an informed position from which usefully to guide their patients.

Future research will help define the conditions (medical, psychological, physical) under which effects are most likely to be measurable, mechanisms by which healing may occur, target systems that are most amenable, the common denominators and necessary factors for distant healing interventions, the relationship between spiritual issues and distant healing outcomes and whether individuals can be trained to improve their distant healing abilities.

Future research might unveil that at the base of healing and prayer effects lies a completely different category of effects we have not even thought of before. Hence, research in such effects is not only another branch of CAM research, but also has important foundational and paradigmatic consequences.

SUMMARY

- The double-blind RCT is the gold standard for trials of prayer and distant healing.
- It presupposes that a stable, causal agent is operative in healing that can be isolated through repeated experimentation; researchers should be aware that the subject matter of distant healing might violate these very presuppositions.
- Adequate blinding and randomization procedures should be followed and documented.
- The intervention must be well defined (including frequency, amount of time and training and/or experience level of healers).
- Baseline information, including psychological status, beliefs about prayer and healing and other sources of prayer and healing, should be collected from subjects in clinical trials. This should be examined as part of the final data analysis for contribution to outcomes.
- Objectively measurable outcomes with adequate variability should be chosen.
- Subject study participation activities, such as clinical interviews, travelling to special sites, journalling or meditation should be minimized to avoid washing out a small effect.
- In clinical trials subjects should be asked if they believed they were in the treatment group and this information should be entered as a co-variate for data analysis.
- Healers/those praying should be treated in a collegial and respectful way. Their healing efforts (time, location, method) should be documented in a log and they should be periodically contacted and encouraged by experimenters if the study is taking place over an extended period of time.
- Observational and outcomes research can add an important dimension to healing research.
- Qualitative studies may also make an important contribution and help guide the development of future controlled trials or understand conflicting data from current studies.

REFERENCES

Abbot, N.C., Harkness, E.F., Stevinson, C., et al., 2001. Spiritual healing as a therapy for chronic pain: a randomized, clinical trial. Pain 91, 79–89.

Astin, J.A., Stone, J., Abrams, D.I., et al., 2006. The efficacy of distant healing for human immunodeficiency virus – Results of a randomized trial. Altern. Ther. Health Med. 12, 36–41.

Attevelt, J.T.M., 1988. Research into paranormal healing. State University of Utrecht.

Aviles, J.M., Whelan, E., Hernke, D.A., et al., 2001. Intercessory prayer and cardiovascular disease progression in a coronary care unit population: a randomized controlled trial. Mayo Clinics Proceedings 76, 1192–1198.

Barnes, P.M., Powell-Griner, E., McFann, K., et al., Complementary and alternative medicine use among adults: United States, 2002. Center for Disease Control: Advance Data from Vital and Health Statistics. 2004 (343) (May 27).

Baumann, S., Lagle Stewart, J., Roll, W.G., 1986. Preliminary results from the use of two novel detectors for psychokinesis. In: Weiner, D.H., Radin, D.I. (Eds.), Research in Parapsychology. Scarecrow, Metuchen, NJ, pp. 59–62.

Bengston, W.F., 2004. Methodological difficulties involving control groups in healing research: parallels between laying on of hands for the treatment of induced mammary cancers in mice to research in homeopathy? J. Altern. Complement. Med. 10, 227–230.

Bengston, W.F., Krinsley, D., 2000. The effect of the 'Laying on of Hands' on transplanted breast cancer in mice. Journal of Scientific Exploration 14, 353–364.

Bengston, W.F., Moga, M., 2007. Resonance, placebo effects, and Type II errors: Somo implications from healing research for experimental methods. J. Altern. Complement. Med. 13, 317–327.

Benor, D.J., 1992. Healing Research. Holistic Energy Medicine and Spirituality. vol. 1, Research in Healing. Helix, Munich.

Benor, D.J., 2001. Spiritual Healing: Scientific Validation of a Healing Revolution. Vision Publications, Southfield, Mi.

Benson, H., Dusek, J.A., Sherwood, J.B., et al., 2006. Study of the Therapeutic Effects of Intercessory Prayer (STEP) in cardiac bypass patients: A multicenter randomized trial of uncertainty and certainty of receiving intercessory prayer. Am. Heart J. 151, 934–942.

Beutler, J.J., 1988. Paranormal Healing and Hypertension. Br. Med. J. 296, 1491–1494.

Braud, W., 1989. Distant mental influence on rate of hemolysis. In: Roll, W.G., Morris, R.L., Morris, J.D. (Eds.), Research in parapsychology. Scarecrow, Metuchen, NJ, pp. 1–6.

Braud, W., Schlitz, M., 1983. Psychokinetic influence on electrodermal activity. J. Parapsychol. 47, 95–119.

Braud, W.G., Schlitz, M.J., 1991. Conscious interactions with remote biological systems: Anomalous intentionality effects. Subtle Energies 2, 1–46.

Brennan, B., 1987. Hands of Light. Bantam, New York.

Byrd, R.C., 1988. Positive therapeutic effects of intercessory prayer in a coronary care unit population. South. Med. J. 81, 826–829.

Chen, K.W., Shiflett, S.C., Ponzio, N.M., et al., 2002. A preliminary study of the effect of externa Qigong on lymphoma growth in mice. J. Altern. Complement. Med. 8, 615–621.

Cooperstein, M.A., 1992. The myths of healing: A summary of research into transpersonal healing experiences. Journal of the American Society for Psychical Research 86, 99–133.

Dossey, L., 1993. Healing Words: The Power of Prayer and the Practice of Medicine. Harper, San Francisco.

Dossey, L., 1997. Running scared: how we hide from who we are. Altern. Ther. Health Med. 3, 8–15.

Dossey, L., 2002. The dark side of consciousness and the therapeutic relationship. Altern. Ther. Health Med. 8 (6), 12–16.

Galton, F., 1872. Statistical inquiry into the efficacy of prayer. Fortnightly Review 68, New Series(August 1), 125–135.

Grad, B., 1965. Some biological effects of the 'Laying on of Hands': a review of experiments with animals and plants. Journal of the American Society for Psychic Research 59, 95–129.

Greyson, B., 1996. Distance healing of patients with major depression. Journal of Scientific Exploration 10, 447–465.

Halifax, J., 1979. Shamanic voices: a survey of visionary narratives. Arkana Books, New York.

Harris, W.S., Gowda, M., Kolb, J.W., et al., 1999. A randomized, controlled trial of the effects of remote, intercessory prayer on outcomes in patients admitted to the coronary care unit. Arch. Intern. Med. 159, 2273–2278.

Kennedy, J.E., Taddonio, J.L., 1976. Experimenter effects in parapsychological research. J. Parapsychol. 40, 1–33.

Krieger, D., 1975. Therapeutic touch: the imprimatur of nursing. Am. J. Nurs. 7, 784–787.

Krippner, S., Villoldo, A., 1979. The Realms of Healing. Celestial Arts, Milbrae, CA.

Krucoff, M.W., Crater, S.W., Green, C.L., et al., 2001. Integrative noetic therapies as adjuncts to percutaneous intervention during unstable coronary syndromes: Monitoring and Actualization of Noetic Training (MANTRA) feasibility study. Am. Heart J. 142, 760–767.

Krucoff, M.W., Crater, S.W., Gallup, D., et al., 2005. Music, imagery, touch, and prayer as adjuncts to interventional cardiac care: the Monitoring and Actualisation of Noetic Trainings (MANTRA) II randomised study. Lancet 366, 211–217.

Lucadou, W.V., Römer, H., Walach, H., 2007. Synchronistic Phenomena as Entanglement Correlations in Generalized Quantum Theory. Journal of Consciousness Studies 14, 50–74.

O'Laoire, S., 1997. An experimental study of the effects of distant, intercessory prayer on self-esteem, anxiety, and depression. Altern. Ther. Health Med. 3, 38–53.

Quinn, J.F., 1989. Therapeutic touch as energy exchange: replication and extension. Nurs. Sci. Q. 2 (2), 79–87.

Radin, D., Taft, R., Yount, G., 2004. Effects of healing intention on cultured cells and truly random events. J. Altern. Complement. Med. 10, 103–112.

Rauscher, E.A., Rubik, B., 1983. Human volitional effects on a modal bacterial system. Psi Research 2 (1), 38.

Rosenthal, R., 1976. Experimenter Effects in Behavioral Research. Irvington Publishers, New York.

Rosenthal, R., 1984. Interpersonal expectancy effects and psi: Some communalities and differences. New Ideas in Psychology 2, 47–50.

Rubik, B., 1995. Energy medicine and the unifying concert of information. Altern. Ther. Health Med. 1 (1), 34–36.

Schlitz, M., Braud, W., 1997. Distant intentionality and healing: Assessing the evidence. Altern. Ther. Health Med. 3, 38–53.

Schmeidler, G.R., 1998. Parapsychology and psychology. Mc Farland, Jefferson, N.C.

Schmidt, S., Schneider, R., Utts, J., et al., 2004. Remote intention on electrodermal activity – Two meta-analyses. Br. J. Psychol. 95, 235–247.

Sicher, F., Targ, E., Moore, D., et al., 1998. A randomized double-blind study of the effect of distant healing in a population with advanced AIDS. Report of a small scale study. West. J. Med. 169, 356–363.

Snel, F.W.J., Hol, P.R., 1983. Psychokinesis experiments in casein-induced amyloidosis of the hamster. J. Parapsychol. 5 (1), 51–76.

Snel, F.W.J.J., Van Der Sijde, P.C., 1995. The effect of paranormal healing on tumor growth. Journal of Scientific Exploration 9, 209–221.

Taft, R., Moore, D., Yount, G., 2005. Time-lapse analysis of potential cellular responsiveness to Johrei, a Japanese healing technique. BMC Complement. Altern. Med. 5 (1), 2.

Targ, E.F., 1997. Evaluating distant healing: a research review. Altern. Ther. Health Med. 3 (6), 74–78.

Thomson, K.S., 1996. The revival of experiments on prayer. American Science 84, 532–534.

Vickers, A., Cassileth, B., Ernst, E., et al., 1997. How should we research unconventional therapies? Int. J. Technol. Assess. Health Care 13 (1), 10–15.

Walach, H., 2005. Generalized Entanglement: A new theoretical model for understanding the effects of Complementary and Alternative Medicine. J. Altern. Complement. Med. 11, 549–559.

Walach, H., Schmidt, S., 1997. Empirical evidence for a non-classical experimenter effect: An experimental, double-blind investigation of unconventional information transfer. Journal of Scientific Exploration 11, 59–68.

Walach, H., Bösch, H., Haraldsson, E., et al., 2002. Efficacy of distant healing – a proposal for a four-armed randomized study (EUHEALS). Forsch. Komplementärmed. Klass. Naturheilkd. 9, 168–176.

Walach, H., Bösch, H., Lewith, G., et al., 2008. Efficacy of distant healing in patients with chronic fatigue syndrome: A randomised controlled partially blinded trial (EUHEALS). Psychother. Psychosom. 77, 158–166.

Walker, S.R., Tonigan, J.S., Miller, W.R., et al., 1997. Intercessory prayer in the treatment of alcohol abuse and dependense: a pilot investigation. Altern. Ther. Health Med. 3, 79–86.

Walleczek, J. (Ed.), 2000. Self-Organized Biological Dynamics and Nonlinear Control. Toward Understanding Complexity, Chaos and Emergent Function. Cambridge University Press, Cambridge.

Watkins, G.K., Watkins, A.M., 1971. Possible PK influence on the resuscitation of anesthetized mice. J. Parapsychol. 35 (4), 257–272.

Wiseman, R., Schlitz, M., 1997. Experimenter effects and the remote detection of staring. J. Parapsychol. 61, 197–208.

Yount, G.L., Quian, C., Smith, H., 1997. Cell biology meets chi gong. 16th Annual Meeting of the Society for Scientific Exploration, Las Vegas.

Yount, G., Smith, S., Avanozian, V., et al., 2004. Biofield perception: A series of pilot studies with cultured human cells. J. Altern. Complement. Med. 10, 463–467.

Zachariae, R., Hojgaard, L., Zachariae, C., et al., 2005. The effect of spiritual healing on in vitro tumour cell proliferation and viability – an experimental study. Br. J. Cancer. 93 (5), 538–543.

FURTHER READING

Colditz, G., Miller, J.N., Mosteller, F., 1989. How study design affects outcomes in comparisons of therapy. I. Stat. Med. 8, 441–454.

Dossey, L., 1995. How should alternative therapies be evaluated: an examination of fundamentals. Altern. Ther. Health Med. 1 (2), 6–9.

Dossey, L., 1997. The return of prayer. Altern. Ther. Health Med. 3 (6), 10–15.

Kiene, H.A., 1996. Critique of the double-blind clinical trial. Altern. Ther. Health Med. 2 (1), 74–80.

Rubik, B., 1995. Energy medicine and the unifying concept of information. Altern. Ther. Health Med. 1, 34–36.

Schmeidler, G.R., 1988. Parapsychology and psychology. McFarland, Jefferson, NC.

Thomson, K.S., 1996. The revival of experiments on prayer. American Science Journal 84, 532–534.

Vickers, A., Cassileth, B., Ernst, E., Fisher, P., Goldman, P., Jonas, W., et al., 1997. How should we research unconventional therapies? Int. J. Technol. Assess. Health Care. 13 (1), 111–121.

Manipulation

Alan Breen

13

CHAPTER CONTENTS

INTRODUCTION

Manipulation is a mechanical treatment that has often been recommended in national evidence-based guidelines for common musculoskeletal disorders (Agency for Health Care Policy Research 1994; Waddell et al. 1999; (NHMRC) NHaMRC 2003; Airaksinen et al. 2006; van Tulder et al. 2006; Haldeman et al. 2008; NICE 2008). Such is the volume of evidence for its clinical value that it may be reasonable to ask why it is still sometimes regarded as a complementary therapy. However, part of the reason for this probably lies in gaps in the research literature in relation to its role in care. Firstly, manipulative treatment implies a rationale that links a reduction of mechanical dysfunction to improvement in health, but the relevance of mechanical dysfunction models in health remains unclear in the research literature. Secondly, manipulation is not generally practised as a monotherapy, because practitioners usually

DOI: 10.1016/B978-0-443-06956-7.00013-6

provide other interventions along with it (Burton 1981; Huisman & Breen 1990; Pedersen 1994; Wilson 2003; Chown et al. 2008). The effects of manipulation cannot therefore be the only factors in play. This requires us to consider those of the other interventions that may often accompany it (Harvey et al. 2003). Research in this context is relatively new.

The third reason relates to its provision in health care. Manipulation and the other components of the care that surrounds it take a long time to learn if they are to be practised competently. This makes it difficult, if not impossible, to incorporate manipulation into undergraduate medical training. More importantly, the musculoskeletal conditions for which it is mainly used do not fit well into a purely biomedical model of health, even though they do constitute a huge societal cost to industrialized nations (World Health Organization 2001). Instead, they also usually call for a functional approach. Because the health, social and societal costs of musculoskeletal disorders are generally considered separately, their real impact on the gross domestic product of western countries is seldom fully appreciated. Public resources for their care are generally given relatively low priority compared to, for example, cancer and heart disease. Sufferers are also sometimes denigrated as the 'walking wounded' and their practitioners regarded as somewhat marginal (Coulter & Shekelle 2005).

The scope for gaining useful knowledge around this topic through research is therefore very wide and ranges from the most intrinsic to the most global of health issues. This chapter will attempt to provide an overview of these.

WHAT IS MANIPULATION?

Manipulation is most commonly defined as: 'a small amplitude, high velocity movement at the limit of joint range taking the joint beyond its passive range of movement, without exceeding its anatomical integrity' (Sandoz 1969; Figure 13.1). This is therapeutically different from mobilization, which

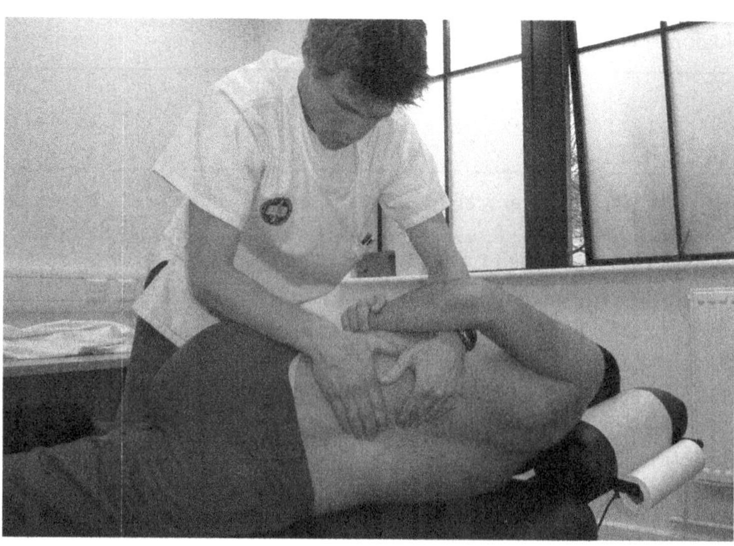

FIGURE 13.1 A lumbar manipulation.

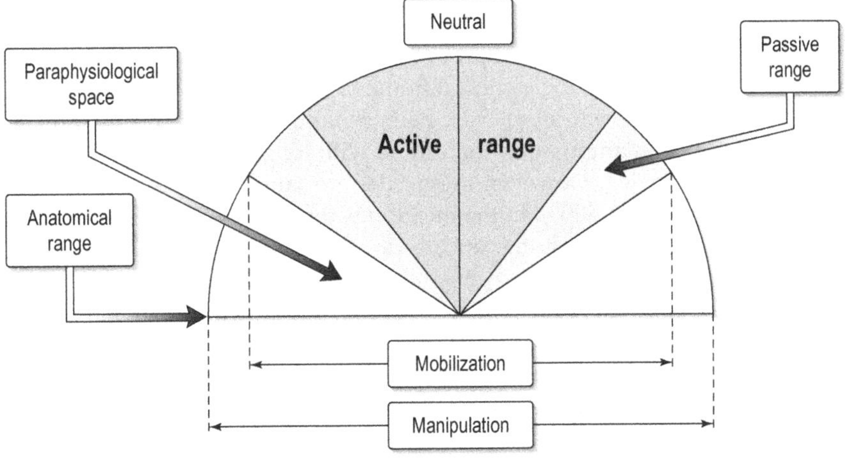

FIGURE 13.2 Theoretical differences between manipulation and mobilization.

is a repetitive passive movement (i.e. within the passive range) (Harvey et al. 2003) (Figure 13.2). Manipulation is sometimes accompanied by an audible pop, or cavitation (Unsworth et al. 1971). However it has been argued that this is not necessary to qualify as a successful procedure (Flynn et al. 2003). Apparently, when it does occur, it may also come from multiple surrounding joints (Ross et al. 2004). The possible effects of cavitation manipulation on the mechanics of joints have been extensively discussed (Evans 2002; Evans & Breen 2007), but useful experimental studies in living subjects are difficult to perform (Reeves et al. 2007).

THE MECHANICAL DYSFUNCTION MODEL

Until relatively recently, the mechanical dysfunction model of health was portrayed as an alternative paradigm, propounded by heterodox practitioners who offered it for all manner of conditions (Hewitt & Wood 1975). However, we now know that such care is used by the public more to complement conventional practice than to replace it (Eisenberg et al. 1993; Thomas et al. 2001), mainly for common musculoskeletal complaints and especially for low-back pain (Breen 1977; Burton 1981; Pedersen 1994). Trial evidence reviews have shown that spinal manipulation, which depends on such a model, has moderately positive effects for low-back pain (Assendelft et al. 2004). The problem is that this evidence is not consistent, which tempts a certain amount of selective reporting by reviewers. It also reflects the heterogeneity of the samples, interventions, trial designs and outcome measures. Nonetheless, its recommendation as a treatment in most back pain guidelines (European Commission CBMC 2006; Chou & Huffman 2007; Hurwitz et al. 2008) is on the basis of reducing pain and disability in people who are not recovering spontaneously from acute back pain (van Tulder et al. 2006) or are suffering exacerbations of chronic back pain (Airaksinen et al. 2006). More research has been called for to identify the kinds of patients who will benefit most from manipulation (van Tulder et al. 2006).

THE ESTABLISHMENT OF SUBGROUPS

One approach to identifying subgroups has been to develop and test prediction rules based on accessible clinical findings (Childs et al. 2004). For example, patients with recent-onset back pain, without leg pain, are thought to respond better to manipulation than those with longer-duration pain which radiates down the leg. However, these rules are said to require further validation (Hancock et al. 2008). In the meantime, the accepted model of care for people who are not recovering, once serious pathology has been excluded, is to adopt a psychosocial and general physical fitness approach (Waddell 1998). Despite reasonable rationales for a relationship between biomechanics and spinal pain, therefore, we lack scientific explanation of how manipulation confers benefit. Furthermore biomechanical measures themselves are seldom recommended for use for assessing outcomes (Pincus et al. 2008a).

How then could manipulation contribute to reduction in pain and disability for such conditions? It is common to refer to laboratory studies of cadaveric spines (White & Panjabi 1990) to try to understand how mechanical interventions reduce spinal pain and disability. These studies have shown, for example, that during trunk movement, stiff segments transfer mechanical stress to adjacent ones, causing abnormal force concentrations there (Bowden et al. 2008). Motion segments that become lax may repeatedly tug at their attachments during unguarded movements. It makes sense to think that this could result in pain and a variety of other neuromuscular effects (Panjabi 1992a, b; Panjabi et al. 1992). It is not difficult to imagine how spinal manipulation could influence this, but there is no good clinical evidence that it happens in patients and is related to pain.

HOW DO WE INVESTIGATE THE MECHANICAL DYSFUNCTION MODEL?

Part of the rationale for manipulation is to increase intervertebral motion and reduce painful deformation of intervertebral discs and ligaments (Haldeman 1996). For example, there is some evidence that manipulation may increase overall range in the cervical spine (Nansel et al. 1989; Cassidy et al. 1992; Nilsson et al. 1996). However, increasing range of motion has not been confirmed as being associated with reduced disability or pain (Nattrass et al. 1999) and evidence that the manipulation of spinal segments actually does increase their range is rare. This is largely due to poor reliability in the measurement of intervertebral motion from the end-of-range radiographs that are traditionally used for this (Shaffer et al. 1990; Panjabi et al. 1992; Mayer et al. 1995). The field of spine stabilization surgery suffers from similar problems (Reeves et al. 2007) and we have long needed an objective and reliable way of measuring spine kinematics in living subjects. However, this is gradually becoming possible using quantitative fluoroscopy, which is a combination of digital fluoroscopy and image processing (Teyhen et al. 2005; Breen et al. 2006; Wong et al. 2006) where hundreds of digital X-ray images are recorded as the patient is moved and the motions of the vertebrae are tracked and recorded using computer programs (Figure 13.3). A graphical example of increased range of motion following lumbar manipulation is shown using this technology in Figure 13.4.

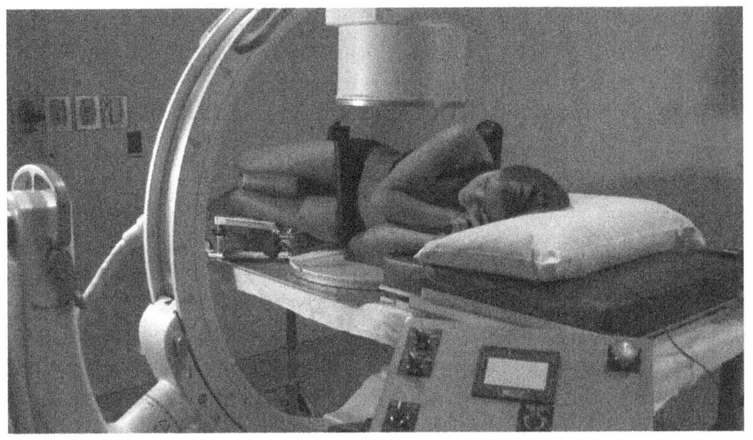

FIGURE 13.3 Quantitative fluoroscopy image acquisition. *With kind permission of Ortho Kinematics, Inc, USA.*

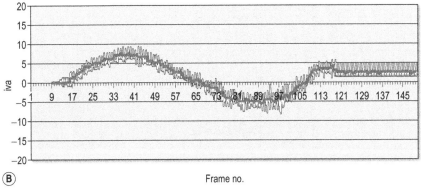

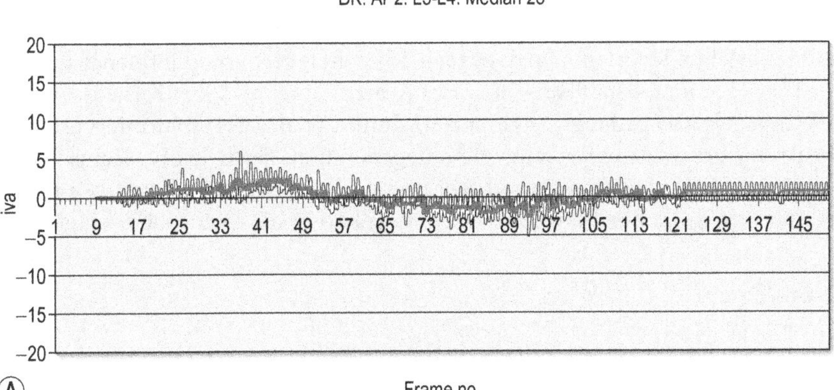

FIGURE 13.4 Increase in intervertebral side-bending motion (iva) after manipulation (from quantitative fluoroscopic studies). A Pre-manipulation; B post-manipulation.

These quantitative fluoroscopic studies have the potential to reveal what previously only cadaveric studies could show. Since most back and neck pain is not associated with either serious pathology or nerve compression, subgrouping of 'non-specific' spinal pain is essential and some of these subgroups may be mechanical ones.

'INSTABILITY'

Perhaps the most popular model of pain-producing mechanical dysfunction of the spine is segmental 'instability', which until recently has only been quantifiable in specimens (Reeves et al. 2007). The term 'instability' is probably inappropriate in relation to non-traumatic mechanical spinal disorders and investigators have traditionally used alternatives such as 'hypermobility' (Van Akkerveeken et al. 1979) and 'laxity' (Fernandez-Bermego et al. 1993). However, given the wide variation of the normal range of intervertebral motion, 'hypermobility', taken as increased range alone, would be difficult to associate with pain. Laxity, however, may be another matter. A lax joint does not necessarily move too far under normal physiological stresses – it moves too fast. This distinction is embedded in Panjabi's 'neutral zone' theory (Panjabi 1992a, b), in which pain is generated when tissues fail to restrain their vertebrae near the neutral position (Figure 13.5), causing altered loading during motion and irritation at its end-range. It is a small step to imagine how manual therapies, aimed at the vertebral levels involved, or their adjacent levels, could influence this.

There are long-established theories (Gertzbein et al. 1985; Kirkaldy-Willis 1992), as well as cadaveric evidence (Mimura et al. 1994) that intervertebral laxity occurs with early-stage disc degeneration. Such laxity seems to be caused by loss of normal intradiscal pressure, which, under load, is a major restraining influence between vertebrae (Zhao et al. 2005). Early-stage disc

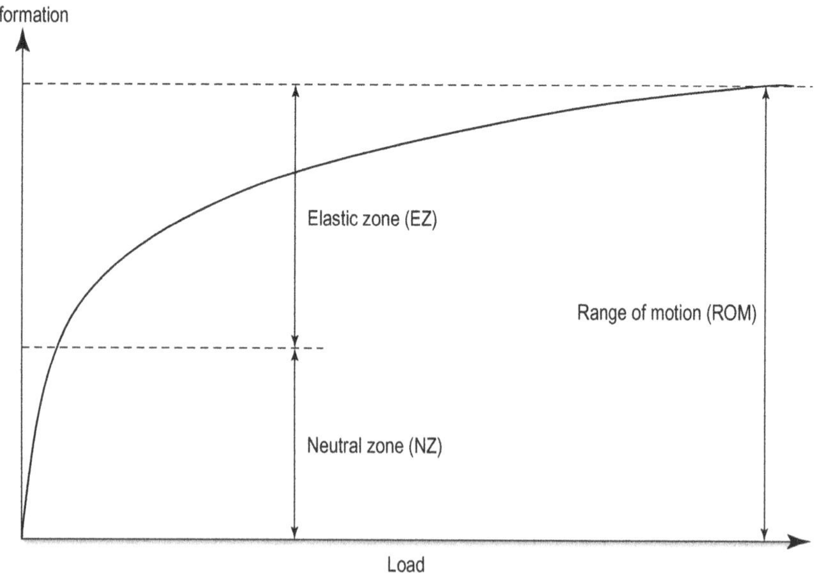

FIGURE 13.5 The neutral zone (Panjabi 1992b).

degeneration is much more readily detectible with magnetic resonance than with plain X-rays (Pfirrmann et al. 2001) but there is emerging evidence, also from magnetic resonance studies, of an association between aberrant (paradoxical) intervertebral motion and disc degeneration as detected by magnetic resonance (Fowler et al. 2006), adding weight to the concept of aberrant motion as a source of mechanical pain.

Recent quantitative fluoroscopy research has moved this model of mechanical dysfunction from the realm of theory to that of biomechanical measurement and from cadaveric to patient studies. Separate from this, and using cadaveric studies, Mimura et al. (1994) and Zhao et al. (2005) established a relationship between laxity and early disc degeneration, expressing it as the proportion of overall intervertebral range that is achieved in the neutral zone. Using quantitative fluoroscopy, Wong et al. (2004) and Breen et al. (2000a) then measured it in living subjects. The latter also demonstrated lax appearance in the motion patterns of lumbar motion segments adjacent to surgically stabilized ones (Figure 13.6).

It is important to have a practical measurement of laxity to use in patient studies. Wong et al. (2004) used the slope of intervertebral motion against trunk motion to express laxity (Figure 13.7). Mellor et al. (2008) used both the slope of intervertebral to trunk motion and the proportion of the intervertebral range in the first 10° of trunk motion. Such studies are gradually accumulating normative reference information with which to compare patient data.

What this amounts to is the capability to measure intervertebral laxity and the influence that physical therapies may have upon it in living subjects. This is a new horizon in research into spinal manipulation that could lead to better trials of efficacy. It should then also be possible to establish whether manipulation does, as in Figure 13.4, restore mobility to stiff spinal joints. This old concept of the mechanism of spinal manipulation (Haldeman 1992; Peterson & Bergmann 2002; Liebenson 2006; Morris 2006) would then at last be testable. However, this is just the beginning. The mechanical effects of manipulation could also be explained by changes in muscle activity and length (Sihvonen et al. 1991; Kaigle et al. 1998; Mannion 1999; Lariviere et al. 2002) and by neurological and circulatory effects (Sandoz 1978; Wyke 1985). This adds further levels of complexity and calls for even more sophistication in study design.

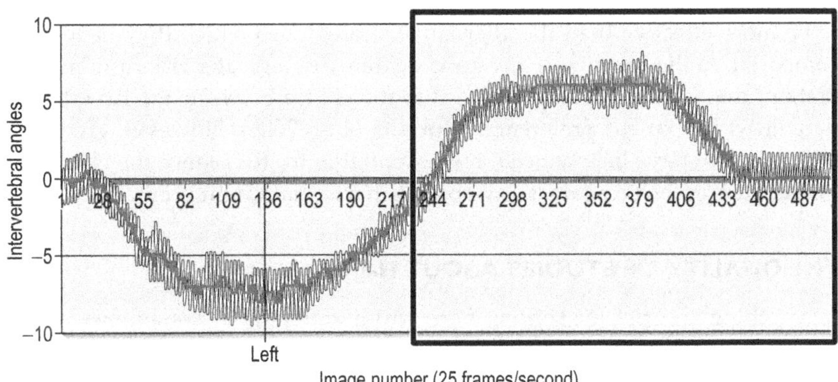

FIGURE 13.6 Example of intervertebral laxity in right lateral bending in a patient *(from quantitative fluoroscopic studies).*

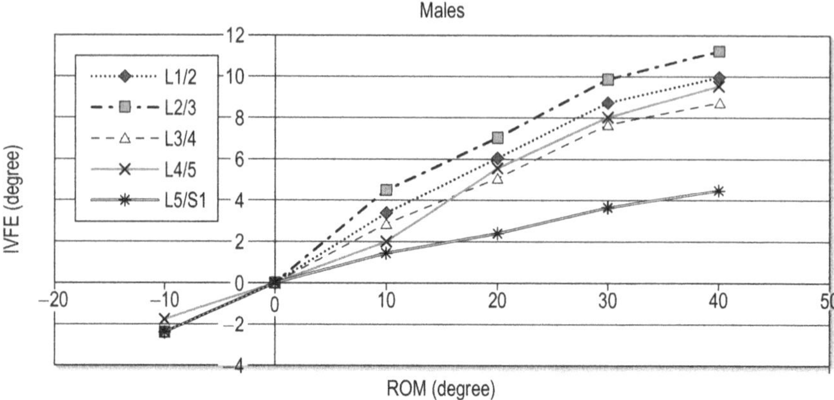

FIGURE 13.7 Intervertebral flexion–extension (IVFE) motion against trunk range of motion (ROM) in 100 healthy volunteers measured by quantitative fluoroscopy (Wong et al. 2004).

HOW SAFE IS MANIPULATION?

Given the higher range of motion intended with manipulation, there are implications for both clinical effectiveness and patient safety. Mainly used for low-back pain, the risk of serious adverse effects is thought to be extremely low in skilled hands, therefore guidelines generally stipulate only that practitioners should be adequately trained (van Tulder et al. 2006).

The second most frequent use of manipulation is for neck pain (Pedersen 1994), where there have been reports in the research literature, plus considerable press speculation, about the (rare) occurrence of postmanipulation stroke (Ernst 2002). In a recent prospective study of 529 chiropractic patients who received neck manipulation, the main adverse effects, albeit transient, were reported to be headache or a temporary worsening of neck symptoms (Rubinstein et al. 2008). Even the most severe of these did not have long-term effects. In a subsequent large prospective cohort study of 50 275 neck manipulations (Thiel et al. 2007) no serious adverse effects were reported.

The Neck Pain Task Force of the World Health Organization found that neck mobilization and manipulation have similar degrees of effectiveness (Gross et al. 2005; Hurwitz et al. 2008). Combined with exercise, they are reported to be more effective than the alternative strategies to which they have been compared. In the absence of any good evidence of a greater risk from manipulation, the authors recommended that the choice between the two should be guided by patient preference (Hurwitz et al. 2008). However, given the concerns that have been voiced, it is essential to try to balance the good that manual therapies do against any possible harm that might occur.

THE QUALITY OF STUDIES ABOUT HARM

Researching the risk of serious harm from a treatment sometimes brings researchers into contact with stakeholders with strong ontic commitment to certain conceptions of the physical system in play (Martin 1962). Where the research question and the interpretation of evidence are also difficult, there is great pressure on investigators. It therefore makes sense to choose the best methodology to determine whether there is a significant risk of stroke as a result of manipulation and there are a range of approaches to choose from. These include: hypothetical estimates of absolute risk (Klougart et al. 1996), retrospective surveys of practices (Dvorak & Orelli 1985), reviews of case reports (Ernst 2002), case-control studies (Rothwell et al. 2001; Smith et al. 2003; Cassidy et al. 2008), prospective cohort studies without controls (Thiel et al. 2007; Rubinstein et al. 2008) and prospective cohort studies with controls. Whichever technique is chosen, the rigour of both the research design and its execution will determine the authority with which the result is ultimately regarded (Levine et al. 1994). At the low end are estimates from numbers of patients treated against incidence from other studies. Then come estimates from case reports. Then probably come retrospective surveys of practices and unblinded prospective cohort studies without controls. Close to the top, as far as quality is concerned, are case-control studies that allow the inference of causation (and which give us our current best evidence) and, finally, prospective cohort studies with controls (of which none yet exist).

To study risk in a prospective cohort would probably be most feasible in a community stroke study, where strokes and transient ischaemic attacks, reported in primary care and confirmed by a neurologist, are investigated for exposure, or otherwise, to manipulation. (This would be superior to a study based on hospital discharge because many patients with mild strokes are never hospitalized.) These would then be compared with a matched population from the community, who have not had strokes, for exposure to manipulation. This helps to avoid errors in case ascertainment and failure to include all relevant cases (such as carotid strokes) as in retrospective hospital discharge studies (Cassidy et al. 2008). It also ensures that study populations are relevant and avoids having to use controls who have had other kinds of strokes (Smith et al. 2003). Finally, and importantly, it helps to avoid comparing cases and controls with different risk factors for cerebrobasilar stroke (Rothwell et al. 2001).

Such an opportunity did once present itself in a 10-year follow-up to the Oxford Community Stroke Study (Bamford et al. 1990), but was not taken up. In the meantime, although case-control studies do seem consistently to suggest that there is a relationship between manipulation and stroke, especially in younger patients with neck pain or headaches (Rothwell et al. 2001; Smith et al. 2003; Cassidy et al. 2008); although it seems to have been established that the manipulation is unlikely to be causal. This was found by concurrently investigating the relationship to general practitioner visits and finding it to be similar. In other words (and as suggested 6 years before: Breen 2002), patients who are about to have a cerebrobasilar stroke may visit either their manipulation practitioner or their general practitioner and thereafter suffer the same event as part of natural history and not as a result of seeing either practitioner.

Nevertheless, this does not make the problem go away. Some people may not discriminate between manipulation causing a stroke and manipulation being associated with it for another reason. Others may ignore the evidence base and remain bound to their own preconceptions. The question may, therefore, continue to be raised in the popular press. Replication of the Cassidy study (Cassidy et al. 2008) may therefore be necessary before minds are set at rest and we can focus more on research that would help the

Table 13.1 *Risk factors for cervical artery dissection*

Risk factor	Odds ratio (95% CI)
Aortic root diameter >34 mm	14.2 (3.2–63.6)
Carotid artery diameter change during cardiac cycle	10.0 (1.8–54.2)
Migraine	3.6 (1.5–8.6)
Trivial trauma (neck manipulation)	3.8 (1.3–11.0)
Recent infection	1.6 (0.7–3.8)
Homocysteine	(unknown) (1.1–1.5)

CI, confidence interval.
Reproduced from Rubinstein et al. (2005).

patients who are at risk. This research should address the question of what good it would do to be able to recognize these patients in primary care practice. Are there interventions that could minimize progression to infarction if the risks were recognized in time? Are the risk factors sufficiently well known and accessible to be detected by practitioners? Could they be? A systematic review of risk factors for cervical artery dissection (Rubinstein et al. 2005) (Table 13.1) suggests that the main ones (increased aortic root diameter and change in carotid arterial diameter) could not be detected without vascular imaging studies, although the lesser ones (minor trauma, classical migraine and recent infection) certainly could.

THE MANIPULATION ‘PACKAGE OF CARE’

For people with spinal problems, the reduction of pain and the return to normal activity may also benefit any concurrent cardiovascular, mental and general health problems (Ong et al. 2004; Waddell & Burton 2004). This approach in rehabilitation implies that the practitioner who uses manipulation should also engage with the psychological and social factors that influence the course of chronic pain (Truchon 2001). This is very much in keeping with the wider biopsychosocial understanding of health that has come to be expected of most practitioners who deal with musculoskeletal conditions (Weigl et al. 2006). Thus, manipulation is not the mainstay of treatment for either of these conditions, but a useful addition to evidence-based care. This evidence-based management comes with a few simple messages:

- A case history and physical examination should be carried out.
- People should be given information and person-specific advice about how to manage pain and recover.
- Progress should be reviewed and management revised as needed.
- Most people are best managed in primary care.

If a person consults early in the course of the problem, the main consideration is to control pain while avoiding withdrawal and inactivity. If the patient's condition is chronic, then practitioners are advised to assess prognostic factors and provide a consistent, cognitive behavioural approach.

ADHERENCE TO THE EVIDENCE AND DOING IT BETTER

The practice styles of many manipulation practitioners already reflect this closely, but manipulation may be overutilized by them while pain control is underutilized. This may be rooted in the natural healing tradition of the professions and an in-principle aversion to drugs. However, there is evidence that many manipulation practitioners already have evidence-based care within their traditions. Indeed, before guidelines began to be published, a survey of 1012 chiropractic patients throughout Europe in the early 1990s (Pedersen 1994) had found that virtually all had received a comprehensive case history and examination and an explanation of their symptoms. Within 3 months of their first attendance, 65% of them had had reassessments recorded in their clinical records. Eighty-seven per cent were advised to stay active and only 2% and 5% (respectively) were advised to have bed rest and/or stay off work. However, only 4% were advised to take analgesics to control pain while almost all were given a manual treatment at most attendances. Explanation of symptoms, ergonomic advice and psychological and social advice were consistently provided for patients across the first five visits. In a subsequent study of UK chiropractors (Lauridsen 1999), 98% of respondents were found to use some form of exercises for chronic low-back pain. The use of X-rays, which is not recommended for back and neck pain unless pathology is suspected, has reduced sharply in chiropractic from an estimated 5112 new films annually in 1973 (Breen 1977) to only 158 in 2000 (Breen et al. 2000b).

TAKING ACCOUNT OF SOCIETAL FACTORS

With a few exceptions, therefore, the care traditionally offered by many practitioners of manipulation already reflects the evidence base. This assumes, however, that our biopsychosocial understanding of common health problems is wide enough. The overall cost of back pain alone is thought to be 2–3% of the gross domestic product of western European economies (Nachemson et al. 2000). In the UK in 2007, this was estimated at £1333 billion (National Statistics 2007), which would put this cost in the region of £27bn ($40bn). These are apparently mainly from lost production and other societal costs, especially in chronic cases (Clinical Standards Advisory Group Epidemiology Review 1994), while the total UK health care bill for back pain has been estimated at around £1bn (Maniadakis & Gray 2000). One explanation may be that it is the social and societal spectrum of problems associated with chronic back pain that is generating most of the cost and not just the back pain itself. If this is the case, a biomedical approach to back pain is not only inadequate (Foster et al. 2003), but fundamentally inappropriate. The social and societal factors are:

- work problems (unemployment, job dissatisfaction)
- financial problems (low economic status, low education)

- legal limitations (compensation pending and insurance rules)
- health care system (low priority, poor integration)
- social problems (poor housing, low support, low sense of control) (Pincus et al. 2008b).

These, together with other health problems, multisite pain and psychological problems (distress and depression), help to explain the high impact of back pain-related disability, which is not solvable by physical treatment alone. The sheer size of this impact means that the attention of policy-makers is urgently required and a multidisciplinary, biopsychosocial approach needs to be expected of all who attempt to help the sufferer. Among those who do offer such help are, or course, practitioners who use manipulation. Research has already shown, and may continue to reveal, to what extent practice remains aligned to the evidence, or even improves by addressing this wider spectrum of prognostic factors. Central to this will be whether manipulation remains the focus of their approach or becomes a tool within it.

Regular surveys of practice are crucial if the manipulating professions are to develop themselves optimally. Studies of patient cohorts could reveal the relationship between these new issues, such as the engagement of the practitioner with the wider context of health and its effect on clinical outcomes. However, this also calls for new outcome measures. How do we measure the impact of social and societal factors? To what extent do practitioners who use manipulation in primary care make an explicit attempt to improve them as part of their clinical management? There is reasonable international consensus that the above factors are the main ones (Pincus et al. 2008b) and that the appropriate method for measuring their effect sizes is inception cohort studies. However, we do not have instruments that measure, for example, 'the influence of compensation litigation' or 'employer intransigence'. It is also worth finding out if practice in the private and public sectors is equally effective for patients.

RESEARCHING CLINICAL EFFECTIVENESS

The randomized trial is generally considered to be the best study design for comparing the effectiveness of treatments, but a truly valid comparison is sometimes very difficult, to the extent that some regard the randomized controlled trial as being of dubious value and potentially misleading (Bolton 1997). Koes (2004) outlined the main problems as:

- being able to compare populations that otherwise have the same prognosis
- standardizing the interventions
- blinding patients, therapists and outcome measurement
- recruiting an adequate sample size
- drop-outs and loss to follow-up.

GUIDELINES

The importance of having high-quality trials is that they form a large part of the basis of clinical guidelines. The consequences of adopting misleading conclusions from low-quality clinical trials surface particularly when guidelines based on them are monodisciplinary or based on trial evidence alone, to the exclusion of clinical expertise and patient preference (Sackett et al. 1996). In some back pain guidelines, for example, manipulation is not even mentioned (Philadelphia Panel 2001; Bekkering et al. 2003), despite the amount of evidence that surrounds it.

The potential consequences of low-quality guidelines are:

- poor patient care
- inflexibility
- disruption of practice
- threat to livelihood
- medicolegal liability (if not following) (Breen 2006).

This also makes useful social policy reform difficult and is a reason why guideline appraisal is essential before dissemination and implementation are attempted (AGREE 2001). Although manipulation is seldom administered as a monotherapy (Pedersen 1994), none of the individual components of the packages of care that include it have large therapeutic effects in populations (Assendelft et al. 2004). Some recent trials of physical therapy have sought to compare some components of such packages against others, or with the whole, but with little or no difference detected (Frost et al. 2004; Klaber Moffett et al. 2005) and scholars often disagree about the level of causation that trials of physical therapies could reasonably be expected to reveal (Cornwall & Murrell 1993). Certainly attenuation or enhancement of treatment effects could be related to trial design and it is useful to consider how such systematic effects could influence outcomes and some ways in which to avoid these pitfalls.

THE QUALITY OF MANIPULATION TRIALS

Key quality criteria for clinical trials of manual therapies have been offered in a previous edition of this chapter (Breen 2001) as: adequate randomization, blinding of outcome assessment, no exclusions from analysis and numbers and reasons for drop-out and withdrawal recorded (Table 13.2). These are principally aimed at eliminating assessor bias. However, there may be others that could affect results to the extent that any attempt to infer causation could be dubious (Phillips & Goodman 2004). These other quality criteria mainly relate to what actually happened to the subjects. For example, patients with musculoskeletal disorders may have strong preferences for one or other of the treatments (Meade et al. 1990), increasing the danger of selective drop-out or cross-over. 'Intention-to-treat' analysis, which is a standard quality requirement, will only tell us which group assignment was the most successful and not necessarily which treatment was superior. Because blinding is often impossible and patients generally prefer to be in the treatment group than the control group, intention-to-treat analysis may show an inflated level of effectiveness for controls if there are high levels of cross-over to manipulation treatment. It has therefore been suggested that an 'as treated' analysis should also be conducted to compare the effectiveness of the treatments themselves and not just the 'intention' to use them (M Campbell, personal communication).

Table 13.2 ***Methodological quality grading for clinical trials***

Criterion	Points
Randomization	
Randomized	+1
Method described and appropriate[a]	+1
Method inappropriate[a]	−1
Blinding of outcome assessment[b]	
Double-blind	+1
Masking described and appropriate	+1
Method inappropriate	−1
Intention-to-treat analysis[c]	**+1**
Drop-outs and withdrawals	
Numbers and reasons for withdrawal reported	+1
Maximum total points	**6**

[a]Random numbers generated by computer, random numbers table, shuffled cards or tossed coins and minimization. Randomization clearly (authors explicitly state method) and adequately concealed from treatment and assessment.

[b]Outcome evaluators shielded from knowledge of treatment assignments.

[c]No exclusions from analysis regardless of whether they: (1) deviated from protocol; (2) withdrew; (3) dropped out; (4) were lost to follow-up.

Adapted from: Schulz et al. (1995) and Moher et al. (1998).

DOES IT REALLY MAKE A DIFFERENCE?

Emphasis is traditionally placed on the statistical significance of differences found in trials (Bouter et al. 1998; van Tulder et al. 2003; Ferrer et al. 2006). This is generally placed at the 95% level with at least 80% power to show the expected difference. However there have been calls for the application of minimum clinically important differences (MCID) to the outcome. A good example of this has evolved for the Roland and Morris Back Pain Disability Questionnaire (Roland & Morris 1983), which has a 24-point scale, and is among the most commonly used disability measures in manipulation trials. For such trials, the MCID could be considered as the lowest score in patients who improve according to their scores on a concurrently applied pain transition scale (Stratford et al. 1996a). Studies in the UK have determined that this is around 2.5 points out of the 24 (Klaber-Moffett et al. 1999; UK BEAM TT 2004). For clinical practice, as opposed to research use, this has been recommended as the change score reached at the lower 95% confidence interval of the mean scores in a group of patients (Stratford et al. 1996b), or, alternatively, a change score of more than 30% of their initial score in patients who say they have improved. The higher the MCID is taken to be, the more relevant will be the results of treatment for the patients for whom it is achieved, but the more difficult it will be to achieve in the first place. This is a challenge to all interventions for common musculoskeletal problems, which have so far shown only modest improvements at most. However, lower levels of improvement may also be important, given the huge costs of these conditions (UK BEAM TT 2004). Future research will have to demonstrate a credible trade-off between these two priorities.

Finally, recommendations for improved methodology in trials of non-pharmacologic interventions have been made in an extension of the Consolidated Standards of Reporting Trials (CONSORT) statement (Altman et al. 2001; Moher et al. 2001; Boutron et al. 2008a, b). This suggests that, although the practitioners who apply interventions such as manipulation cannot be blinded to treatment allocation, any others who supply co-interventions, such as exercises, should at least be blinded. Further, the expertise of care providers, and any clustering thereof in factorial design trials, need also to be taken into account.

RESEARCH AND ACCESS TO MANIPULATION IN THE UK

Chiropractors and osteopaths, the main practitioners of manipulation, provide the most sought-after of complementary interventions by the public in England, but not the most commissioned by the National Health Service (NHS) on its behalf (Thomas et al. 2001). This reflects a continuing lack of acceptance that is difficult to explain. Before manipulation became accepted in health care, its practitioners were widely viewed with scepticism by mainstream colleagues and people sought manipulative treatment late in the course of their conditions (Breen 1977; Burton 1981). More recently, however, they have tended to consult much earlier (Pedersen 1994). Yet despite the public recognition and regulation of chiropractic and osteopathy, only 4–10% of these professionals' services are available through the UK NHS (Wadsworth 1998). This is consistent with evidence that a different part of society receives manipulation for back pain from chiropractors and osteopaths than from physiotherapists (Ong et al. 2004). These former are the higher wage earners with better general health and are apparently well motivated to recover from their problems (Langworthy & Breen 2007).

The continuing isolation of manipulation practitioners may be in part caused by their own mistrust of the health care system and of each other and be a reason why a minority of them may continue treatment when patients are not responding in preference to referring into what may be perceived as an abyss (Pincus et al. 2006). The answer to why they are rather less welcomed than might be expected may also lie in poor communication in primary care, or in competing priorities in general practice, where the greatest proportion of musculoskeletal patients seek help (Parsons et al. 2007). It is unlikely to be because GPs are adverse to receiving patient reports from them, but perhaps more because they find their terminology confusing (Brussee et al. 2000, 2001). Such reports may, however, be infrequent and therefore miss the opportunity to familiarize GPs with the context of manipulation in the community. Much more research is needed into the relationships, and potential relationships, of practitioners of manipulation with mainstream health care.

MANIPULATION AND THE TRANSITION TO MAINSTREAM HEALTH CARE

There appear also to be barriers to commissioning manipulation services in the NHS. Despite the low-tech, evidence-based service that guidelines call for, care pathways are not always compatible with ways of working in primary care. Referrals for musculoskeletal problems may be poorly documented in practice databases and it may therefore be difficult to locate a starting point for innovatory change. Patients may be averse to an evidence-based approach if they have already set their minds on sick certification, X-rays or consultant referral. There may also be other factors, for example, managerial policies of 'no return until fully fit', that conflict, or legal or insurance coverage provisions that work against a supported rehabilitation programme. Finally and importantly, evidence-based management of musculoskeletal problems is not included within the NHS Quality and Outcomes Framework. These are major reasons for poor uptake of guidelines (Bird 2000; Langworthy et al. 2002, 2005) and will continue to be until they are addressed as health and social policy issues.

CONCLUSION

Research relating to manipulation needs to include the mechanisms of action, the trends in practice and the influence of the settings and social circumstances in which the therapy is used. Clinical value is generally understood to be based on clinical outcomes, functional outcomes, satisfaction and cost factors (Nelson et al. 1996). Yet, for example, there may be little association between patient satisfaction with care and recovery (Breen & Breen 2003). This may require uncomfortable trade-offs in service arrangements.

We may also now have new opportunities to investigate the mechanical effects of the intervention. This will depend on further technological innovations in biomechanical measurement in vivo and, in particular, defining the limits of normality of new, but relevant, physiological values. We may then be able to determine whether there is any relationship between biomechanics and health measures such as pain and disability. This would allow the long-awaited explanatory trials of manipulation in returning biomechanics to normal to be carried out.

Pragmatic trials of optimized packages of care that include manipulation are also needed. For example, previous trials have not generally included the manipulator as a prescriber of pain control and exercise, yet these are important parts of evidence-based care with which manipulation is normally associated. There also needs to be greater clarity about the importance of short-term relief. This is often important to patients and there are sometimes conflicts between providing interventions that last, but take time to act, and those that may act quickly, even if recovery is to be expected eventually, without any intervention. Future trials could also usefully control for the presence of prognostic factors, such as multisite pain (Carnes et al. 2007), distress, high pain at onset and minor comorbidity (Breen et al. 2005).

The UK's Musculoskeletal Services Framework (Department of Health 2006) calls for practitioners who can provide evidence-based assessment and management of people with common musculoskeletal disorders to supply the expertise for the interface between primary and secondary care. This raises intriguing questions for primary care commissioning, as well as for health care quality improvement. These could be investigated using carefully designed qualitative outcomes and health service utilization studies involving primary and secondary care practitioners and commissioners. To do justice to the problem, however, these will require the cooperation and active participation of the chiropractors, osteopaths and specialist physiotherapists who provide manipulation. The role of these practitioners in the management of chronic pain is by no means clear. The stumbling block is bound up with understanding and providing a 'multi-disciplinary bio-psychosocial intervention' (Karljalainen et al. 2001). Commissioners have begun to articulate what this might involve (NHS 2008), but given the number of stakeholders, implementation will always be challenging.

The overall message of the evidence for common musculoskeletal problems is a simple one. In populations, the effects of the best interventions are on average only moderate and these interventions are not high-tech ((NHMRC) NHaMRC 2003; European Commission CBMC 2006). Seen in this light, it makes sense to make service arrangements that allow patients to have access to all of these interventions from one practitioner, if possible. It will help if we work, through research, to determine where manipulation has the strongest rationale for care and where other physical or psychosocial interventions do.

REFERENCES

Agency for Health Care Policy Research, 1994. Clinical practice guidelines no.14 – acute low back pain problems in adults. Report No.: 14. Agency for Health Care Policy Research, US Department of Health and Human Services, Washington DC.

A.G.R.E.E, 2001. Appraisal of guidelines for research and evaluation. St George's Hospital Medical School, London.

Airaksinen, O., Brox, J.I., Cedraschi, C., et al., 2006. European guidelines for the management of chronic nonspecific low back pain. Eur. Spine J. 15, S192–S300.

Altman, D.G., Schulz, K.F., Moher, D., et al., 2001. The revised CONSORT statement for reporting randomized trials: explanation and elaboration. Ann. Intern. Med. 134 (8), 663–694.

Assendelft, W.J.J., Morton, S.C., Yu, E.I., et al. (Eds.), 2004. Spinal manipulative therapy for low back pain (Cochrane Review). John Wiley, Chichester, UK.

Bamford, J., Sandercock, P., Dennis, M., et al., 1990. A prospective study of acute cerebrovascular disease in the community: the Oxfordshire Community Stroke Project – 1981–86 1. Incidence, case fatality rates and overall outcome at one year of cerebral infarction, primary intracerebral and subarachnoid haemorrihage. J. Neurol. Neurosurg. Psychiatry 53, 16–22.

Bekkering, G.E., Hendriks, H.J.M., Koes, B.W., et al., 2003. Dutch physiotherapy guidelines for low back pain. Physiotherapy 89 (2), 82–96.

Bird, C., 2000. Commissioned R&D Programmes: Implementation of low back pain guidelines in North Thames. NHS Executive London Regional Office, London.

Bolton, J.E., 1997. Future directions for outcomes research in back pain. European Journal of Chiropractic 45, 57–64.

Bouter, L.M., van Tulder, M.W., Koes, B.W., 1998. Methodologic Issues in Low Back Pain Research in Primary Care. Spine 23 (18), 2014–2020.

Boutron, I., Moher, D., Altman, D.G., et al., 2008a. Methods and Processes of the CONSORT Group: Example of an Extension for Trials Assessing Nonpharmacologic Treatments. Ann. Intern. Med. 148 (4), 61–66.

Boutron, I., Moher, D., Altman, D.G., et al., 2008b. Extending the CONSORT Statement to Randomized Trails of Nonpharmacologic Treatment: Explanation and Elaboration. Ann. Intern. Med. 148 (4), 295–309.

Bowden, A.E., Guerin, H.L., Villarraga, M.L., et al., 2008. Quality of motion considerations in numercial analysis of motion restoring implants of the spine. Clin. Biomech. 23, 536–544.

Breen, A.C., 1977. Chiropractors and the treatment of back pain. Rheumatol. Rehabil. 16, 46–53.

Breen, A.C., 2001. Manual Therapies. In: Lewith, G., Jonas, W.B., Walach, H. (Eds.), Clinical Research in Complementary Therapies. Churchill Livingstone, Edinburgh, pp. 247–261.

Breen, A.C., 2002. Manipulation of the neck and stroke: time for more rigorous evidence. Med. J. Aust. 176 (15 April), 363–364.

Breen, A., 2006. From guidelines to practice: what is the practitioner's role? In: Liebenson, C. (Ed.), Rehabilitation of the Spine, second ed. Lippincott, Williams & Wilkins, Philadelphia, pp. 933–945.

Breen, A., Breen, R., 2003. Back pain and satisfaction with chiropractic treatment: What role does the physical outcome play? Clin. J. Pain 19, 263–268.

Breen, A.C., Langworthy, J., Vogel, S., et al., 2000a. Primary care audit toolkit: acute low back pain. Institute for Musculoskeletal Research and Clinical Implementation, Bournemouth.

Breen, A., Carrington, M., Collier, R., et al., 2000b. Communication between general and manipulative practitioners: a survey. Complement. Ther. Med. 8, 8–14.

Breen, A., Langworthy, J., Bagust, J., 2005. Improved early pain management for musculoskeletal disorders: Health and Safety Executive. Report No: 399. Available online at http://www.hse.gov.uk/research/rrhtm/rr399.htm.

Breen, A., Muggleton, J., Mellor, F., 2006. An objective spinal motion imaging assessment (OSMIA): reliability, accuracy and exposure data. BMC Musculoskelet. Disord. 7 (1), 1–10.

Breen, A., Fowler, J., Mellor, F., 2007. Adjacent segment motion and posterior lumbar spine instrumention: a comparison of patient groups. Spine Arthroplasty Society Global Symposium on Motion Preservation Technology. Berlin.

Brussee, W.J., Assendelft, W.J.J., Breen, A.C., 2001. Communication between general practitioners and chiropractors. J. Manipulative Physiol. Ther. 24 (1), 12–16.

Burton, A.K., 1981. Back pain in osteopathic practice. Rheumatol. Rehabil. 20, 239–246.

Carnes, D., Parsons, S., Ashby, D., et al., 2007. Chronic musculoskeletal pain rarely presents in a single body site: results from a UK population study. Rheumatology 46 (1), 1168–1170.

Cassidy, J.D., Lopes, A.A., Yong-Hing, K., 1992. The immediate effect of manipulation versus mobilisation on pain and range of motion in the cervical spine: a randomised controlled trial. J. Manipulative Physiol. Ther. 15 (9), 570–575.

Cassidy, J.D., Boyle, E., Cote, P., et al., 2008. Risk of Vertebrobasilar Stroke and Chiropractic Care: Results of a Population-Based Case-Control and Case-Crossover Study. Spine 33 (4S), Neck Pain Task Force(Supplement): S176–S183.

Childs, J.D., Fritz, J.M., Flynn, T.W., et al., 2004. A clinical prediction rule to identify patients with low back pain most likely to benefit from spinal manipulation: a validation study. Ann. Intern. Med. 141 (12), 920–928.

Chou, R., Huffman, L.H., 2007. Nonpharmacologic Therapies for Acute and Chronic Low Back Pain: A Review of the Evidence for an American Pain Society/American College of Physicians Clinical Practice Guideline. Ann. Intern. Med. 147 (7), 492–504.

Chown, M., Whittamore, L., Rush, M., et al., 2008. A prospective study of patients with chronic back pain randomised to group exercise, physiotherapy or osteopathy. Physiotherapy 94, 21–28.

Clinical Standards Advisory Group Epidemiology Review, 1994. The epidemiology and cost of back pain. Report of a Clinical Standards Advisory Group Committee on Back Pain. Department of Health, London.

Cornwall, M.W., Murrell, P., 1993. Pre-experimental, Experimental and Quasi-experimental Research Designs. Handbook of Physical Therapy Research. J.B. Lippincott, Philadelphia, 143–175.

Coulter, I.D., Shekelle, P.G., 2005. Chiropractic in North America: a descriptive analysis. J. Manipulative Physiol. Ther. 28, 83–89.

Department of Health, 2006. The Musculoskeletal Services Framework. Department of Health, London.

Dvorak, J.O., Orelli, F.V., 1985. How dangerous is manipulation to the cervical spine? Manual Medicine 2, 1–4.

Eisenberg, D.M., Kessler, R.C., Foster, C., et al., 1993. Unconventional medicine in the United States: prevalence, costs and patterns of use. N. Engl. J. Med. 328 (4), 246–252.

Ernst, E., 2002. Manipulation of the cervical spine: a systematic review of case reports of serious adverse events, 1995–2001. Med. J. Aust. 176 (15 April), 376–380.

European Commission CBMC, 2006. COST B13: European Guidelines for the management of low back pain. Eur. Spine J. 15 (Suppl. 2).

Evans, D.W., 2002. Mechanisms and effects of spinal high-velocity, low-amplitude thrust manipulation: previous theories. J. Manipulative Physiol. Ther. 25, 251–262.

Evans, D.W., Breen, A.C., 2006. A biomechanical model for mechanically efficient caitation production during spinal manipulation: prethrust position and the neutral zone. J. Manipulative Physiol. Ther. 29 (1), 72–82.

Fernandez-Bermego, E., Garcia-Jimenez, M.A., Fernandez-Palomeque, C., et al., 1993. Adolescent idiopathic scoliosis and joint laxity: a study with somatosensory evoked potentials. Spine 18 (7), 918–922.

Ferrer, M., Pellise, F., Escudero, O., et al., 2006. Validation of a Minimum Outcome Core Set in the Evaluation of Patients With Back Pain. Spine 31 (12), 1372–1379.

Flynn, T.W., Fritz, J., Wainner, R.S., et al., 2003. The audible pop is not necessary for successful spinal high-velocity thrust manipulation in individuals with low back pain. Arch. Phys. Med. Rehabil. 84, 1057–1060.

Foster, N.E., Pincus, T., Underwood, M.R., et al., 2003. Editorial: Understanding the process of care for musculoskeletal conditions – why a biomedical approach is inadequate. Rheumatology 42, 401–403.

Fowler, J., Mellor, F., Muggleton, J., et al., 2006. Abnormal inter-vertebral motion is associated with chronic low back pain and MR disc degeneration. Spine Society of Europe Annual Meeting. Istanbul.

Frost, H., Lamb, S.E., Doll, H.A., Carver, P.T., Stewart-Brown, S., 2004. Randomised controlled trial of physiotherapy compared with advice for low back pain. Br. Med. J. 329, 708–711.

Gertzbein, S.D., Seligman, J., Holtby, K., 1985. Centrode patterns and segmental instability in degenerative disc disease. Spine 10 (3), 257–261.

Gross, A.R., Hoving, J.L., Haines, T.A., et al., 2005. Manipulation and mobilisation for mechanical neck disorders (Review). The Cochrane Library. http://wwwthecochranelibrarycom. (2).

Haldeman, S. (Ed.), 1992. Principles and Practice of Chiropractic, second ed. Norwalk, Connecticut, Appleton & Lange.

Haldeman, S.D., 1996. Spinal manipulation: when, how and who? Bulletin: Hospital for Joint Diseases 55 (3), 135–137.

Haldeman, S., Carroll, L., Cassidy, J.D., et al., 2008. The Bone and Joint Decade 2000–2010 Task Force on Neck Pain and Its Associated Disorders: Executive Summary. Spine 33 (4S), Neck Pain Task Force(Supplement): S5–S7.

Hancock, M.J., Maher, C.G., Latimer, J., et al., 2008. Independent evaluation of a clinical prediction rule for spinal manipulative therapy: a randomised controlled trial. Eur. Spine J. 17, 936–943.

Harvey, E., Burton, A.K., Moffett, J.K., et al., 2003. Spinal manipulation for low-back pain: a treatment package agreed by the UK chiropractic, osteopathy and physiotherapy professional associations. Man. Ther. 8 (1), 46–51.

Hewitt, D., Wood, P.H., 1975. Heterodox Practitioners and the availability of specialist advice. Rheumatol. Rehabil. 14 (3), 191–199.

Huisman, M., Breen, A., 1990. The Changing Face of British Chiropractic. Contact 4 (2), 11–12.

Hurwitz, E.L., Carragee, E.J., van der Velde, G., et al., 2008. Treatment of Neck Pain: Noninvasive Interventions: Results of the Bone and Joint Decade 2000–2010 Task Force on Neck Pain and Its Associated Disorders. Spine 33 (4S), Neck Pain Task Force(Supplement): S123–S152.

Kaigle, A.M., Wesberg, P., Hansson, T.H., 1998. Muscular and kinematic behavior of the lumbar spine during flexion-extension. J. Spinal Disord. 11 (2), 163–174.

Karljalainen, K., Malmivaara, A., van Tulder, M., et al., 2001. Multidisciplinary biopsychosocial rehabilitation for subacute low-back pain among working age adults. Spine 26, 262–269.

Kirkaldy-Willis, W.H., 1992. Pathology and pathogenesis of low back pain. In: Kirkaldy-Willis, W.H., Burton, C.V. (Eds.), Managing Low Back Pain. Churchill Livingstone, New York, pp. 49–79.

Klaber-Moffett, J., Torgerson, D., Bell-Syer, S., et al., 1999. Randomised controlled trial of exercise for low back pain: clinical outcomes, costs and preferences. Br. Med. J. 319, 279–283.

Klaber Moffett, J.A., Jackson, D.A., Richmond, S., et al., 2005. Randomised trial of a brief physiotherapy intervention compared with usual physiotherapy for neck pain patients: outcomes and patients' preference. Br. Med. J. 330, 75–78.

Klougart, N., Leboeuf-Yde, C., Rasmussen, L.R., 1996. Safety in chiropractic practice. Part II: Treatment to the upper neck and the rate of cerebrovasulcar incidents. J. Manipulative Physiol. Ther. 19 (9), 563–569.

Koes, B.W., 2004. How to evaluate manual therapy: value and pitfalls of randomized clinical trials. Man. Ther. 9, 183–184.

Langworthy, J., Breen, A., 2007. Psychosocial factors and their predictive value in chiropractic patients with low back pain: a prospective inception cohort study. Chiropractic & Osteopathy 15 (1), 5.

Langworthy, J.M., Breen, A.C., Vogel, S., et al., 2002. Chiropractic and the National Health Care system: a basis for partnership in the UK. J. Manipulative Physiol. Ther. 25 (1), 21–33.

Langworthy, J., Clow, W., Breen, A., 2005. Low back pain: barriers to effective clinical governance. Clinical Governance: An International Journal 10 (4), 281–290.

Lariviere, C., Gagnon, D., Loisel, P., 2002. A biomechanical comparison of lifting techniques between subjects with and without chronic low back pain during freestyle lifting and lowering tasks. Clin. Biomech. 17 (2), 89–98.

Lauridsen, H., 1999. Are chiropractors in the United Kingdom using intensive physical training programmes for patients with chronic low back pain? MSc thesis. Anglo-European College of Chiropractic.

Levine, M., Walter, S., Lee, H., et al., 1994. Users' guides to the medical literature – IV. How to use an article about harm. JAMA 271 (20), 1615–1619.

Liebenson, C., 2006. Rehabilitation of the Spine: a practitioner's manual. Lippincott, Williams & Wilkins, Philadelphia.

Maniadakis, N., Gray, A., 2000. The economic burden of back pain in the UK. Pain 84 (1), 95–103.

Mannion, A.F., 1999. Fibre type characteristics and function of the human paraspinal muscles: normal values and changes in association with low back pain. J. Electromyogr. Kinesiol 9, 363–377.

Martin, R.M., 1962. On denotation and ontic commitment. Philos. Stud. 13 (3), 35–39.

Mayer, R.S., Chen, I.H., Lavender, S.A., et al., 1995. Variance in the Measurement of Sagittal Lumbar Spine Range of Motion Among Examiners, Subjects, and Instruments. Spine 20 (13), 1489–1493.

Meade, T.W., Dyer, S., Browne, W., et al., 1990. Low back pain of mechanical origin: randomised comparison of chiropractic and hospital outpatient treatment. Br. Med. J. 300, 1431–1437.

Mellor, F., Muggleton, J.M., Bagust, J., et al., 2008. Mid-lumbar lateral flexion stability measured in healthy volunteers by in-vivo fluoroscopy. Spine 34, E811–E817.

Mimura, M., Panjabi, M.M., Oxland, T.R., et al., 1994. Disc Degeneration Affects the Multidirectional Flexibility of the Lumbar Spine. Spine 19 (12), 1371–1380.

Moher, D., Pham, B., Jones, A., 1998. Does quality of reports of randomized trials affect estimates of intervention efficacy reported in meta-analyses? Lancet 352, 609–613.

Moher, D., Schulz, K.F., Altman, D., 2001. The CONSORT Statement: Revised recommendations for improving the quality of reports of parallel-group randomized trials. J. Am. Med. Assoc. 285 (15), 1987–1991.

Morris, C.E., 2006. Low Back Syndromes: Integrated clinical management. McGraw-Hill Medical, New York.

Nachemson, A., Carlsson, C.A., Englund, L., et al. (Eds.), 2000. Back pain, Neck pain: an evidence based review – Summary and conclusions. Swedish Council on Technology Assessment in Health Care, Stockholm.

Nansel, D., Cremata, E., Carlson, J., et al., 1989. Effect of unilateral spinal adjustments on goniometrically-assessed cervical lateral-flexion end-range asymmetries in otherwise asymptomatic subjects. J. Manipulative Physiol. Ther. 12 (6), 419–427.

National Statistics, 2007. Available online at: http://www.statistics.gov.uk/cci/nugget.asp?id=192.

Nattrass, C.L., Nitschke, J.E., Disler, P.B., et al., 1999. Lumbar spine range of motion as a measure of physical and functional impairment: an investigation of validity. Clin. Rehabil. 24, 211–218.

Nelson, E.C., Mohr, J.J., Batalden, P.B., et al., 1996. Improving Health Care, Part 1: The Clinical Value Compass. Journal on Quality Improvement 22 (4), 243–256.

(NHMRC) NHaMRC, 2003. Evidence-based management of acute musculoskeletal pain. Australian Acute Musculoskeletal Pain Guidelines Group. University of Queensland and the Commonwealth Department of Health and Ageing, Brisbane.

NHS, 2008. Service Development and Commissioning Directives: Chronic, Non-Malignant Pain. Cardiff, Welsh Assembly Government.

NICE, 2008. Low back pain: the acute management of patients with chronic (longer than 6 weeks) non-specific low back pain (consultation version). National Institute of Health and Clinical Excellence, London.

Nilsson, N., Christensen, H.W., Hartvigsen, J., 1996. Lasting changes in passive range of motion after spinal manipulation: a randomised, blind, controlled trial. J. Manipulative Physiol. Ther. 19 (3), 165–168.

Ong, C.K., Doll, H., Bodeker, G., et al., 2004. Use of osteopathic or chiropractic services among people with back pain: a UK population survey. Health and Social Care in the Community 12 (3), 265–273.

Panjabi, M.M., 1992a. The stabilising system of the spine – Part 1: Function, dysfunction, adaptation and enhancement. J. Spinal Disord. 5 (4), 383–389.

Panjabi, M.M., 1992b. The stabilising system of the spine – Part 2: Neutral zone and instability hypothesis. J. Spinal Disord. 5 (4), 390–397.

Panjabi, M., Chang, D., Dvorak, J., 1992. An analysis of errors in kinematic parameters associated with in vivo functional radiographs. Spine 17 (2), 200–205.

Parsons, S., Harding, G., Breen, A., et al., 2007. The Influence of Patients' and Primary Care Practitioners' Beliefs and Expectations About Chronic Musculoskeletal Pain on the Process of Care. Clin. J. Pain. 23 (1), 91–98.

Pedersen, P., 1994. A survey of chiropractic practice in Europe. European Journal of Chiropractic 42 (S), 3–28.

Peterson, D.H., Bergmann, T.F., 2002. Chiropractic technique: principles and procedures, second ed. Mosby, St Louis, Missouri.

Pfirrmann, C.W.A., Metzdorf, A., Zanetti, M., et al., 2001. Magnetic resonance classification of lumbar intervertebral disc degeneration. Spine 26 (17), 1873–1878.

Philadelphia Panel, 2001. Philadelphia Panel evidence-based clinical practice guidelines on selected rehabilitation interventions for neck pain. Phys. Ther. 81 (10), 1701–1717.

Phillips, C.V., Goodman, K.J., 2004. The missed lessons of Sir Austin Bradford Hill. Epidemiologic Perspectives and Innovations 1 (3).

Pincus, T., Vogel, S., Breen, A., et al., 2006. Persistent back pain – why do physical therapy practitioners continue treatment? A qualitative study of chiropractors, osteopaths and physiotherapists. Eur. J. Pain 10, 67–76.

Pincus, T., Santos, R., Breen, A., et al., 2008a. A review and proposal for a core set of factors for prospective cohorts in low back pain: A consensus statement. Arthritis Rheum. 59 (1), 14–24.

Pincus, T., Santos, R., Breen, A., et al., 2008b. A Review and Proposal for a Core Set of Factors for Prospective Cohorts in Low Back Pain: A Consensus Statement. Arthritis Rheum. 59 (1), 14–24.

Reeves, N.P., Narendra, K.S., Cholewicki, J., 2007. Spine stability: The six blind men and the elephant. Clin. Biomech. 22, 266–274.

Roland, M., Morris, R.A., 1983. Study of the natural history of pack pain: Part I – development of a reliable and sensitive measure of disability in low back pain. Spine 8 (2), 141–144.

Ross, J.K., Bereznick, D.E., McGill, S.M., 2004. Determining cavitation location during lumbar and thoracic spinal manipulation. Is spinal manipulation accurate and specific. Spine 29 (13), 1452–1457.

Rothwell, D.M., Bondy, S.J., Williams, J.I., 2001. Chiropractic manipulation and stroke: a population-based case-control study. Stroke 32 (10), 1054–1060.

Rubinstein, S.M., Peerdeman, S.M., van Tulder, M.W., et al., 2005. A systematic review of the risk factors for cervical artery dissection. Stroke 36, 1575–1580.

Rubinstein, S.M., Leboeuf-Yde, C., Knol, D.L., et al., 2008. Predictors of Adverse Events Following Chiropractic Care for Patients With Neck Pain. J. Manipulative Physiol. Ther. 31 (2), 94–103.

Sackett, D.L., Rosenberg, W.M.C., Gray, J.A.M., et al., 1996. Evidence based medicine; what it is and what it isn't. Br. Med. J. 312, 71–72.

Sandoz, R., 1969. The significance of the manipulative crack and of other articular noises. Annals of the Swiss Chiropractors. Association 4, 47–68.

Sandoz, R.W., 1978. Some reflex phenomena associated with spinal derangements and adjustments. Annals of the Swiss Chiropractors. Association VII, 45–65.

Schulz, K.F., Chalmers, I., Hayes, R.J., et al., 1995. Review: empirical evidence of bias. J. Am. Med. Assoc. 273, 408–412.

Shaffer, W.O., Spratt, K.F., Weinstein, J.D., et al., 1990. Volvo Award in Clinical

Sciences: The Consistency and Accuracy of Roentgenograms for Measuring Sagittal Translation in the Lumbar Vertebral Motion Segment: An Experimental Model. Spine 15 (8), 741–750.

Sihvonen, T., Partanen, J., Hanninen, O., et al., 1991. Electric behavior of low back muscles during lumbar pelvic rhythm in low back pain patients and health controls. Arch. Phys. Med. Rehabil. 72, 1080–1087.

Smith, W.S., Johnston, S.C., Skalabrin, E.J., et al., 2003. Spinal manipulative therapy is an independent risk factor for vertebral artery dissection. Neurology 60, 1424–1428.

Stratford, P.W., Binkley, J., Solomon, P., et al., 1996a. Defining the minimum level of detectable change for the Roland-Morris Questionnaire. Phys. Ther. 76 (4), 359–365.

Stratford, P.W., Finch, E., Solomon, P., et al., 1996b. Using the Roland-Morris Questionnaire to make decisions about individual patients. Physiother. Can. 48 (2), 107–110.

Teyhen, D.S., Flynn, T.W., Bovik, A.C., et al., 2005. A new technique for digital fluoroscopic video assessment of sagittal plane lumbar spine motion. Spine 30 (14), E406–E413.

Thiel, H.W., Bolton, J.E., Docherty, S., et al., 2007. Safety of chiropractic manipulation of the cervical spine; A prospective national survey. Spine 32 (21), 2375–2378.

Thomas, K.J., Nicholl, J.P., Coleman, P., 2001. Use and expenditure on complementary medicine in England: a population based survey. Complement. Ther. Med. 9, 2–11.

Truchon, M., 2001. Determinants of chronic disability related to low back pain: Towards an integrative biopsychosocial model. Disability & Rehabilitation. 23 (17), 758–767.

UK BEAM TT, 2004. United Kingdom back pain exercise and manipulation (UK BEAM) randomised trial: cost effectiveness of physical treatments for back pain in primary care. Br. Med. J. 329, 1377–1384.

Unsworth, A., Dowson, D., Wright, V., 1971. 'Cracking Joints'. A bioengineering study of cavitation in the metacarpophalangeal joint. Ann. Rheum. Dis. 30, 348–358.

Van Akkerveeken, P.F., O'Brien, J.P., Park, W.M., 1979. Experimentally induced hypermobility in the lumbar spine: a pathologic and radiologic study of the posterior ligament and annulus fibrosus. Spine 4 (3), 236–241.

van Tulder, M., Furlan, A., Bombardier, C., et al., 2003. Updated Method Guidelines for Systematic Reviews in the Cochrane Collaboration Back Review Group. Spine 28 (12), 1290–1299.

van Tulder, M., Becker, A., Bekkering, T., et al., 2006. Chapter 3: European guidelines for the management of acute nonspecific low back pain in primary care. Eur. Spine J. 15 (Suppl. 2), s169–s191.

Waddell, G., 1998. The Back Pain Revolution. Churchill Livingstone, Edinburgh.

Waddell, G., McIntosh, A., Hutchinson, A., et al., 1999. Low back pain evidence review. Royal College of General Practitioners, London.

Waddell, G., Burton, A., 2004. Concepts of rehabilitation for the management of common health problems. The Stationery Office, London.

Wadsworth, R., 1998. Commissioning complemerntary medicine. Quality in Complementary Medicine: A Meeting of the Forum on Quality in Health Care of the Royal Society of Medicine. Royal Society of Medicine, London, pp. 22–24.

Weigl, M., Ciezam, A., Kostanjsek, N., et al., 2006. The ICF comprehensively covers the spectrum of health problems encountered by health professionals in patients with musculoskeletal conditions. Rheumatology 45, 1247–1254.

White, A.A., Panjabi, M.M., 1990. Clinical Biomechanics of the Spine. JB Lippincott, Philadelphia.

Wilson, F., 2003. A survey of chiropractors in the United Kingdom. European Journal of Chiropractic 50 (3), 185–198.

Wong, K.W.N., Leong, J.C.Y., Chan, M-K., et al., 2004. The flexion–extension profile of lumbar spine in 100 healthy volunteers. Spine 29 (15), 1636–1641.

Wong, K., Luk, K., Leong, J., et al., 2006. Continuous dynamic spinal motion analysis. Spine 31 (4), 414–419.

World Health Organization, 2001. ICF (International Classification of Functioning, Disability and Health) – Revision of the International Classification of Impairments, Disabilities and Handicaps (ICIDH). Resolution no. WHA54.21. World Health Organization, Geneva.

Wyke, B.D., 1985. Articular neurology and manipulative therapy. In: Glasgow, E.F., Twomey, L.T., Scull, E.R., Kleyham, A.M., et al. (Eds.), Aspects of Manipulative Therapy. Churchill Livingstone, London, pp. 72–77.

Zhao, F., Pollintine, P., Hole, B.D., et al., 2005. Discogenic Origins of Spinal Instability. Spine 30 (23), 2621–2630.

Mind–body medicine approaches

14

Enrique Auba • Albert Yeung • Pedro Huertas
Jeffrey A. Dusek • Herbert Benson • Gregory L. Fricchione

CHAPTER CONTENTS

INTRODUCTION

The National Center for Complementary and Alternative Medicine (NCCAM) defines mind–body medicine as an approach that 'focuses on the interactions among the brain, mind, body and behavior, and on the powerful ways in which emotional, mental, social, spiritual, and behavioral factors can directly affect health' (NCCAM National Institutes of Health 2008). Thus, it refers to the power of the mind to modify bodily functions and physical health. More concretely, mind–body medicine encompasses an array of heterogeneous techniques among which we can highlight the relaxation techniques, meditation, biofeedback, guided imagery, hypnosis, yoga, tai chi, qigong and autogenic training. In the present chapter we will try to point out the common elements of these techniques and the core elements of the mind–body approach.

Mind–body medicine is both a philosophical conception of healing and health as well as a group of techniques. Most of these techniques come from eastern cultural traditions, mainly from China and India. They may have a religious foundation with a particular conceptualization of human life, different from those in the occidental culture. In fact, these eastern approaches are frequently considered 'whole medical systems'. This is one of the reasons why many people have doubts about mind–body medicine, considering it a mysterious and non-rationalist perspective. However, even though some people will feel attracted by the religious aspects, they are not essential for everyone. Throughout this chapter we will attempt to show how recent research is providing evidence on the effectiveness of these treatments, establishing their scientific value and facilitating their integration into mainstream medicine.

DOI: 10.1016/B978-0-443-06956-7.00014-8

The role of mind–body medicine will be mainly complementary to current allopathic therapies, but for some conditions it may also be efficient alone. These approaches imply an integrative and holistic concept of mind–body interaction, which complements the medical mission to care for the whole person. In this way, it contributes to the transition from an exclusively reductionistic biomedical model to a not only biopsychosocial but also a biopsychosocial spiritual integrative model (Puchalski 2007).

When we look at our society today, we realize there is a huge demand for stress management therapies in general, and for mind–body approaches in particular. Concurrently, the number of centres offering these therapies is growing, most of them associated with first-order hospitals or universities. However, many physicians and health professionals are still reluctant to incorporate or recognize the clinical effectiveness of mind–body therapies. There are many reasons for this. On the one hand, the integration and transition from research to clinical practice is slow and gradual, as happens in many other areas of medicine (Lenfant 2003). At the same time, it is true that mind–body medicine research has intrinsic difficulties, as we will describe later on. Nevertheless, there is already enough evidence of the clinical efficacy of the mind–body techniques to make them viable options for patients who want to improve their self-care. As has been described in a recent study (Astin et al. 2005), the main barriers among health professionals for the integration of mind–body medicine are the lack of knowledge of existing evidence, a perception that psychological factors are beyond their competency, and a dualistic conception of the mind–body relationship. Thus, there is a significant epistemological barrier, manifested as prejudices and a priori negative attitude.

STRESS PHYSIOLOGY

Mind–body medicine deals with the effects of stress on the body. Stress has become one of the pillars in the aetiopathogenic understanding of disease, and numerous theories and models centred on stress have been developed in recent years. The current clinical practice in mind–body medicine is based on the perceived importance of the integration of biological, psychological, social and spiritual dimensions, and it has its own reflection in research. Psychoneuroendocrinology and psychoneuroimmunology provide a scientific framework and have become important axes of the new mind–body medicine.

Stress has been defined as a state of disharmony or of threatened homeostasis (Chrousos & Gold 1992). It refers to a disruption of the dynamic equilibrium among the person's biological, psychological and social dimensions, as a result of the perceived presence of an external or internal threat. Different alterations or disorders in the environment may provoke a physiological response mediated by several interconnected physiological systems constituting the denominated stress system. Stressors, stress system and stress response are the three key elements to the process we will briefly analyse step by step.

The stress system is composed of elements of the central nervous system, the hypothalamic–pituitary–adrenal (HPA) axis, the autonomic nervous system and the immune system. These systems constitute a complex matrix with overlapping boundaries. This coordinated system maintains homeostasis by regulating different bodily functions. The system controls the administration, distribution and use of energy, adapting the level of functioning of different organs to the global corporeal needs under each specific circumstance. It is constantly functioning, at varying levels of intensity, autoregulated by negative-feedback mechanisms. It can also be overactivated by the presence of stressors, in order to adapt to new conditions. It is at this point that we talk about the stress response, which can be overwhelming in the face of an enormous stressor or chronic in the setting of persistent unrelenting ones.

The physiology of the stress response has been well described (Tsigos & Chrousos 2002). When the stress response is activated, some functions can be stimulated, such as metabolism, cardiac output, vascular tone, respiration and muscle contraction. Other functions can be suppressed, such as the excretory system and gastrointestinal and reproductive activity. Different chemical mediators are implicated in the stress response, among which the most important ones are catecholamines and cortisol. In consequence, an increased heart rate, increased breathing rate, increased metabolism, increased oxygen consumption and increased brain wave activity are produced. These characteristics define the so-called 'flight or fight' response, described by Walter Cannon early in the 20th century in the physiology laboratories at Harvard Medical School (Cannon 1929).

The central nervous system plays an important role in the regulation of the stress response (McEwen 2007). On the one hand, we must look at the cognitive dimension which is regulated by the brain. A psychosocial stressor is a stressor only when it is perceived as such. At this first level, we determine what is stressful, what is threatening. Different events will be considered stressful depending on the cognitive appraisals we apply to them. Depending on our appraisal, the mediators of the stress response may or may not emerge (Lazarus & Folkman 1984). In fact, it has been shown that anticipatory cognitive appraisal is an important determinant of the cortisol stress response (Gaab et al. 2005). On the other hand, the brain also determines the physiological and behavioural responses to stress. The limbic system is a set of structures related to the control of emotional responses, behaviour and long-term memory. The main structures involved are the hippocampus and the amygdala. The limbic system has connections with the prefrontal cortex, related to attention and motivation, and with the hypothalamus, which regulates endocrine and autonomic system functioning. At the same time, the hippocampus is a target of stress hormones. Chronic increase in cortisol level may induce structural remodelling and selective atrophy of hippocampus, associated with altered behavioural and physiological responses (McEwen 1999).

The immune system also plays an important role in the stress response, and it is completely integrated in the psychoneuroendocrinological system. Both catecholamines and glucocorticoids control the amplitude of immune response by negative-feedback mechanisms. In physically threatening situations, inflammatory cytokines, mainly interleukin-6, stimulate the HPA axis, and the elevation of cortisol levels induces the suppression of the immune/inflammatory reaction. Simultaneously, the sympathetic system causes systemic secretion of cytokines which will eventually suppress the immune system (Stratakis & Chrousos 1995). Thus we see how the activation of the HPA axis helps to regulate the activity of the immune response, and in the case of psychological distress, the immune system can be suppressed.

These aspects of the immune response's physiology hypothetically have relevance in the genesis or progression of multiple diseases. An increased HPA axis activity, as in chronic stress, may have a tendency to increase susceptibility to infections or neoplasias. And a defective HPA axis response, as happens in post chronic stress situations, will tend to increase susceptibility to autoimmune/inflammatory diseases.

The modification of the global activity of the immune system also depends on the time and the type of stressor. Stressors differ one from another not only in intensity but also in temporal and qualitative properties. This has been referred to as the specificity of the stress response (Pacak & Palkovits 2001). Different types of stressor will affect the immune response in diverse ways, leading to different disorders. A meta-analysis (Segerstrom & Miller 2004) suggests that acute stressors are associated with suppression of specific humoral immunity, brief naturalistic stressors tend to suppress cellular immunity, while chronic stressors are associated with suppression of both cellular and humoral measures, which coincides with a non-specific inflammation.

This discussion on the type of stressors leads us to stop and briefly consider the meaning of the 'flight or fight' response. To understand it fully we need to adopt an evolutionary developmental perspective. The stress response is an adaptive preservationary phenomenon. Biologically, the 'flight or fight' response is a primitive response, a reflection of early stages in our species' development, and thus, it is not well suited to deal with the type of stressors we face nowadays. To understand how the stress response evolutionarily designed to help us survive can also hurt us, we will employ two useful concepts: allostasis and allostatic load.

Allostasis, a concept incorporated into medicine by Sterling & Eyer (1988), is the ability to achieve stability through change. It refers to the biological mechanisms that protect the body from internal and external stress, to maintain the internal balance of homeostasis. But sometimes, the stress system cannot maintain the internal balance for different reasons. Selye (1946) had described the general adaptation syndrome by identifying three stages: the alarm stage, the stage of resistance and the state of exhaustion. This process describes the pathophysiology of those disorders in which the body is overwhelmed by sustained stressors. But, in the presence of chronic stress, other mechanisms must be taken into consideration, and it is important to realize that the overactivation of the allostatic systems can lead to different disorders or diseases. This long-term effect of the physiologic response to stress has been called allostatic load – the metabolic wear and tear on the organism that occurs as the price for maintaining allostasis of physiological systems (McEwen & Stellar 1993; McEwen 1998). Several physiological parameters that reflect levels of activity of different systems have been described (Seeman et al. 1997). This allows us to conceptualize allostatic load as a cumulative measure of dysregulation across these regulatory systems.

This allostatic load process can be studied also at a cellular level. It is now increasingly clear that psychosocial stress can be translated into metabolic activation and processed at the cellular level as oxidative stress (McEwen & Seeman 1999). Oxidative stress refers to potentially pathogenic effects of the mitochondrial breakdown products (oxidative metabolites and free radicals) produced as a result of the overactivity of cellular oxidative metabolism in the face of physical and psychosocial stressors (Maes 2009). Recently it has been shown how chronic psychosocial stress can lead to a pathogenic process because of cellular oxidative stress (Epel et al. 2006), associated with telomere length shortening in peripheral blood mononuclear cell and low telomerase activity (Epel et al. 2004). The proinflammatory transcription factor NF-κB has been identified as a potential critical bridge between stress and oxidative cellular activation (Bierhaus et al. 2004). Studies show that NF-κB is activated by different types of stressor (Nagabhushan et al. 2001; Bierhaus et al. 2003), and this activation is correlated with an increase in catecholamines and cortisol.

These oxidative stress processes also correlate with modifications in gene expression (Madrigal et al. 2002). NF-κB then binds to DNA and activates transcription of genes for cytokines and other inflammatory mediators, and enhances the survival of tumour cells by upregulating antiapoptotic genes (Schottelius & Dinter 2006). Furthermore, allostatic loading can lead to oxidative and nitrosative stress with the resultant production of free radicals and gene expression/production of stress-sensitive heat shock protein (Billack et al. 2002), a regulator of oxidative stress. As we will see later on, all these findings on this potential stress–pathology link will aid research into whether stress reduction therapies can also influence cellular activities (Bierhaus et al. 2003).

These mechanisms we have just addressed constitute a plausible explanation of how stress is implicated in the genesis and progression of multiple disorders. The statistical association between stress and these disorders is clear. Although more research is required to establish a causal link unequivocally, consistent evidence suggests that this causal relation exists (Cohen et al. 2007). The increasing prevalence of allostatic load disorders, such as metabolic syndrome, leads one to wonder whether stress is really increasing in the last few decades. Due to conceptual and methodological reasons, it is difficult to compare today's stress levels accurately with levels in the past. However, there are some indicators that suggest both objective and subjective stress levels are increasing along with their physiological manifestations. In fact, studies suggest that around 70% of all primary care visits are related to psychological factors or stress-related conditions (Strosahl 1998). What interests us next is that mind–body interventions (MBIs) can constitute an approach which specifically counteracts the harmful effects of stress.

THE RELAXATION RESPONSE

In the same building at Harvard Medical School where Cannon's 'flight or fight' response was described years earlier, Dr Herbert Benson (2000) described a physiological response which became known as the 'relaxation response' (RR). The RR refers to a physiological state observed in people while meditating, characterized by decreased metabolism, decreased heart rate, decreased blood pressure, decreased rate of breathing and slower brain waves. The RR is, in a sense, the opposite of the stress response, but while the stress response occurs automatically when one experiences stress, the RR is elicited voluntarily.

More specifically, the RR is a hypometabolic physiological state usually brought about by an altered state of consciousness. It implies both a deeply relaxed physical condition and a focused, clear and alert mental state. Such a physiological state turns off the 'inner dialogue' and thereby decreases the arousal of the sympathetic nervous system. The RR is composed of several integrated physiological mechanisms and adjustments that counteract the stress response. Much research has been done reporting evidence on the physiology of the RR. This research documented decreased oxygen consumption and carbon dioxide production (Beary & Benson 1974; Benson et al. 1978a), reduced sympathetic nervous system responsivity (Hoffman et al. 1982), reduction in frontal electroencephalogram beta activity (Jacobs et al. 1996a), increased liberation and exhalation of nitric oxide (Stefano et al. 2001a) and functional activation of neural structures involved in attention and control of the autonomic nervous system, particularly the hippocampus (Lazar et al. 2000).

Benson developed a simplified method to elicit the RR, based on experience and on a detailed analysis of the efficacious elements common to different techniques. This method consists of two steps: breaking the train of everyday thoughts and repetition of a word, thought or movement, with passive return to the repetitive pattern when daily thoughts intrude. This proposed method, frequently associated with the physiological response elicited, has led some researchers to classify the RR as a relaxation technique (Astin et al. 2003) or as a meditation technique (Barrows & Jacobs 2002). However, since its definition, the RR has been understood as an underlying mechanism present in diverse techniques, and several physiological parameters support the existence of the RR during the practice of different techniques (Hassed 2007).

Concretely, the RR is present in relaxation therapies (e.g. progressive muscle relaxation), different forms of meditation (transcendental meditation, mindfulness meditation and others), autogenic training, corporal therapies (yoga, tai chi, qigong), hypnosis and guided imagery. The RR is a common element in these techniques, though they may all offer special features. The specific method used usually reflects the preferred approach of the person eliciting the RR, and it is important to point out that it is not necessary to adopt a specific theoretical approach or a particular religious orientation to achieve the RR. Indeed, the RR can also be achieved with repetitive physical exercise, repetition of a word or other repetitive patterns.

Nevertheless meditation is possibly the most powerful way of eliciting the RR (Hassad 2006). In every religion or culture, meditation has a particular meaning and purpose. Beyond that meaning are the physiological effects of this 'self-regulation of attention'. There are multiple forms of meditation, and it can be difficult to classify them for research purposes. Different definitions of meditation, like those of Manocha (2000) or Cardoso et al. (2004), can be helpful to describe authentic and specific meditation techniques. However, they can be too constrictive and, according to our experience, a wider concept of meditation may be needed so as to extend its benefits to a broader population, without the necessity of adopting any particular religious attitude. Arias and colleagues (2006) propose a multidimensional classification system, which allows for comparison and differentiation among the different types of meditation. The system includes several dimensions, including physical and mental activity, goals and also the ability to elicit the RR.

The therapeutic effect of the RR resides in its ability to reduce sympathetic nervous activation and increase parasympathetic system activity, restoring the balance and mitigating the effects of overactivation of the stress response and of the inflammatory response syndrome (Hoffman et al. 1982; Tracey 2007). The knowledge of stress physiology and its relation to oxidative stress and inflammatory processes lead us to consider new potential therapeutic mechanisms of the RR. As we saw earlier, the extent of NF-κB activation in peripheral blood mononuclear cells, which when activated become macrophages, correlates with oxidative stress and it has been shown that it can be reduced by therapeutic interventions that decrease oxidative stress (Hoffmann et al. 1999). Patients with altered downregulation of the NF-κB activation may be more vulnerable to stress. One way to address this issue is to stabilize the association of I-kappa B-alpha with NF-κB, reducing the production of protein activators of oxidative stress as well as proinflammatory cytokines (Stefano et al. 2001b). The RR and other mental activities may be able to effect such stabilization through enhancement of constitutive nitric oxide mechanisms. Nitric oxide is a gaseous transmitter, which in its constitutive form relaxes vascular endothelium, retards endothelial cell ageing and enhances neural long-term potentiation-based memory, among other effects on the body and brain (Stefano et al. 2001b). The RR stabilization effect may be reflected in the correlation of exhaled nitric oxide with decreased oxygen consumption in individuals taught the RR (Dusek et al. 2006). In addition our team was recently able to show that novice subjects after 8 weeks of RR training National Academies Press, showed blood gene activation profiles consistent with reduced oxidative stress and reduced NF-κB activation (Dusek et al. 2008).

The regular elicitation of the RR has been shown to result in long-term physiological changes that counteract the harmful effects of stress (Hoffman et al. 1982). Thus, it has been reported to alleviate many stress-related medical disorders (Mandle et al. 1996; Jacobs 2001; Esch et al. 2003). The regular elicitation of the RR has been found to be efficacious in the treatment of hypertension, arrhythmias (Benson et al. 1975), chronic pain (Caudill et al. 1991), insomnia (Jacobs et al. 1993, 1996b), anxiety and mild and moderate depression (Benson et al. 1978b), premenstrual syndrome (Goodale et al. 1990) and infertility (Domar et al. 1990).

In a clinical setting, the RR is not offered alone but in the context of integrated stress management and resiliency enhancement programmes. These approaches (Nakao et al. 2001a) include instruction in a combination of behavioural interventions such as nutrition, exercise, sleep hygiene, cognitive restructuring and social support. These dimensions are not independent but rather components of an overall approach (Friedman et al. 1995) for the benefit of the patient. They are addressed to patients with chronic illnesses and stress-related conditions, and help them manage the consequences of stress more effectively. This multidimensional context of the RR-based mind–body approach helps us to understand better psychosomatic balance and its therapeutic implications. It suggests that a mind–body medicine equation hypothesis can be derived from the research described above (Albee 1982; Ting & Fricchione 2006). In this equation the propensity to health is defined by a relationship between the stress burden (allostatic load) and genetic vulnerability as denominator and all those personal resources which help us to cope better with the stressors (resilience) and genetic endowment as numerator. As numerator of the equation we must include all the mentioned self-management skills regarding the ability to elicit the RR, cognitive skills, social support, prosocial behaviour, positive psychology and spiritual beliefs. Gene expression changes, likely induced epigenetically, may form the links within the numerator between genes and resiliency and within the denominator between genes and stress (Dusek et al. 2008). Thus, MBIs, by promoting a secure attachment style and enriched environment, are effective in buffering against stress and in building resilience.

USE AND EFFICACY OF THE MIND–BODY TECHNIQUES

Before looking at the clinical efficacy of MBIs, it may be interesting to consider briefly how many people use these approaches, what particular interventions they use, and for what conditions. The interest in mind–body medicine among the general population has grown over the years, as has been documented in a national survey in the USA (Eisenberg et al. 1998; Wolsko et al. 2004). Around 20% of the population has used an MBI of some kind in the last year. Meditation and relaxation techniques were the most highly endorsed. This figure coincides with another study in which health professionals manifested higher interest in learning these approaches and lower interest in biofeedback and hypnosis (Sierpina et al. 2007a). Mind–body therapies were most frequently used for different chronic conditions, such as anxiety, depression, chronic pain, insomnia, gastrointestinal disorders and fatigue, for which currently available therapies are not entirely satisfactory. In fact, anxiety and pain have been proposed as the symptoms that best predict the public's search for alternative therapies (Hassed 2006). However, the main reason why people use these kinds of interventions is not dissatisfaction with conventional medicine but because they have found these interventions to be more consistent with their own beliefs, values and personal philosophy (Astin 1998).

Despite the difficulties inherent in this particular clinical research, evidence for the efficacy of MBIs is becoming stronger (Ernst et al. 2007). According to Astin and colleagues (2003), there is strong to moderate evidence of MBI efficacy in the following medical conditions: cardiovascular disease (Linden et al. 1996; Dusseldrop et al. 1999), hypertension (Jacob et al. 1991; Linden & Chambers 1994), insomnia (Morin et al. 1994; Wang et al. 2005), low-back pain (van Tulder et al. 2000), headache (Holroyd & Penzien 1990; Haddock et al. 1997; Sierpina et al. 2007b), arthritis self-care (Lorig & Holman 1993; Superio-Cabuslay et al. 1996), incontinence (Burgio et al. 1998; Glavind et al. 1998; Hirsch et al. 1999), surgical outcomes (Johnston & Vogele 1993; Dreher 1998) and cancer treatment tolerance (Redd et al. 2001). Pelletier (2004) reports that for acute pain (Seers & Carroll 1998) and fibromyalgia (Hadhazy et al. 2000) there is also strong evidence, and adds a number of other conditions where research is less definitive but current randomized controlled trials indicate positive efficacy: allergies (Watkins 1994), asthma (Castes et al. 1999; McQuaid & Nassau 1999; Smyth et al. 1999), dermatological disorders (Kabat-Zinn et al. 1998), diabetes (Aikens et al. 1997; Henry et al. 1997; Jablon et al. 1997), human immunodeficiency virus (HIV) progression (Cruess et al. 1999; Robinson et al. 1999), irritable bowel syndrome

(Schwarz et al. 1990; Blanchard & Malamood 1996; Galovski & Blanchard 1998; Vollmer & Blanchard 1998), poststroke rehabilitation (Moreland et al. 1998), peptic ulcer (Levenstein et al. 1999), pregnancy outcomes (Scott et al. 1999), chronic obstructive pulmonary disease (Devine & Pearcy 1996) and tinnitus (Andersson & Lyttkens 1999).

Looking at these conditions, we understand that they are related to allostatic loading and stress physiology at different levels: autonomic nervous system, endocrinological axes and immune system. Many other disorders are also likely to respond to MBIs, but sufficient studies have not yet been done. The role of stress has been widely discussed in the disorders of anxiety and depression (Esch et al. 2002; Swaab et al. 2005) and MBIs have been shown to be effective (Benson et al. 1978b; Kabat-Zinn et al. 1992), though there are methodological limitations (Pilkington et al. 2005; Toneatto & Nguyen 2007). Anxiety and depression are important comorbid conditions with somatic symptoms, and it is not easy to say whether they are an intermediate step in the aetiopathology of somatic symptoms or whether both somatic and psychological symptoms are a manifestation of an underlying common pathophysiology. In any case, both anxiety and depression play a role in the prognosis of somatic conditions, and while the level of depression is related to the reporting of somatic symptoms (Nakao et al. 2001b), anxiety appears to be a good indicator for somatic symptom reduction using MBIs (Nakao et al. 2001c).

Other aspects must also be considered regarding the clinical effectiveness of MBIs. Because they promote self-care (Benson et al. 1974), MBIs also seem to be cost-effective. It has been documented (Sobel 2000) that these approaches reduce ambulatory visits, post surgical days in the hospital, unnecessary procedures and medical costs. As part of the cost-effectiveness analysis, MBIs also improve patient satisfaction, sense of control and quality of life (Sobel 1995). We must also highlight that, despite the effectiveness described, MBIs are not panaceas (Jacobs 2001), and in most cases, they are to be used as complementary therapies in combination with conventional medical procedures. Research will also have to define the role of mind–body medicine in primary prevention (Astin 2004), considering that stress plays a role in the onset of some diseases and MBIs lead to modifications in lifestyle.

THEORIES OF MECHANISMS OF ACTION

It is not yet possible to describe accurately the mechanisms of MBIs. At the same time we must be aware that mind–body therapies, like many other interventions, can demonstrate efficacy without our fully understanding the mechanisms of action (Astin 2002). Nevertheless, we will mention some hypotheses that have been suggested and psychophysiological models that help to explain some of the effects of these approaches. Although space does not allow us to be systematic, given biopsychosocial spiritual integration and according to the structure and components of the human stress system, we will consider different levels of action of mind–body therapies.

The contribution of the placebo effect to our understanding of mind–body effects in general is sizeable. The placebo effect is inherent to the doctor–patient relationship, and it is present in all MBIs, as it is in other therapeutic interventions (see Chapter 16). However it would be a mistake to think that the whole effect of MBIs comes down to the placebo effect. Usually, the placebo effect has negative connotations with regard to research because of its supposed non-specificity. Actually, the placebo effect may well be a constitutive and critical element of the mind–body therapies themselves (Astin 2004). However, in a clinical context we welcome the placebo effect as a powerful example of the healing power of the mind. MBIs try to take advantage of this non-specific innate capacity of the organism in a therapeutic and specific way.

The placebo effect represents the manifestation of a 'proactive mind–body link that evokes an innate protective response' (Stefano et al. 2001b). Motivation, suggestion, positive expectations and beliefs of the patient, which are enhanced and used in MBIs, can constitute a stimulus that elicits this protective response. The underlying mechanisms of this response are not clear, but there is consistent evidence (Lazar et al. 2000; Stefano et al. 2001b; Mayberg et al. 2002; Ploghaus et al. 2003; Raz et al. 2005) that the prefrontal cortex is activated under conditions of conscious positive expectation. It is known that the prefrontal cortex is particularly related to attention, and it is part of the brain motivation and reward circuitry, which is also involved in the placebo effect. The prefrontal cortex establishes connection through corticostriatal tracts with corpus striatum and ventral tegmentum and with structures in the limbic system (amygdala and hippocampus) and hypothalamus, involved in learning and memory, motivation and arousal/autonomic control. Simultaneously, in these natural proactive processes, molecular mechanisms are involved, including opioid neuropeptides and nitric oxide. Endorphins and enkephalins are associated with analgesia, a sense of well-being, and also help modulate the immune system. Constitutive nitric oxide is an immune, vascular and neural signalling molecule that performs vital physiological activities. Both these mechanisms provide possible links between stress, cognitive processes and the central nervous system on the one hand, and the autonomic nervous system, endocrinological axes and immune system on the other. In comparing the RR and the placebo effect, we find they are related and share common mechanisms. In fact, the RR has been defined as the physical learned component of the placebo effect (Stefano et al. 2001b). But the placebo effect can act without eliciting the RR, and the RR can be elicited without special expectation or beliefs, through the use of focused attention and with processes of active and passive repetition. Placebo response may emerge in the light of the meaning that comes with positive expectation, which then produces a version of the RR (Moerman & Jonas 2002).

Another specific mechanism of action of MBIs, especially of the meditation techniques, is constituted by a special focusing of attention. Attention plays an important role in filtering both external and internal stimuli. This mechanism is implicated in different somatic disorders, both in the perception of the symptoms and in the feedback mechanisms involved in the genesis and maintenance of the symptoms. Common health complaints are normal for most people, but intolerable for some (Ursin & Eriksen 2007). In fact, somatoform disorders can be understood as disorders in the perception of bodily signals (Rief & Barsky 2005). Reasons for these misperceptions can be amplified sensory signals, reduced filtering capacities or further factors influencing the strength of the signal or the capacity of the sensory filters. This may be explained by psychobiological sensitization within neural loops maintained by sustained attention, as it is described in the cognitive activation theory of stress (Ursin & Eriksen 2004). Sustained high levels of arousal lead to sensitization processes, in which the same signals can lead to more and more amplified perceptions.

MBIs specifically address these mechanisms in different ways. Firstly, they develop a focused attention that helps to filter both external and internal stimuli efficiently, thus reducing perceived stress. This enhances a detached observation which may in turn cause an uncoupling of the affective and sensory dimensions of the pain experience (Kabat-Zinn 1982). Secondly, the RR present in many MBIs results in a hypometabolism state that produces an attenuation of stress reactivity (Astin 2004). The physiological state of hypoarousal (RR) may serve to diminish pain and its related emotional symptoms directly. It reduces sensitivity to catecholamines (Morrell & Hollandsworth 1986) and decreases sympathetic nervous system reactivity (Hoffman et al. 1982). Nitric oxide also counteracts noradrenaline (norepinephrine) activity and sympathetic responsivity directly (Stefano et al. 2001a). And thirdly, in developing a better sense of bodily control and awareness of emotional processes, these interventions can increase the feedback and improve the autoregulation processes (Astin 2004). Both sense of control and feedback permit the organism to reduce its level of arousal (Ursin & Eriksen 2004). The process of auto-observing present in MBIs may result in a deconditioning of the alarm reactivity to primary sensations. Through these mechanisms, individuals become more aware of their cognitive/emotional patterns and ways of reacting and recognition of the automatic and unconscious nature of stress reactivity facilitates greater control while enlarging the repertoire of possible responses to daily stressors. Thus, coping with stress is facilitated and is performed more effectively.

MBIs also facilitate coping with stress by building cognitive skills and enhancing social support, prosocial behaviour and spirituality. On the one hand, social support is associated with lower rates of mortality and morbidity (Uchino 2006), and beneficial changes in cardiovascular, neuroendocrine and immune function have been described. Emotional attachment and social integration are included in the concept of social support (Rosengren et al. 2004). Perceived social support has a direct effect on NK cells so that increased social support might be accompanied by high natural immunity (Miyazaki et al. 2003). Spirituality implies a sense of connectedness to something larger than oneself, to one's deepest self, to other people and to all regarded as good, and it urges us to share qualities such as love, empathy, caring and compassion with others. Spirituality thus implies a sense of meaning and purpose, and it constitutes a unifying force which harmonizes the physical, mental, emotional and social aspects and dimensions of health. It has been shown that patients who are more spiritual may use their beliefs in coping with stress, tend to have better recovery from illness and surgery, and tend to live longer (Puchalski 2001). Spirituality enhances a secure style of attachment, which lowers separation stress and thus is very relevant to stress-buffering and health-strengthening.

Finally, from the developmental perspective, mind–body medicine interventions are effective in buffering against the effects of stress and building resilience. Resilience is a multidimensional construct that refers to the ability to maintain positive adaptation under significant adversity or challenging life conditions (Luthar et al. 2000). Despite the fact that the concept has been criticized for its loose definition, it provides a framework for thinking about development, is useful in understanding the adjustment to stress as a dynamic process and helps us to integrate the different elements of mind–body medicine. Resiliency refers to cognitive, behavioural and emotional capacities that reduce our vulnerability to the pathogenic effects of allostatic loading. Resiliency factors such as RR ability, social support, cognitive skills, positive psychology with optimism, meaning and purpose, and spirituality can be enhanced with MBIs and will help in diverse adaptational domains. From a neurobiological perspective, resilience is directly related to allostasis and the same biological mediators (Seeman et al. 1997) of allostatic load may contribute to resiliency or vulnerability. Charney (2004) identifies three neural mechanisms that are relevant to the character traits associated with resiliency: (1) the mesolimbic-mesocortical dopamine pathways and the nucleus accumbens and ventral pallidum involved in reward, motivation, hedonia and optimism; (2) the structures of the limbic system (mainly the amygdala and hippocampus) and its connections with prefrontal cortex, hypothalamus and brainstem, relevant in learning, memory and fear responsiveness; and (3) the circuitries involving the anterior cingulate and affiliative neuropeptide neuromodulation (oxytocin and vasopressin), relevant to altruism, attachment and adaptive social behaviour.

CONCLUSIONS

In summary, we can say that stress has a huge impact in many conditions and disorders. These conditions are increasing nowadays in our society, both because of lifestyle and because of a lack of personal resources. Available conventional treatments fail in their attempt to improve stress-related symptoms and, as a result, patients suffer greatly and go on to develop chronic conditions. These disorders are also a burden for health systems. Mind–body medicine and RR-based approaches specifically counteract the impact of stress both on the cognition and on the physiology of the individual, and they encourage a breaking of the negative stress cycle and a fostering of healthy behaviours. As we have described in this chapter, there is now enough evidence to suggest the efficacy of these interventions supporting their application in mainstream practice, in most cases as adjunctive or complementary treatments (Astin 2004). Much research is still to be done and we will now point out some areas in which research in mind–body medicine is particularly relevant.

Research must continue to address the specificity of MBIs. Astin (2004) points out that it is necessary to identify clearly which strategies are effective under what conditions and for which patients. One intrinsic difficulty consists of the fact that the natural context for MBIs is really a package of interventions, so it is neither easy nor natural to address the efficacy of each intervention independently. And furthermore, another difficulty is that each intervention can include in itself components of other techniques, so the mechanisms are not exclusive to each intervention. Thus, future research will need to assess the efficacy of multicomponent interventions for specific conditions, and at the same time, examine the mechanisms of actions of each technique.

The best efficacy studies are double-blind, randomized, placebo-controlled trials, which are necessary to assess the specific effect of the intervention. However, these methodologies may be especially difficult to carry out in mind–body medicine (Astin 2004; Berman & Straus 2004) because it is exceedingly difficult to blind patients and controls, and because, as we have seen, the placebo effect is one of the important mechanisms of action of these interventions. Similar difficulties are found for controlled trials in psychotherapy, and we should minimize bias using supportive no-treatment controls (Miller et al. 2004).

A particular difficulty in mind–body research stems from the fact that compliance with the treatment doesn't necessarily mean that the intervention is being administered properly (Caspi & Burleson 2005), because we must also monitor the quality and intensity of the intervention. At the same time, not all techniques evoke the RR in the same way. It has been shown that, with practice, deeper relaxation states are achieved, associated with more therapeutic effect. Long-term or expert meditation practitioners also showed more functional magnetic resonance imaging activation of brain regions involved in sustained attention than those with little practice (Brefczynski-Lewis et al. 2007). Different methods can be useful to quantify the intensity of the RR. Oxygen consumption levels have been used as an indicator, and exhaled nitric oxide has been proposed as a good parameter that co-varies with reductions in oxygen consumption during RR (Stefano et al. 2001a). However, more research must be done to determine the operative way to use these indicators clinically.

Mind–body medicine research must also be open to a variety of research challenges. We have previously commented on the necessity of assessing the efficacy of these interventions in primary prevention (Astin 2004), as well as evaluating cost-effectiveness with clinical trials (Pelletier 2004) of these approaches. Important new study designs (Caspi & Burlseon 2005) can be used in mind–body research. For example, mixed methods (Cunningham 2002), integrating qualitative into quantitative studies, can be used in such a way that participants' experiences and attributions are taken into consideration not only for clinical purposes but also with regard to research aims. In addition, pragmatic clinical trials, a concept recently introduced (Tunis et al. 2003), can be useful in analysing the real efficacy and cost-effectiveness of mind–body treatments. Future research in mind–body medicine must also be performed in what has been called psychosocial genomics (Rossi 2002). Allostatic loading and MBIs are likely to modify gene expression, constituting short-term changes compatible with a developmental understanding. In this regard, recently, a study using RR and a study using qigong both showed distinctive gene expression profile changes in genes associated with oxidative metabolism, apoptosis and inflammatory response modulation (Dusek et al. 2008).

REFERENCES

Aikens, J.E., Kiolbasa, T.A., Sobel, R., 1997. Psychological predictors of glycemic change with relaxation training in non-insulin-dependent diabetes mellitus. Psychother. Psychosom. 66 (6), 302–306.

Albee, G.W., 1982. Preventing psychopathology and promoting human potential. Am. Psychol. 37 (9), 1043–1050.

Andersson, G., Lyttkens, L., 1999. A meta-analytic review of psychological treatments for tinnitus. Br. J. Audiol. 33 (4), 201–210.

Arias, A.J., Steinberg, K., Banga, A., et al., 2006. Systematic review of the efficacy of meditation techniques as treatments for medical illness. J. Altern. Complement. Med. 12 (8), 817–832.

Astin, J.A., Goddard, T.G., Forys, K., 2005. Barriers to the integration of mind–body medicine: perceptions of physicians, residents, and medical students. Explore (NY) 1 (4), 278–283.

Astin, J.A., 1998. Why patients use alternative medicine: results of a national study. JAMA 279 (19), 1548–1553.

Astin, J.A., 2002. Complementary and alternative medicine and the need for evidence-based criticism. Acad. Med. 77 (9), 864–868. discussion 869–875.

Astin, J.A., 2004. Mind–body therapies for the management of pain. Clin. J. Pain 20 (1), 27–32.

Astin, J.A., Shapiro, S.L., Eisenberg, D.M., et al., 2003. Mind–body medicine: state of the science, implications for practice. J. Am. Board Fam. Pract. 16 (2), 131–147.

Barrows, K.A., Jacobs, B.P., 2002. Mind–body medicine. An introduction and review of the literature. Med. Clin. North Am. 86 (1), 11–31.

Beary, J.F., Benson, H., 1974. A simple psychophysiologic technique which elicits the hypometabolic changes of the relaxation response. Psychosom. Med. 36 (2), 115–120.

Benson, H., 2000. The relaxation response. Avon Books, New York.

Benson, H., Beary, J.F., Carol, M.P., 1974.The relaxation response. Psychiatry 37 (1), 37–46.

Benson, H., Alexander, S., Feldman, C.L., 1975. Decreased premature ventricular contractions through use of the relaxation response in patients with stable ischaemic heart-disease. Lancet 2 (7931), 380–382.

Benson, H., Dryer, T., Hartley, L.H., 1978a. Decreased VO_2 consumption during exercise with elicitation of the relaxation response. J. Human Stress 4 (2), 38–42.

Benson, H., Frankel, F.H., Apfel, R., et al., 1978b. Treatment of anxiety: a comparison of the usefulness of self-hypnosis and a meditational relaxation technique. An overview. Psychother. Psychosom. 30 (3–4), 229–242.

Berman, J.D., Straus, S.E., 2004. Implementing a research agenda for complementary and alternative medicine. Annu. Rev. Med. 55, 239–254.

Bierhaus, A., Wolf, J., Andrassy, M., et al., 2003. A mechanism converting psychosocial stress into mononuclear cell activation. Proc. Natl. Acad. Sci. U S A 100 (4), 1920–1925.

Bierhaus, A., Humpert, P.M., Nawroth, P.P., 2004. NF-kappaB as a molecular link between psychosocial stress and organ dysfunction. Pediatr. Nephrol. 19 (11), 1189–1191.

Billack, B., Heck, D.E., Mariano, T.M., et al., 2002. Induction of cyclooxygenase-2 by heat shock protein 60 in macrophages and endothelial cells. Am. J. Physiol. Cell Physiol. 283 (4), C1267–C1277.

Blanchard, E.B., Malamood, H.S., 1996. Psychological treatment of irritable bowel syndrome. Professional Psychology: Research and Practice 27 (3), 241–244.

Brefczynski-Lewis, J.A., Lutz, A., Schaefer, H.S., et al., 2007. Neural correlates of attentional expertise in long-term meditation practitioners. Proc. Natl. Acad. Sci. U S A 104 (27), 11483–11488.

Burgio, K.L., Locher, J.L., Goode, P.S., et al., 1998. Behavioral vs drug treatment for urge urinary incontinence in older women: a randomized controlled trial. JAMA 280 (23), 1995–2000.

Cannon, W., 1929. Bodily changes in pain, hunger, fear, and rage. Appleton, New York.

Cardoso, R., de Souza, E., Camano, L., et al., 2004. Meditation in health: an operational definition. Brain Res. Brain Res. Protoc. 14 (1), 58–60.

Caspi, O., Burleson, K.O., 2005. Methodological challenges in meditation research. Adv. Mind Body. Med. 21 (1), 4–11.

Castes, M., Hagel, I., Palenque, M., et al., 1999. Immunological changes associated with clinical improvement of asthmatic children subjected to psychosocial intervention. Brain Behav. Immun. 13 (1), 1–13.

Caudill, M., Schnable, R., Zuttermeister, P., et al., 1991. Decreased clinic use by chronic pain patients: response to behavioral medicine intervention. Clin. J. Pain 7 (4), 305–310.

Charney, D.S., 2004. Psychobiological mechanisms of resilience and vulnerability: implications for successful adaptation to extreme stress. Am. J. Psychiatry 161 (2), 195–216.

Chrousos, G.P., Gold, P.W., 1992. The concepts of stress and stress system disorders. Overview of physical and behavioral homeostasis. JAMA 267 (9), 1244–1252.

Cohen, S., Janicki-Deverts, D., Miller, G.E., 2007. Psychological stress and disease. JAMA 298 (14), 1685–1687.

Cruess, D.G., Antoni, M.H., Kumar, M., et al., 1999. Cognitive-behavioral stress management buffers decreases in dehydroepiandrosterone sulfate (DHEA-S) and increases in the cortisol/DHEA-S ratio and reduces mood disturbance and perceived stress among HIV-seropositive men. Psychoneuroendocrinology 24 (5), 537–549.

Cunningham, A.J., 2002. A new approach to testing the effects of group psychological therapy on length of life in patients with metastatic cancers. Adv. Mind Body Med. 18 (2), 5–9.

Devine, E.C., Pearcy, J., 1996. Meta-analysis of the effects of psychoeducational care in adults with chronic obstructive pulmonary disease. Patient Educ. Couns. 29 (2), 167–178.

Domar, A.D., Seibel, M.M., Benson, H., 1990. The mind/body program for infertility: a new behavioral treatment approach for women with infertility. Fertil. Steril. 53 (2), 246–249.

Dreher, H., 1998. Mind–body interventions for surgery: evidence and exigency. Adv. Mind Body Med. 14 (3), 207–222.

Dusek, J.A., Chang, B.H., Zaki, J., et al., 2006. Association between oxygen consumption and nitric oxide production during the relaxation response. Med. Sci. Monit. 12 (1), CR1–CR10.

Dusek, J.A., Otu, H.H., Wohlhueter, A.L., et al., 2008. Genomic counter-stress changes induced by the relaxation response. PLoS ONE 3 (7), e2576.

Dusseldorp, E., van Elderen, T., Maes, S., et al., 1999. A meta-analysis of psychoeduational programs for coronary heart disease patients. Health Psychol. 18 (5), 506–519.

Eisenberg, D.M., Davis, R.B., Ettner, S.L., et al., 1998. Trends in alternative medicine use in the United States, 1990–1997: results of a follow-up national survey. JAMA 280 (18), 1569–1575.

Epel, E.S., Blackburn, E.H., Lin, J., et al., 2004. Accelerated telomere shortening in response to life stress. Proc. Natl. Acad. Sci. U S A 101 (49), 17312–17315.

Epel, E.S., Lin, J., Wilhelm, F.H., et al., 2006. Cell aging in relation to stress arousal and cardiovascular disease risk factors. Psychoneuroendocrinology 31 (3), 277–287.

Ernst, E., Pittler, M.H., Wider, B., et al., 2007. Mind–body therapies: are the trial data getting stronger? Altern. Ther. Health Med. 13 (5), 62–64.

Esch, T., Stefano, G.B., Fricchione, G.L., et al., 2002. The role of stress in neurodegenerative diseases and mental disorders. Neuro. Endocrinol. Lett. 23 (3), 199–208.

Esch, T., Fricchione, G.L., Stefano, G.B., 2003. The therapeutic use of the relaxation response in stress-related diseases. Med. Sci. Monit. 9 (2), RA23–RA34.

Friedman, R., Sobel, D., Myers, P., et al., 1995. Behavioral medicine, clinical health psychology, and cost offset. Health Psychol. 14 (6), 509–518.

Gaab, J., Rohleder, N., Nater, U.M., et al., 2005. Psychological determinants of the cortisol stress response: the role of anticipatory cognitive appraisal. Psychoneuroendocrinology 30 (6), 599–610.

Galovski, T.E., Blanchard, E.B., 1998. The treatment of irritable bowel syndrome with hypnotherapy. Appl. Psychophysiol Biofeedback 23 (4), 219–232.

Glavind, K., Laursen, B., Jaquet, A., 1998. Efficacy of biofeedback in the treatment of urinary stress incontinence. Int. Urogynecol. J. Pelvic. Floor Dysfunct. 9 (3), 151–153.

Goodale, I.L., Domar, A.D., Benson, H., 1990. Alleviation of premenstrual syndrome symptoms with the relaxation response. Obstet. Gynecol. 75 (4), 649–655.

Haddock, C.K., Rowan, A.B., Andrasik, F., et al., 1997. Home-based behavioral treatments for chronic benign headache: a meta-analysis of controlled trials. Cephalalgia 17 (2), 113–118.

Hadhazy, V.A., Ezzo, J., Creamer, P., et al., 2000. Mind–body therapies for the treatment of fibromyalgia. A systematic review. J. Rheumatol. 27 (12), 2911–2918.

Hassed, C., Mind–body medicine: science, practice and philosophy. [updated 2006 October; cited 2007 December 15]. Available online from: http://www.gawler.org/files/5WE1GZCXQL/MBM%20revised%2006.pdf.

Henry, J.L., Wilson, P., Bruce, D., et al., 1997. Cognitive-behavioural stress management for patients with non-insulin dependent diabetes mellitus. Psychol. Health Med. 2 (2), 109–118.

Hirsch, A., Weirauch, G., Steimer, B., et al., 1999. Treatment of female urinary incontinence with EMG-controlled biofeedback home training. Int. Urogynecol. J. Pelvic. Floor Dysfunct. 10 (1), 7–10.

Hoffman, J.W., Benson, H., Arns, P.A., et al., 1982. Reduced sympathetic nervous system responsivity associated with the relaxation response. Science 215 (4529), 190–192.

Hofmann, M.A., Schiekofer, S., Isermann, B., et al., 1999. Peripheral blood mononuclear cells isolated from patients with diabetic nephropathy show increased activation of the oxidative-stress sensitive transcription factor NF-kappaB. Diabetologia 42 (2), 222–232.

Holroyd, K.A., Penzien, D.B., 1990. Pharmacological versus non-pharmacological prophylaxis of recurrent migraine headache: a meta-analytic review of clinical trials. Pain 42 (1), 1–13.

Jablon, S.L., Naliboff, B.D., Gilmore, S.L., et al., 1997. Effects of relaxation training on glucose tolerance and diabetic control in type II diabetes. Appl. Psychophysiol. Biofeedback 22 (3), 155–169.

Jacobs, G.D., 2001. Clinical applications of the relaxation response and mind–body interventions. J. Altern. Complement. Med. 7 (Suppl. 1), S93–S101.

Jacob, R.G., Chesney, M.A., Williams, D.M., et al., 1991. Relaxation therapy for hypertension: Design effects and treatment effects. Ann. Behav. Med. 13 (1), 5–17.

Jacobs, G.D., Rosenberg, P.A., Friedman, R., et al., 1993. Multifactor behavioral treatment of chronic sleep-onset insomnia using stimulus control and the relaxation response. A preliminary study. Behav. Modif. 17 (4), 498–509.

Jacobs, G.D., Benson, H., Friedman, R., 1996a. Topographic EEG mapping of the relaxation response. Biofeedback Self Regul. 21 (2), 121–129.

Jacobs, G.D., Benson, H., Friedman, R., 1996b. Perceived benefits in a behavioral-medicine insomnia program: a clinical report. Am. J. Med. 100 (2), 212–216.

Johnston, M., Vogele, C., 1993. Benefits of psychological preparation for surgery: A meta-analysis. Ann. Behav. Med. 15 (4), 245–256.

Kabat-Zinn, J., Massion, A.O., Kristeller, J., et al., 1992. Effectiveness of a meditation-based stress reduction program in the treatment of anxiety disorders. Am. J. Psychiatry 149 (7), 936–943.

Kabat-Zinn, J., Wheeler, E., Light, T., et al., 1998. Influence of a mindfulness meditation-based stress reduction intervention on rates of skin clearing in patients with moderate to severe psoriasis undergoing phototherapy (UVB) and photochemotherapy (PUVA). Psychosom. Med. 60 (5), 625–632.

Kabat-Zinn, J., 1982. An outpatient program in behavioral medicine for chronic pain patients based on the practice of mindfulness meditation: theoretical considerations and preliminary results. Gen. Hosp. Psychiatry 4 (1), 33–47.

Lazar, S.W., Bush, G., Gollub, R.L., et al., 2000. Functional brain mapping of the relaxation response and meditation. NeuroReport 11 (7), 1581–1585.

Lazarus, R., Folkman, S., 1984. Stress, appraisal and coping. Springer, New York.

Lenfant, C., 2003. Shattuck lecture – clinical research to clinical practice – lost in translation? N. Engl. J. Med. 349 (9), 868–874.

Levenstein, S., Ackerman, S., Kiecolt-Glaser, J.K., et al., 1999. Stress and peptic ulcer disease. JAMA 281 (1), 10–11.

Linden, W., Chambers, L., 1994. Clinical effectiveness of non-drug treatment for hypertension: A meta-analysis. Ann. Behav. Med. 16 (1), 35–45.

Linden, W., Stossel, C., Maurice, J., 1996. Psychosocial interventions for patients with coronary artery disease: a meta-analysis. Arch. Intern. Med. 156 (7), 745–752.

Lorig, K., Holman, H., 1993. Arthritis self-management studies: a twelve-year review. Health Educ. Q. 20 (1), 17–28.

Luthar, S.S., Cicchetti, D., Becker, B., 2000. The construct of resilience: a critical evaluation and guidelines for future work. Child. Dev. 71 (3), 543–562.

Madrigal, J.L., Hurtado, O., Moro, M.A., et al., 2002. The increase in TNF-alpha levels is implicated in NF-kappaB activation and inducible nitric oxide synthase expression in brain cortex after immobilization stress. Neuropsychopharmacology 26 (2), 155–163.

Maes, M., 2009. Inflammatory and oxidative and nitrosative stress pathways underpinning chronic fatigue, somatization and psychosomatic symptoms. Curr. Opin. Psychiatry 22 (1), 75–83.

Mandle, C.L., Jacobs, S.C., Arcari, P.M., et al., 1996. The efficacy of relaxation response interventions with adult patients: a review of the literature. J. Cardiovasc. Nurs. 10 (3), 4–26.

Manocha, R., 2000. Why meditation? Aust. Fam. Physician 29 (12), 1135–1138.

Mayberg, H.S., Silva, J.A., Brannan, S.K., et al., 2002. The functional neuroanatomy of the placebo effect. Am. J. Psychiatry 159 (5), 728–737.

McEwen, B.S., 1998. Protective and damaging effects of stress mediators. N. Engl. J. Med. 338 (3), 171–179.

McEwen, B.S., 1999. Stress and hippocampal plasticity. Annu. Rev. Neurosci. 22, 105–122.

McEwen, B.S., 2007. Physiology and neurobiology of stress and adaptation: central role of the brain. Physiol. Rev. 87 (3), 873–904.

McEwen, B.S., Seeman, T., 1999. Protective and damaging effects of mediators of stress. Elaborating and testing the concepts of allostasis and allostatic load. Ann. N Y Acad. Sci. 896, 30–47.

McEwen, B.S., Stellar, E., 1993. Stress and the individual. Mechanisms leading to disease. Arch. Intern. Med. 153 (18), 2093–2101.

McQuaid, E.L., Nassau, J.H., 1999. Empirically supported treatments of disease-related symptoms in pediatric psychology: asthma, diabetes, and cancer. J. Pediatr. Psychol. 24 (4), 305–328.

Miller, F.G., Emanuel, E.J., Rosenstein, D.L., et al., 2004. Ethical issues concerning research in complementary and alternative medicine. JAMA 291 (5), 599–604.

Miyazaki, T., Ishikawa, T., Iimori, H., et al., 2003. Relationship between perceived social support and immune function. Stress and Health: Journal of the International Society for the Investigation of Stress 19 (1), 3–7.

Moerman, D.E., Jonas, W.B., 2002. Deconstructing the placebo effect and finding the meaning response. Ann. Intern. Med. 136 (6), 471–476.

Moreland, J.D., Thomson, M.A., Fuoco, A.R., 1998. Electromyographic biofeedback to improve lower extremity function after stroke: a meta-analysis. Arch. Phys. Med. Rehabil. 79 (2), 134–140.

Morin, C.M., Culbert, J.P., Schwartz, S.M., 1994. Nonpharmacological interventions for insomnia: a meta-analysis of treatment efficacy. Am. J. Psychiatry 151 (8), 1172–1180.

Morrell, E.M., Hollandsworth Jr., J.G., 1986. Norepinephrine alterations under stress conditions following the regular practice of meditation. Psychosom. Med. 48 (3–4), 270–277.

Nagabhushan, M., Mathews, H.L., Witek-Janusek, L., 2001. Aberrant nuclear expression of AP-1 and NFkappaB in lymphocytes of women stressed by the experience of breast biopsy. Brain Behav. Immun. 15 (1), 78–84.

Nakao, M., Myers, P., Fricchione, G., et al., 2001a. Somatization and symptom reduction through a behavioral medicine intervention in a mind/body medicine clinic. Behav. Med. 26 (4), 169–176.

Nakao, M., Yamanaka, G., Kuboki, T., 2001b. Major depression and somatic symptoms in a mind/body medicine clinic. Psychopathology 34 (5), 230–235.

Nakao, M., Fricchione, G., Myers, P., et al., 2001c. Anxiety is a good indicator for somatic symptom reduction through behavioral medicine intervention in a mind/body medicine clinic. Psychother. Psychosom. 70 (1), 50–57.

NCCAM National Institutes of Health, Mind–body medicine: an overview. [updated 2007; cited 2008 February 26]. Available online from: http://nccam.nih.gov/health/backgrounds/mindbody.htm.

Pacak, K., Palkovits, M., 2001. Stressor specificity of central neuroendocrine responses: implications for stress-related disorders. Endocr. Rev. 22 (4), 502–548.

Pelletier, K.R., 2004. Mind–body medicine in ambulatory care: an evidence-based assessment. J. Ambul. Care Manage. 27 (1), 25–42.

Pilkington, K., Kirkwood, G., Rampes, H., et al., 2005. Yoga for depression: the research evidence. J. Affect. Disord. 89 (1–3), 13–24.

Ploghaus, A., Becerra, L., Borras, C., et al., 2003. Neural circuitry underlying pain modulation: expectation, hypnosis, placebo. Trends Cogn. Sci. 7 (5), 197–200.

Puchalski, C.M., 2001. The role of spirituality in health care. Proc. (Bayl Univ Med Cent) 14 (4), 352–357.

Puchalski, C.M., 2007. Spirituality and the care of patients at the end-of-life: an essential component of care. Omega (Westport) 56 (1), 33–46.

Raz, A., Fan, J., Posner, M.I., 2005. Hypnotic suggestion reduces conflict in the human brain. Proc. Natl. Acad. Sci. U S A 102 (28), 9978–9983.

Redd, W.H., Montgomery, G.H., DuHamel, K.N., 2001. Behavioral intervention for cancer treatment side effects. J. Natl. Cancer Inst. 93 (11), 810–823.

Rief, W., Barsky, A.J., 2005. Psychobiological perspectives on somatoform disorders. Psychoneuroendocrinology 30 (10), 996–1002.

Robinson, F.P., Mathews, H.L., Witek-Janusek, L., 1999. Stress and HIV disease progression: psychoneuroimmunological framework. J. Assoc. Nurses AIDS Care 10 (1), 21–31.

Rosengren, A., Wilhelmsen, L., Orth-Gomer, K., 2004. Coronary disease in relation to social support and social class in Swedish men. A 15 year follow-up in the study of men born in 1933. Eur. Heart J. 25 (1), 56–63.

Rossi, E.L., 2002. Psychosocial genomics: gene expression, neurogenesis, and human experience in mind–body medicine. Adv. Mind Body Med. 18 (2), 22–30.

Schottelius, A.J., Dinter, H., 2006. Cytokines, NF-kappaB, microenvironment, intestinal inflammation and cancer. Cancer Treat Res. 130, 67–87.

Schwarz, S.P., Taylor, A.E., Scharff, L., et al., 1990. Behaviorally treated irritable bowel syndrome patients: a four-year follow-up. Behav. Res. Ther. 28 (4), 331–335.

Scott, K.D., Berkowitz, G., Klaus, M., 1999. A comparison of intermittent and continuous support during labor: a meta-analysis. Am. J. Obstet. Gynecol. 180 (5), 1054–1059.

Seeman, T.E., Singer, B.H., Rowe, J.W., et al., 1997. Price of adaptation – allostatic load and its health consequences. MacArthur studies of successful aging. Arch. Intern. Med. 157 (19), 2259–2268.

Seers, K., Carroll, D., 1998. Relaxation techniques for acute pain management: a systematic review. J. Adv. Nurs. 27 (3), 466–475.

Segerstrom, S.C., Miller, G.E., 2004. Psychological stress and the human immune system: a meta-analytic study of 30 years of inquiry. Psychol. Bull 130 (4), 601–630.

Selye, H., 1946. The general adaptation syndrome. J. Clin. Endocrinol. 6, 177.

Sierpina, V., Levine, R., Astin, J., et al., 2007a. Use of mind–body therapies in psychiatry and family medicine faculty and residents: attitudes, barriers, and gender differences. Explore (NY) 3 (2), 129–135.

Sierpina, V., Astin, J., Giordano, J., 2007b. Mind–body therapies for headache. Am. Fam. Physician 76 (10), 1518–1522.

Smyth, J.M., Stone, A.A., Hurewitz, A., et al., 1999. Effects of writing about stressful experiences on symptom reduction in patients with asthma or rheumatoid arthritis: a randomized trial. JAMA 281 (14), 1304–1309.

Sobel, D.S., 1995. Rethinking medicine: improving health outcomes with cost-effective psychosocial interventions. Psychosom. Med. 57 (3), 234–244.

Sobel, D.S., 2000. The cost-effectiveness of mind–body medicine interventions. Prog. Brain Res. 122, 393–412.

Stefano, G.B., Fricchione, G.L., Slingsby, B.T., et al., 2001a. The placebo effect and relaxation response: neural processes and their coupling to constitutive nitric oxide. Brain Res. Brain Res. Rev. 35 (1), 1–19.

Stefano, G.B., Murga, J., Benson, H., et al., 2001b. Nitric oxide inhibits norepinephrine stimulated contraction of human internal thoracic artery and rat aorta. Pharmacol. Res. 43 (2), 199–203.

Sterling, P., Eyer, J., 1988. Allostasis: a new paradigm to explain arousal pathology. In: Fisher, S., Reason, J. (Eds.), Handbook of life stress, cognition and health. John Wiley, New York.

Stratakis, C.A., Chrousos, G.P., 1995. Neuroendocrinology and pathophysiology of the stress system. Ann. N Y Acad. Sci. 771, 1–18.

Strosahl, K., 1998. Integrating behavioural health and primary care services: the primary mental health care model. In: Blount, A. (Ed.), Integrated primary care: the future of medical and mental health collaboration. Norton, New York.

Superio-Cabuslay, E., Ward, M.M., Lorig, K.R., 1996. Patient education interventions in osteoarthritis and rheumatoid arthritis: a meta-analytic comparison with nonsteroidal antiinflammatory drug treatment. Arthritis Care Res. 9 (4), 292–301.
Swaab, D.F., Bao, A.M., Lucassen, P.J., 2005. The stress system in the human brain in depression and neurodegeneration. Ageing Res. Rev. 4 (2), 141–194.
Ting, W., Fricchione, G., 2006. The heart mind connection. McGraw Hill, New York.
Toneatto, T., Nguyen, L., 2007. Does mindfulness meditation improve anxiety and mood symptoms? A review of the controlled research. Can. J. Psychiatry 52 (4), 260–266.
Tracey, K.J., 2007. Physiology and immunology of the cholinergic antiinflammatory pathway. J. Clin. Invest. 117 (2), 289–296.
Tsigos, C., Chrousos, G.P., 2002. Hypothalamic–pituitary–adrenal axis, neuroendocrine factors and stress. J. Psychosom. Res. 53 (4), 865–871.
Tunis, S.R., Stryer, D.B., Clancy, C.M., 2003. Practical clinical trials: increasing the value of clinical research for decision making in clinical and health policy. JAMA 290 (12), 1624–1632.
Uchino, B.N., 2006. Social support and health: a review of physiological processes potentially underlying links to disease outcomes. J. Behav. Med. 29 (4), 377–387.
Ursin, H., Eriksen, H.R., 2004. The cognitive activation theory of stress. Psychoneuroendocrinology 29 (5), 567–592.
Ursin, H., Eriksen, H., 2007. Cognitive activation theory of stress, sensitization, and common health complaints. Ann. N Y Acad. Sci. 1113, 304–310.
van Tulder, M.W., Ostelo, R., Vlaeyen, J.W., et al., 2000. Behavioral treatment for chronic low back pain: a systematic review within the framework of the Cochrane Back Review Group. Spine 25 (20), 2688–2699.
Vollmer, A., Blanchard, E.B., 1998. Controlled comparison of individual versus group cognitive therapy for irritable bowel syndrome. Behav. Ther. 29 (1), 19–33.
Wang, M.Y., Wang, S.Y., Tsai, P.S., 2005. Cognitive behavioural therapy for primary insomnia: a systematic review. J. Adv. Nurs. 50 (5), 553–564.
Watkins, A.D., 1994. The role of alternative therapies in the treatment of allergic disease. Clin. Exp. Allergy 24 (9), 813–825.
Wolsko, P.M., Eisenberg, D.M., Davis, R.B., et al., 2004. Use of mind–body medical therapies. J. Gen. Intern. Med. 19 (1), 43–50.

FURTHER READING

Benson, H., Klipper, M.Z., 2000. The Relaxation Response. twentyfifth ed Harper Paperbacks, New York.
Harrington, A., 2008. The Cure Within. A History of Mind Body Medicine. WW Norton, New York.
Kabat-Zinn, J., 1990. Full Catastrophe Living. Using the Wisdom of Your Body and Mind to Face Stress, Pain and Illness. Delta, New York.
McEwen, B., 2002. The End of Stress as We Know It. National Academies Press, Washington, DC.

SECTION III
APPLYING RESEARCH STANDARDS IN CAM

SECTION CONTENTS

Inspiration and perspiration: what every researcher needs to know before they start

15

Andrew J. Vickers

CHAPTER CONTENTS

DOI: 10.1016/B978-0-443-06956-7.00015-X

INTRODUCTION

Art, we are often told, is 10% inspiration and 90% perspiration. The moment of brilliance on stage, or on the art gallery wall, is the result of thousands of hours of learning, planning, rehearsal and laborious attention to fine detail.

A similar adage for science might be: '10% statistics, 90% logistics'. As a clinical researcher, I spend less time devising protocols, analysing results and writing papers than I do organizing staff, checking work that I have delegated, sorting out financial administration and programming databases.

Research is a practical business, and unless you get the practicalities right, your research will fail, no matter how brilliant its design or conception. Unfortunately, few methodology books will tell you this. This chapter will review some of the practical aspects of research. My aim is to give some simple advice and guidelines based on my own personal experience as a researcher specializing in quantitative research. Some, though not all, of these considerations will also be relevant to qualitative research.

QUESTIONS

DEFINING THE QUESTION

Research is a tool for answering questions. Unless you know what your question is, you will be unable to design your research. Novice researchers are often unable to frame a question to illustrate their research interest, even after repeated prompting. For example, a researcher at a conference reported that his question was 'to demonstrate the effectiveness of herbal medicine for cystitis'; another cited a wish 'to investigate massage for cancer patients'. These are clearly not questions.

There are three general guidelines for defining a research question: (1) questions should be in four parts; (2) questions should be focused; (3) questions should be explicit.

Questions should be in four parts

Often, research questions are at first stage too general to be useful. It is helpful to make them more precise. When analysed carefully, many questions in health research can be formulated in four parts.

1. an intervention
2. a comparison
3. an outcome measure
4. a population.

Each of these four parts can be seen easily in this question for a clinical trial: 'What are the effects of acupuncture compared to no acupuncture on headache, health status, days off sick and resource use in patients with headache in primary care?' The four-part question can be applied to many other types of research, including prognosis (e.g. 'What proportion of coronary heart disease patients who develop heart failure will die compared to those who do not develop heart failure?') and diagnosis ('What is the reproducibility of IgG/IgE testing for food intolerance in patients with chronic disease?'). In the last case, the 'intervention' is IgG/IgE testing and the 'comparison' is a second test.

Not all forms of research involve a comparison and in these cases the four-part question becomes a three-part question. Examples include case series ('What is the average reduction in pain scores [outcome measure] in pain clinic patients [population] undertaking an integrated package of care [intervention]?') or surveys ('What proportion of UK adults [population] have seen a practitioner [outcome measure] of complementary medicine [intervention]?') Some research questions, particularly qualitative studies, are difficult to put in the three- or four-part format; nonetheless, the format remains a useful rule of thumb.

Questions should be focused

A colleague of mine was once asked to advise a researcher who wanted to know 'What forms of discourse were used by doctors in discussing cancer with their patients, what did patients think of this and what were the effects on outcome of the different styles of discourse?' A vague question of this sort will often produce a vague answer and, accordingly, research which benefits no one. Your question must be focused. A quick test of focus: give an imaginary answer to your question; the shorter the answer, the more focused your question (note that a possible exception to this rule of thumb is qualitative research, the results of which can sometimes be difficult to summarize).

Questions should be explicit

A quick test of explicitness: a research question is explicit if it immediately suggests a research design.

ONE QUESTION AT A TIME

Research, like a 'journey of a thousand miles', goes one step at a time. Broad questions such as 'Does hypnosis work?' or 'What are the effects of patient expectations on outcome?' will not be resolved by a single research study. The researcher needs to break down large, global questions into manageable stages: a series of questions each associated with a single study.

BUILD ON EXISTING RESEARCH

Science is a cumulative enterprise. A review of the background can help you define a study topic, identify appropriate research designs and avoid the mistakes of previous workers. Locate as many studies as possible on both the therapy and the condition under investigation and look up other examples of the type of research that you would like to conduct (have a look at some classic surveys if you want to conduct a survey, for instance). Indepth reading of the research literature is one of the most important preparatory steps for a prospective researcher.

KEEP THINGS SIMPLE

Given that research will almost inevitably turn out much more complicated than you could possibly imagine, it is a good idea to keep things simple to start with. Studies involving multiple endpoints, complex designs or large numbers of participants should be avoided by all but the most experienced researchers.

One 'red flag' to watch out for: if anyone comes up to you while you are planning your research and says 'wouldn't it be nice to know …', panic! Of course it would be 'interesting to know' all sorts of things. The point is that you cannot answer all of them in your research. This seems a particular problem in questionnaire surveys, where the temptation is always to add just one more question. The problem is that, the longer a questionnaire is, the less likely you are to get good-quality data from any particular respondent.

The importance of keeping things simple is often inadequately recognized at present in the medical research community. For example, a first-time researcher was recently told by a funding committee to change a simple comparison of a physical therapy technique to no extra treatment to a complex three-way trial of the physical therapy technique, contact with the physical therapist but no use of the technique, and no contact. This was on the grounds that 'it would be interesting to know' which components of the physical therapy technique were of value: was it the actual technique itself or just the time and touch of the teacher? This more than doubled the cost of the trial, and because the funding committee was unwilling to provide the extra money, the trial was never conducted. My own view is that the initial two-arm trial should have been funded with further research questions addressed subsequently.

PROTOCOLS

WHAT IS A STUDY PROTOCOL?

A study protocol is a precise description of all methodologically pertinent features of a study. An example of a protocol is given in the further reading section, below. The point of a protocol is that it should provide a complete guide to all aspects of trial management and analysis. It should be extremely detailed and explicit: a protocol I recently wrote, for instance, was nearly 8000 words long. As an illustration, here is a short section, chosen more or less at random, which describes the rules for data entry if data are ambiguous:

- chronicity: rounded to nearest year; if a range is given, the highest number will be taken
- age: rounded to nearest year on date of recruitment
- severity: if two tick boxes are marked, take the higher.

Many protocols are inadequately detailed, particularly the plan for statistical analysis. Examples I have seen recently include: 'we expect to measure the proportion experiencing pain relief of at least 35–50%' and 'the main outcome measure will be forced expiratory volume'. Compare this to 'the primary outcome measure will be the change in mean daily headache score between baseline and the 1-year follow-up'. This is an absolutely explicit guide: you do not have to guess whether to choose 35% or 50% as a cut-off nor guess at which follow-up point forced expiratory volume should be assessed.

In centres conducting many studies, certain aspects of methodology can be defined by standard operating procedures (SOPs). SOPs describe certain aspects of research, such as how to chase up missing data by telephone, or how to deal with ambiguous data. The SOPs can be summarized in a single, standalone document that is then referred to in protocols.

CHECKLISTS

A good way to make sure that you have incorporated all appropriate detail in your protocol is to use a methodological checklist. An example of a checklist, in this case for clinical trials, is given in Box 15.1. One useful trick is to go through the checklist a second time, this time asking 'who?' rather than 'what?' (e.g. 'What measurements will be taken before treatment?' becomes 'Who will take measurements on participants before treatment?').

BOX 15.1 Methodological checklist for clinical trials

- From where will patients be recruited?
- How many patients will be recruited and what is the justification for this sample size?
- What are the criteria for including patients?
- What are the criteria for excluding patients?
- How will ethical approval for the study be obtained?
- How will informed consent be obtained?
- What control group will be used?
- How will patients be assigned to treatment and control groups?
- For a randomized trial: What method will be used to generate the randomization schedule? What method will be used to conceal allocation until participant is entered into the trial? What method will be used to ensure that treatment allocation cannot be changed after participant had been entered into trial?
- What measurements will be taken before treatment?
- What other information will be taken before treatment?
- What is the treatment to be given to patients in each group?
- Will treatment be standardized, or might it vary?
- How many treatments can be given over what length of time?
- Who will give the treatment? Are providers of treatment sufficiently trained and qualified?
- How will the quality be ensured of any medicines used?
- Is there evidence that the treatment used will be effective in the patients?
- Will patients be blinded to their treatment allocation? If so, how?
- How will blinding be checked?
- Will statistical analysis be conducted blind?
- Will the researcher assessing outcome be blinded to patient treatment allocation? If so, how?
- What outcome measures will be used?
- When will the outcome measurement be made?
- What is the primary outcome measure?
- How will you monitor flow of participants through the trial: number eligible; number randomized; number receiving intended intervention; number not receiving intended intervention; number providing data for each outcome measure; number withdrawing for each of the following reasons: intervention thought harmful or ineffective, lost to follow-up (e.g. moved away), other; number completing trial
- What will you do about missing or illegible data?
- What statistical methods will be used to test each of the study hypotheses?

GETTING THE BASICS RIGHT

There has been a good deal of discussion about the importance of adapting research methodologies to the 'special needs' of the therapy under consideration. Though I do believe that this is important, I also believe the foundations of any research study have to be absolutely sound. Research with basic methodological flaws is as good as worthless: if you are undertaking a survey, make sure you get a high response rate; if you conduct a randomized trial, make sure you randomize properly; if you analyse any numerical data, make sure that you have a good statistician on hand. You should have a thorough understanding of the criteria used to assess methodological rigour for the type of research you wish to undertake well before you start.

PEOPLE

COLLABORATION

A wide range of skills is needed for research

Research requires specialist skills and knowledge. More often than not, you will need skills or knowledge that you do not have. Here are some of the areas of skill or knowledge that might be needed for a typical acupuncture clinical trial:

1. searching bibliographic databases: to find relevant background material
2. clinical trial design: to write the protocol
3. acupuncture: to advise of the acupuncture content of the protocol
4. primary care: to understand the perspective of the doctors in the trial
5. practice management: to access practice databases for recruitment
6. consumer perspective: to ensure that the trial meets consumer needs
7. statistics: to aid protocol design and analyse data
8. typing and word-processing: to put together the funding application
9. financial administration: to prepare estimates of costs for the funding application
10. database programming: to design the databases to manage trial data
11. questionnaire design: to design or choose from existing questionnaires
12. typesetting: to produce questionnaires
13. general practice computer systems: to search for data needed for the trial.

If we did not have these skills on the study team, we would not be able to undertake the trial. The most difficult thing for most first-time researchers is that they have few skills. For example, few, if any, of the researchers I have advised had good knowledge and experience of statistics; similarly, very few have programmed a database. How are you going to analyse your results if you are not confident with statistics? How are you going to manage the huge amounts of data which a study produces without a database? The answer is that you need to collaborate, particularly with experienced researchers.

Indepth knowledge is needed for research

I am often asked to talk at 'research days' which aim to teach clinicians how to do research. I sometimes start by saying: 'I am a researcher but I have become interested in [say] surgery. Could you quickly show me in a day or so how to do surgery?' Just as it takes many years of training and practice to become a good clinician, so it takes many years to become a good researcher.

I would expect any researcher to have formal training in research design and statistics; a research-related higher degree; a track record of publishing original research in health-related, peer-reviewed journals; and at least 3 years' experience of original research. This seems a fairly basic requirement: as an analogy, would it be unreasonable to expect a surgeon to have formal training in medical diagnosis and treatment, surgical board certification, a track record of satisfied patients and at least 3 years' experience of giving treatments?

Anyone considering research should either fulfil these criteria or work with someone who does.

STUDY MANUAL

A study manual describes, in detail, the practical procedures for a trial. It includes information on issues such as running the study databases, how to file and check study materials, interviewing participants and the like. Box 15.2 includes some example sections from a study manual of a

BOX 15.2 Example of the contents of a study manual

Preparing for interviews

1. Add data from 'patients agreeing to interview form' to the database. As data for each participant are added, tick by the patient's name. Double-check that the data on screen match the data on the form and then write the date added and your initials on each sheet. File in the 'pain trial recruitment pre-interview' folder.
2. On Friday of every week, run the macro 'information letters needed' on the database (the green icon). This finds recruits who have not been sent confirmation of their interview date and prints out a cover letter and audit sheet of letters sent, changes trial status field to 'information letters sent (date)'. Send these letters on hospital headed note paper with a patient information sheet (blue) and the map showing how to get to the hospital. File audit sheet in 'pain trial recruitment folder' stapled to appropriate 'participants agreeing to interview' form.
3. On Friday of each week, run macro 'print out study appointment sheets' (the blue icon). This prints out the appointment details and contact details for each patient scheduled to attend a recruitment interview in the next week. Give these to the study nurse.
4. On Friday of every week, run the macro 'reminder calls to make' (the red icon). This prints out a list of forthcoming appointments with participant names and numbers.
5. Every day, check whether there are any reminder calls to make. The day before each recruitment interview, call relevant participants and say:

'My name is ... and I am calling from the pain trial. You may remember that you have an appointment tomorrow at .... a.m. / p.m. This is partly a reminder call and partly a chance to check if you have any questions or difficulties.'

If the patient is unable to come, or wants to come at a different time, write a note to the study nurse specifying the person's name and the time of the appointment. Do not make changes to the database (do this when you get the study appointment sheets back).

trial I recently completed. To give an idea of the sort of detail you need to go into, the study manual of this relatively simple trial was nearly 5000 words long.

MANAGEMENT

Research requires careful management. There should be regular team meetings where problems are discussed and progress reviewed. The principal investigator needs to keep careful track of financial expenditure and recruitment. There is also a need for monitoring of a trial, to check that what should be happening is happening. The following is an excerpt from a study protocol about trial monitoring:

The principal investigator will conduct an internal audit at the study centre every 3 months to ensure: confidentiality and integrity of databases; effectiveness of database backup systems; confidentiality and integrity of paper records; reconciliation of enquiries with enquiry outcome; number of treatments received by each patient; data entry procedures; minimization algorithm and numbers allocated to each group; comparison of paper records and electronic records. Each month, the principal investigator will review the progress of recruitment by recording number of letters sent, number of enquiries received, number of calls made, number of patients entered, number of migraine patients randomized, number of patients without migraine randomized.

THE DRY RUN

I always undertake a 'dry run' of a study to test all procedures before involving any patients. I get the study team to go through the trial day by day ('OK, it is now Monday 15 November 2010') with imaginary participants ('Joe Blow has now completed treatment') and imaginary events ('Jo Schmo has telephoned to say that she has decided not to take part'). We add appropriate data to the study databases, print off letters and forms, fill in questionnaires and role-play interviews. One particularly important aspect of the dry run is to play devil's advocate. We imagine situations such as: What do you do if a patient withdraws after baseline but before randomization? What if a patient telephones to say that he will be on holiday during follow-up? Or: What happens if a patient forgets to send back a questionnaire? We then see what, if any, problems this causes our procedures.

DATA

DATABASES

Research involves managing large amounts of data. This applies not only to results and outcomes but also to details of participants' names and addresses, the stage they are at in the study, their doctor's name and so on. It is absolutely essential to manage this data with a computer database. You need a good computer, good software (I personally recommend Filemaker Pro) and someone experienced at database design.

One of the best things about databases is that they can be used to maintain study quality. For example, you can program a database to prompt you to send out follow-up questionnaires at the right time or print out the telephone numbers of participants who are late returning data. You can also program a database to check your data for you (see section on data checking, below).

A word of warning, however: it is all too easy to end up with a database with hundreds of fields, dozens of macros and scores of layouts, many of which you have forgotten what they do and why you added them. When you are working on a database you should document your design in what is known as a 'codebook'. This contains the name of a field, macro or layout and a description of its function. For example: 'field name: 'date q2 late'. Type of field: calculation date field. Description: created by calculation from the field 'date q2 sent' plus 16 days. Contains the date on which questionnaire 2 should be received by the office. Used in the macro 'find all late questionnaires'.'

DON'T TAKE TOO MUCH DATA

Researchers often design studies without sufficient consideration of how they will analyse the information once it has been collected. An easy trap is to ask too many questions and take too much data. For example, an eight-item questionnaire completed daily for 10 weeks by 30 subjects will generate 16 800 data points. Who will type in all this information? How will it be analysed?

RANDOMIZATION

If you wish to conduct a randomized trial, do make sure that you get randomization right. One of the most important but least understood functions of randomization is to prevent triallists being able to influence treatment assignment. To achieve this, it is important that treatment allocation is concealed. 'Concealment of allocation' means that the researchers and clinicians should not be able to guess the group to which a patient will be randomized before he or she is entered into the trial. If allocation is not concealed, it is possible that researchers may interfere with the randomization process, consciously or otherwise. For example, a surgeon who knew that the next patient to be entered into the trial was to be randomized to surgery might try to avoid recruiting a patient thought to have a poor prognosis. A typical example of unconcealed allocation is when a statistician produces a randomized list using a sophisticated computer program that is then posted in the research office for all to see. There is now good evidence that clinicians involved in a trial often subvert randomization unless it is properly concealed, and that trials without adequate allocation concealment are subject to bias.

Randomization should also be designed in such a way that it should be impossible to change treatment assignments once patients have been entered into the trial. This can prevent the sort of problem reported in one case, where randomization took place by removing a coloured or plain marble from a black bag. The principal investigators found that the study nurses were replacing marbles and choosing again if they felt that patients needed a different treatment to the one assigned.

One common method of randomization is the 'sealed envelope' method. You take 100 pieces of card, write 'treatment group' on 50 and 'control' on the remainder, then place them in 100 opaque envelopes and shuffle. The problem with this method is that there is nothing to stop a researcher opening and resealing an envelope or opening a second envelope if the first contained the 'wrong' allocation.

The best method of randomization is to use a secure database system. In brief, you have two databases: a registration database that records patient details and a randomization database that conducts the random allocation. Investigators can access the registration database, adding the name and details of a patient after informed consent. After these data are entered, the registration database automatically accesses an assignment from the randomization database and reveals the assignment to the triallist. Only the computer programmer and a backup programmer, in case of emergency, have the password to access the randomization database or the ability to make changes to the registration databases. Investigators cannot guess an allocation before registration, because they have no access to the randomization database, and cannot change allocation subsequently because they cannot modify data on the registration database after data entry.

DATA CHECKING

You need to check, double-check and recheck your data. A few hints and tips:

- Sign off on data. When a researcher completes a form, standard procedure should be to check that it is complete, accurate and legible and then date and initial or sign. The signature means: 'I have checked these data'. Similarly, when data (e.g. the name and address of a new participant) are added from a form on to a database, the data entry should be visually checked and the form dated and initialled.
- Double-check critical steps. Certain parts of a study are absolutely critical to its quality. For example, if a researcher slightly misspells a participant's surname on the study database, this is sloppy, but not disastrous. If, however, a researcher needs to add the information that a certain participant has withdrawn from a study, but calls up the wrong participant on the database, the result will be that a participant who should be in the trial is not contacted again, reducing sample size and statistical power. A typical procedure to avoid this type of error might be to add all the results of all patient interviews at one time, have the database to print out a list of the data added, check the list against the interview sheets and sign and date the sheet to confirm that a check has been made.
- Guard your code numbers. In most studies, code numbers rather than names are used to identify participants. Given the importance of code numbers, it is surprising to find them treated in a cavalier fashion by some researchers. In a trial I was asked to advise on, the code numbers were written by hand on to the top sheet of a questionnaire. Once the questionnaires had been photocopied it was impossible to check which participant had filled out any given page 2 of the questionnaire. Moreover, some code numbers were difficult to read. Make sure that code numbers are clearly stamped on every sheet of paper and no patient's code number can be changed on the database.

- Automated consistency checks. It is possible to program a database to find data which are illogical. What I have done in the past is to get the study team to think of all possible inconsistencies in the data (e.g. patients recorded as having returned data but who are not yet in the trial, or those who have had study appointments pending but who are recorded as having withdrawn) and then program suitable searches into the study database. These searches are then run every day to alert the study team to possible errors.
- Automate data entry if possible. In place of written questionnaires, forms can be designed to be read by optical scanners. Patients can also complete questionnaires online or via automatic telephone systems ('Enter 0 for no pain, 1 for mild pain, 2 for moderate pain and 3 for severe pain').
- Data entry rules. Provide those entering data with a complete set of rules for missing, illegible or ambiguous data. You should also provide rules for data which might be presented in different ways. In one study, for instance, we asked runners to report how long it had taken them to complete a marathon. Because I didn't give those entering data sufficient guidance, race time was variously entered as '3 hours and 15 minutes', '3.15' and '315'.
- Double-data entry. Any data (e.g. from questionnaires) that you will analyse and report in the published paper of your research should be entered twice, on two separate databases, with automatic checking set up between the two.
- Make extra checks on group assignments. In controlled trials, make extensive checks that every patient code number has been given the correct allocation (treatment or control) and that any codes you use for treatment assignments (e.g. 1 for treatment, 0 for control) are correct.
- Check your finished paper against the original output from your statistical software. It is not uncommon for an experienced researcher to go to extreme lengths to ensure accuracy of data during a study but then to make a typographical error when typing up the final report.

ANALYSIS

Many statistical software packages are programmable: you can load in a set of analyses and run them on whatever data are in memory. I recommend generating a set of simulated data, programming in your analyses as specified in your study protocol, checking that the analyses do what you want them to do and then saving your work. When it comes to adding the real data from your trial, all you have to do is load up your analysis and press the 'go' button. Incidentally, if you hear anyone say 'it took me ages to analyse my results' it is probable that they were not following a predefined protocol.

Some researchers suggest that you write up the results section of your paper, including tables and graphs, before you have any data, for example: 'Mean pain scores (*x* SD *y*) in the treatment/control group were *z* points (95% confidence interval *a*, *b*) lower than those in the treatment/control group (*c* SD *d*).' This helps to ensure that you are doing the analyses correctly and not merely 'data-dredging' (more colourfully known as 'torturing the data until it confesses').

PATIENTS

Recruitment is generally cited as the number one problem experienced by researchers. A large number of studies run into difficulties because insufficient numbers of participants are recruited. Given below are a few brief hints and tips on study recruitment.

GETTING PARTICIPANTS INTO A STUDY

- Motivating gatekeepers. Many trials rely on a 'gatekeeper', such as a patient's doctor, to refer patients to a study. An extremely common problem is that gatekeepers lose motivation and refer far fewer patients than expected. They forget to tell appropriate patients, or fail to do so because of lack of time or simply decide not to because it is not a priority. It is essential to keep gatekeepers involved, to help them feel ownership of a project: arrange regular face-to-face meetings, send a 'thank you' letter when a patient is referred and send a regular newsletter with information about the progress of the trial.
- Keep things as simple as possible for gatekeepers. Use clear and simple forms with tick boxes and a place for a signature at the bottom.
- Remind gatekeepers about the study. Some studies have used complex reminder systems to prompt doctors to refer patients. These include computerized reminders or placing a reminder sticker on notes of patients who could be eligible for a study. Other studies have used simpler approaches, using cups, pens and posters with the trial logo (e.g. 'MI? < 6 hours? Think ISIS trial').
- Recruitment materials should be attractive and professional. Remember that 'the medium is the message': sending poorly photocopied or badly laid out information will not help recruitment.
- Recruitment materials should be personalized. Participants normally prefer a personalized letter, with their name and address.
- Recruitment materials should be simple. In one trial I worked on, we improved recruitment rates significantly by changing the recruitment letter. We replaced a letter which gave a detailed and complex description of the trial with one which just said: 'we are doing some research and it might interest you; give us a call if you want to find out more.'
- Use the media. A study can be a newsworthy event ('Though arthritis patients have used herbs for thousands of years, it is not really known if they can help. Scientists at the University of London are starting to look into this question…'). Call around journalists and see if any are interested in the story. Ask them to add details of the study telephone line or website.

Keeping participants in a study and getting good-quality data

- Make participants feel important. Study materials should carefully explain why you are doing a study and why the information you will get is important. Recruitment interviews and study materials should include phrases such as: 'Your responses will be very helpful to us' or 'Your responses are very important for the study'.

- Keep in contact with participants. Calling participants ('we just wanted to check you were getting on OK') and sending thank you letters or newsletters are good ways of keeping participants motivated, particularly in longer studies. A hint: in any extended study, ask participants to give you the telephone number of a close friend or relative. If you cannot get hold of the participant (e.g. he or she has moved), you can contact the friend or relative for new contact details.

CONCLUSION

My initial response to someone asking for advice on research is often: 'Think about whether you really want this career change.' Research has to be done properly, or not at all. Research cannot be done properly on an amateur basis, without an impact on the rest of a person's professional life. So if you want to do research, bear in mind first the immediate practical implications for yourself and your work. Often, a good solution is to team up with someone experienced in research.

I believe that research is important and that it has practical benefits which improve the lives of those suffering ill health. That means that all health professionals should support the conduct of research and use the results of research in making decisions. It does not mean, however, that everyone should do research. If you are considering research, think first not about methodology, but about the day-to-day practicalities of managing the complex system of data-gathering and analysis that comprises health research.

FURTHER READING

Reporting of randomized trials, see www.consort-statement.org

Vickers, A.J., 2006. How to measure quality of life in integrative oncology research. J. Soc. Integr. Oncol. 4, 100–103.

Vickers, A.J., 2006. How to randomize. J. Soc. Integr. Oncol. 4 (4), 194–198.

Vickers, A.J., 2006. Multiple assessment in quality of life trials: how many questionnaires? How often should they be given. J. Soc. Integr. Oncol. 4, 135–139.

Vickers, A.J., 2007. How to improve accrual to clinical trials of symptom control 1: recruitment strategies. J. Soc. Integr. Oncol. 5 (1), 38–42.

Vickers, A.J., 2007. How to improve accrual to clinical trials of symptom control 2: design issues. J. Soc. Integr. Oncol. 5 (2), 61–64.

Vickers, A.J., 2008. Basic introduction to research: how not to do research. J. Soc. Integr. Oncol. 6 (2), 82–85.

Placebo, meaning and context issues in research

16

Lene Vase • Wayne B. Jonas • Harald Walach

CHAPTER CONTENTS

It has been known for many years that key elements in healing are the meaning attributed to the treatment and the patient–practitioner relationship as well as the patient's expectations and emotional feelings (Frank 1961). However, with the introduction of the randomized clinical trial (RCT), where a pharmacological active agent is tested against an inactive placebo agent, researchers have tried to eliminate these factors in empirical research in order to isolate the effects of the drug. The placebo condition controls not only for the psychosocial factors related to a healing effect, but also for artifacts such as spontaneous remission, regression to the mean and other potential biases (Beecher 1955; Kienle & Kiene 1996, 1997; Kaptchuk 1998). Therefore, symptom changes in a placebo-treated group or condition do not convey information about all placebo effects. In order to investigate the effects of taking a placebo, the symptom change in a placebo-treated group or condition must be compared to the symptom change in a no-treatment group or condition (Fields & Price 1997). Recently, studies have started to investigate placebo mechanisms in this manner and they are yielding evidence that placebo effects may reveal the self-healing capacities of the body. Since mostly complementary and alternative medical (CAM) approaches try to stimulate self-healing to some degree, this self-healing capacity is their common denominator, and placebo effects may

DOI: 10.1016/B978-0-443-06956-7.00016-1

be the way we can study them scientifically. In this review, we argue that the placebo literature teaches how we could maximize healing by harnessing these factors in any therapeutic context, and discuss implications of this view on study design and conduct.

DEFINITION OF PLACEBO AND THE MEANING RESPONSE

Etymologically 'placebo' means 'I will please' (Andersen 1997). Historically, it is derived from Psalm 116.6, which in its Latin version reads *'placebo Domino in regione vivorum* – I will please the Lord in the land of the living'. It was sung at the death bed, and by the Middle Ages it had become common practice to employ others to sing those 'placebos', introducing the meaning of 'replacement', 'not the real thing'. Hence, traditionally placebo has been conceptualized as 'a commonplace method or medicine' (Shapiro & Morris 1978), which is 'prescribed in order to please the patient and not because of its efficiency' (citation from Ekeland 1999). As the randomized double-blind experiment became a commonly used method, placebo was primarily seen as an inactive agent, e.g. a sugar pill, against which the efficacy of the active agent could be tested (Andersen 1997; Kaptchuk 1998a, b). In the 1970s Shapiro & Morris (1978) defined the placebo effect as the non-specific, psychological or psychophysiological therapeutic effect produced by a placebo. However, it is unclear exactly what demarcates specific and non-specific factors and generally it is problematic to explain how inactive substances lead to an effect (Gotzsche 1994; Andersen 1997; Kaptchuk 1998b).

Recently, these problems have been overcome by changing the focus from the inactive agent to the patient's perception of the agent and of the entire therapeutic intervention (Vase et al. 2004). Moerman & Jonas (2000) have presented a useful definition of placebo effects as meaning responses. The placebo effect is seen as the effect that is due to the meaning of a therapeutic intervention for a particular patient and context. This definition has three virtues:

1. It is a semiotic definition in the sense that it acknowledges that humans are not only deterministic machines reacting to mechanical causes (e.g. pharmacological agents). Rather they are responding to signs and the meaning those signs generate in a highly complex, often self-determined and sometimes unpredictable fashion (Uexküll 1995). The meaning is not fully determined by the external stimuli themselves but arises from the interaction between the external environment and the internal conditions of persons, their history, their genetics, their social circumstances, their individual predilections and their expectations.
2. The meaning response definition allows the context factors of an intervention to enter the stage. This definition underlines the individual differences in response to otherwise similar conditions, and brings into focus the importance of individuality in therapy. This makes plausible why one and the same situation, for instance surgery, may arouse hope in one patient and induce fright in another, with completely different physiological reactions and clinical outcomes.
3. It clarifies why placebo factors contribute to the efficacy of any treatment, conventional or complementary.

THE MAGNITUDE OF PLACEBO ANALGESIA EFFECTS

In 1955, Henry Beecher published one of the first meta-analyses on the magnitude of placebo analgesia termed 'The powerful placebo'. The placebo effect was investigated across 15 studies covering nine different diseases such as pain, anxiety and common cold and it was found that 35.2 ± 2.2% of the patients responded positively to placebo. However, the symptom reduction in a placebo group was not compared with the symptom reduction in a no-treatment control group and therefore a true placebo effect was not measured.

In 2001, Hrobjartsson & Gøtzsche published a meta-analysis entitled, 'Is the placebo powerless?' investigating the magnitude of placebo effects in 114 studies covering 40 different conditions such as pain, marital discord and schizophrenia. In contrast to Beecher's meta-analysis, all the studies in this meta-analysis were RCTs, including a natural history condition, so the results were supposedly a more accurate estimate of the magnitude of placebo effects. The studies were divided into binary and continuous outcome measures. There was no significant effect of placebo within the studies using binary outcome measures (relative risk =0.95, 95% confidence interval (CI) 0.88–1.02) which may at least partly be explained by the circumstance that most diseases do not go away completely. Within the studies with continuous outcome measures, only pain studies with subjective outcome measures showed a small but significant effect (relative risk = 0.28, 95% CI −0.38–0.19). As the effect sizes are small, these results suggest that in clinical trials placebo effects are not therapeutically important. In 2004, Hrobjartsson & Gøtzsche updated the meta-analyses and found similar results.

Although these two meta-analyses are well controlled, they have been criticized with respect to the conceptualization of placebo (Kupers 2001; Lilford & Braunholtz 2001; Miller 2001), the number and quality of studies (Einarson et al. 2001) and the interpretation of the data (Kaptchuk 2001; Shrier 2001). To give an example, several of the trials did not consider whether the placebo intervention was valid. For instance, a study had been included which compared the administration of an analgesic in still unconscious patients after surgery to placebo and no treatment (Sinclair et al. 1988). Given that the placebo effect can be seen as a meaning response it is hardly surprising that in such a setting, which did not even allow for patients to realize that they had been treated, no placebo effect was observed. Along the same lines, no differentiation was made between studies in which the context facilitated placebo effects and studies in which this was not the case.

In 2002, Vase and colleagues conducted two meta-analyses of placebo effects to investigate how the context may influence the magnitude of placebo analgesia. In both meta-analyses pain in the placebo condition was compared to pain in a no-treatment control condition. The first meta-analysis included 23 studies in which placebo was used as a control condition and where patients via the informed consent were told that 'this agent may either be an inert substance or a pain-reducing medication'. In such a setting patients are likely to have uncertain expectations of pain relief and, in agreement with Hrobjartsson & Gøtzsche's finding, a small magnitude of placebo analgesia effects against no-treatment control was found (Cohen's d = 0.15). However, the second meta-analysis included 14 studies in which placebo was the main object of the study and where patients were given suggestions to the effect that 'this agent is known to powerfully reduce pain in some patients'. In such a setting, designed to maximize the placebo effect, patients are likely to have higher expectations of pain relief and a large magnitude of placebo analgesia compared with no treatment was found ($d = 0.95$) (Vase et al. 2002).

A new and updated meta-analysis of 28 studies confirms the finding of a large magnitude of placebo analgesia effects in placebo mechanism studies (Vase et al. 2009). Not only pain studies have reported placebo effects against no-treatment control, but also studies using objective outcomes such as blood pressure (Queneau et al. 2002). Epileptic seizures have been induced by a suggestive placebo (Lancman et al. 1994) and a recent meta-analysis found a sizeable response in the placebo arms of randomized studies of antiepileptics (Rheims et al. 2008). Meta-analyses in relation to depression have also reported large placebo effects (Kirsch & Sapirstein 1998; Kirsch et al. 2008).

These results indicate that placebo effects exist and that the magnitude of placebo effects is variable and depends on contextual factors. Therefore, in order to get a better understanding of placebo effects, it is important to take a further look at the contextual factors that influence the placebo effect as well as the psycho-neuro-physiological factors that may mediate placebo effects.

CONTEXT AND MEANING

The meaning model of the placebo effect suggests that the context within which a treatment is offered modulates how an intervention is perceived and hence the effects of placebos. Several contextual factors have been shown to influence the placebo effect: interaction with the health care provider (Amanzio et al. 2001; Kaptchuk et al. 2008), verbal suggestions for pain relief (Pollo et al. 2001; Vase et al. 2002, 2004; Price et al. 2008), expectation (Montgomery & Kirsch 1996, 1997; Amanzio & Benedetti 1999; Vase et al. 2003), conditioning (Voudouris et al. 1985, 1989, 1990; Benedetti & Amanzio 1997; Amanzio & Benedetti 1999; Price et al. 1999) and emotional feelings (Gryll & Katahn 1978; Petrovic et al. 2005; Vase et al. 2005; Zubieta et al. 2005; Price et al. 2008).

PATIENT–PRACTITIONER RELATIONSHIP AND VERBAL SUGGESTIONS

A study by Amanzio and colleagues (2001) has clearly illustrated how patients' perception of the therapeutic intervention influences the treatment outcome. A total of 278 patients undergoing thoracic surgery were randomized to receive buprenorphine, tramadol, ketorolac and metamizol either openly or by a hidden infusion. In the open condition the doctor came to the bedside, injected the active medication in full view of the patients and gave verbal suggestions to the effect that a powerful painkiller was being administered. In the hidden condition the active medication was administered by means of a computer-programmed drug infusion pump, so the doctor was not present and the patients were unaware of the fact that a treatment was being administered. In the open condition, the patients needed less medication to obtain analgesia and the pain relief occurred sooner. The difference in medication needed for analgesia between the open and hidden injections illustrates a way of conceptualizing and investigating placebo effects (Price 2001; Colloca & Benedetti 2004; Price et al. 2008).

A recent study by Kaptchuk and colleagues (2008) has elegantly shown how factors in the delivery of meaning contribute to this meaning effect. A total of 262 patients suffering from irritable bowel syndrome (IBS) were randomized to receive a 3-week treatment with different rituals. These were waiting-list control (observation), placebo acupuncture alone ('limited ritual') or placebo acupuncture with a patient–practitioner relationship augmented by warmth, attention and confidence ('augmented ritual'). The results showed a progressive improvement in symptoms among the three groups; however, the augmented ritual was more effective than the limited ritual, which again was more effective than waiting list. These findings suggest that factors contributing to the placebo effect can be progressively combined in a manner resembling a graded-dose escalation of component parts and that the patient–practitioner interaction is one of the most robust components in the healing effect.

The more subtle influence of the practitioners' attitudes and beliefs has also been investigated. In a study of dental pain patients, the practitioner knew that one group of patients would receive a placebo whereas the second group would receive either a placebo or the active analgesic agent fentanyl (Gracely et al. 1985). When both groups received placebo, the placebo effect was significantly higher in the second group. This result indicates that the practitioner's belief that a patient may receive a powerful painkiller influences the magnitude of placebo analgesia even when the practitioner does not convey this belief verbally or intentionally.

The patient's knowledge about the probabilities of receiving active versus placebo drug also influences the treatment response. Two separate trials tested the effects of painkillers in postpartum pain, one with paracetamol against placebo, and one with paracetamol against naproxen. Due to informed consent patients knew that in one study they would be receiving placebo with a chance of 50% and in the other study one of two active medications. The difference in effectiveness of paracetamol was 20 mm on a 100-mm visual analogue scale between the trials, although everything else – researchers, setting, time, patient population – was the same (Skovlund 1991; Skovlund et al. 1991a, b). This increased effect from the probability of taking an efficacious treatment may also explain why more frequent dosing increases effects. Migraine trials often use non-symmetrical randomization schemes. In those trials, patients know that the likelihood to receive placebo is not 1:1 as in an ordinary study, but, say, 4:1. It has been shown in a meta-analysis that the placebo effect in these studies increases linearly with the heightened expectation of patients to receive real treatment if the likelihood to receive real treatment was higher than 1:1 (Diener et al. 1999). Also, meta-analyses of acid blockers in ulcers have shown that the frequency with which a drug is taken influences the placebo effect. If a drug is dosed to be taken four times a day, the effect is greater than if the drug is dosed to be taken twice a day (de Craen et al. 1999).

Some studies have directly manipulated the strength of verbal suggestions and tested how they influence treatment outcomes (Price et al. 1999; De Pascalis et al. 2002; Pollo et al. 2002; Verne et al. 2003; Vase et al. 2004). Strong verbal suggestions like 'this is a powerful painkiller' have been shown to lead to more pain relief and fewer requests for analgesics than weaker verbal suggestions like 'this is either an active agent or an inactive agent' (Pollo et al. 2002; Verne et al. 2003; Vase et al. 2004, 2005).

The relative influence of verbal suggestions compared to pharmacologically active substances, such as caffeine, alcohol or cannabis, have been tested in the so-called balanced placebo design (Marlatt & Rohsenow 1980). A 2 by 2 factorial design is used, where one factor is the substance versus placebo, and the other factor is correct versus misleading information. For instance, in studies on sexual arousal, subjects receive either alcohol or an appropriate placebo (normally tonic with a few drops of vodka sprinkled on top) and verbal manipulations and then view stimulating visual material. Here, suggestions of receiving alcohol produce strong effects, independent of the substance actually ingested.

Recently, not only the influence of positive verbal suggestions but also the influence of negative verbal suggestions on treatment outcome have been investigated. Negative verbal suggestions such as 'this agent is known to significantly increase pain in some patients' have been shown to increase pain levels (Vase et al. 2003; Colloca et al. 2008) and this facilitation of pain transmission involves the neurotransmitter cholecystokinin (Benedetti et al. 2007; Colloca & Benedetti 2007; Enck et al. 2008). If the verbal suggestion is to reduce pain, this pain reduction involves a different opioid neurotransmitter blocked by naloxone. Thus, the patient–practitioner relationship and the direct or indirect suggestions for symptom improvement or symptom worsening may influence treatment outcome in positive or negative directions.

EXPECTATION AND EMOTIONAL FACTORS

Verbal suggestions are likely to influence treatment outcome through patients' expectations and emotional feelings. Several studies have shown that especially expectation may influence treatment outcome (Kirsch 1990; Montgomery & Kirsch 1996, 1997; Price et al. 1999; De Pascalis et al. 2002). For instance, Vase and colleagues (2003) conducted a study in which 13 IBS patients were tested under no treatment, rectal placebo and rectal lidocaine (active) condition. Right after the agent had been administered and before it had taken effect, patients were asked to rate expected pain levels and desire for pain relief. Patients' expectations and desires for pain relief accounted for 77% of the variance in the placebo effect and 81% of the variance in the active pharmacological effect. Thus, expectations and desires are important placebo factors and these placebo factors also contribute to the efficacy of pharmacologically active agents.

While expectation is probably one of the best investigated factors in relation to placebo effects, factors such as conditioning may also influence patients' level of expectation. For instance, it has been shown that patients who are conditioned with morphine injections on days one and two have a greater placebo effect when they receive saline injections on day three as compared to a group of patients who receive saline injections on all three days (Amanzio & Benedetti 1999). Furthermore, the pain-relieving effect of the saline injection increased if the conditioning procedure was combined with positive verbal suggestions for pain relief. In agreement with these findings it has been shown that the stronger the conditioning procedure and the verbal suggestions for pain relief, the higher the patients' expectations of a positive treatment outcome and the better the treatment outcome (Price et al. 1999; De Pascalis et al. 2002). Conditioning occurs not only in pain, but also in hypertension with antihypertensive medication. Suchman & Ader (1992) have shown in a cross-over trial that placebo effects after antihypertensive medication were much stronger than before, and this could be used to reduce the use of antihypertensive drugs.

Emotional factors such as anxiety have not been investigated to the same extent as expectation. However, models of coping, motivation and emotional feelings show that the interaction between expectations of an outcome and the desires for an outcome interact to predict a range of emotional responses such as depression, anxiety, relief, disappointment, excitement and satisfaction (Price & Barrell 1984; Price et al. 1985). Recent studies have shown that a small reduction in desire for pain relief along with expectations of pain relief may decrease the patients' levels of anxiety and increase the placebo analgesia effect (Vase et al. 2004; Price et al. 2008). The finding that anxiety reduction may be central to placebo effects is in agreement with previous findings (Benson 1975; Gryll & Katahn 1978) as well as more recent brain imaging studies. For instance, Petrovic and colleagues (2005) have found that expectations of anxiety relief may contribute to placebo effects in relation to perception of unpleasant emotional feelings. These findings suggest that reward processing may be a central part of placebo effects in general.

For a long time it has been assumed that placebo effects are short-lasting. However, recent studies challenge this notion. In a study of IBS patients exposed to clinically relevant pain stimuli, the placebo analgesia effect increased over a 40-minute period (Vase et al. 2005) and in a study by Kupers and colleagues (2007) a placebo effect in chronic low-back pain was maintained for 49 days. In a study of arthroscopic surgery for osteoarthritis (Moseley et al. 2002), pain relief from sham surgery lasted over 2 years!

In a meta-analysis of long-term randomized controlled studies no correlation was found between the duration of the treatment or placebo treatment and the effect size of the placebo (Walach et al. 2005).

Furthermore, McRae and colleagues (2004) tested 30 Parkinson disease patients who received either a human fetal mesencephalic transplantation, which may be a possible treatment for Parkinson disease, or a sham surgery at 4, 8 and 12 months after surgery (McRae et al. 2004). At the 12-month follow-up no significant differences were found between the two groups on several outcome measures such as physical and quality-of-life scores. Interestingly, in this study patients were asked whether they believed that they had received the active treatment (fetal tissue transplantation) or placebo treatment (sham surgery). Patients who believed they received transplanted tissue had significant improvements in both quality of life and motor outcomes, regardless of whether they received sham surgery or fetal tissue implantation. Thus, perceived treatment assignment had a beneficial impact on the overall outcome and the difference was still present 12 months after the surgery.

These findings strongly indicate that the meaning patients attribute to a treatment and the expectations and emotional feelings they have in relation to treatment are very important for treatment outcome and may influence whether treatment effect is maintained (Vase et al. 2004; Benedetti 2008; Price et al. 2008).

PSYCHO-NEURO-PHYSIOLOGICAL MECHANISMS

Several neurobiological studies have found that placebo effects are accompanied by changes in neural activity within brain areas known to process symptoms such as pain, anxiety, depression and Parkinson disease.

PAIN

Brain imaging

In two functional magnetic resonance imaging (fMRI) experiments published in a single study, Wager et al. (2004) found that placebo analgesia was related to decreased neural activity in pain-processing areas of the brain. Pain-related neural activity was reduced within the thalamus, anterior insular cortex and anterior cingulate cortex during the placebo condition as compared with the baseline condition. In addition, the magnitude of these decreases was correlated with reductions in pain ratings. Another important aspect of the study by Wager and colleagues was that they imaged not only the period of pain but also the period of anticipation of pain. They hypothesized increases in neural activity within brain areas involved in expectation. In support of their hypothesis they found significant positive correlations (r = 0.4–0.7) between increases in brain activity in the anticipatory period and decreases in pain and pain-related neural activity during stimulation within the placebo condition. The brain areas showing positive correlations during the anticipatory phase included the orbitofrontal cortex, dorsolateral prefrontal cortex, rostal anterior cingulate cortex (rACC) and midbrain periaductal grey (PAG). The dorsolateral prefrontal cortex has been consistently associated with the representation of and maintenance of information needed for cognitive control, consistent with a role in expectation (Miller & Cohen 2001). On the other hand, the orbitofrontal cortex is associated with functioning in the evaluative and reward information relevant to allocation of control, consistent with a role in affective or motivational responses to anticipation of pain (Dias et al. 1996). Such a role is consistent with results showing that desire for relief is a factor in placebo analgesia.

A limitation of Wager and colleagues' study is that most of the decreases in neural activity within pain-related areas occurred during the period that subjects rated pain, leaving open the possibility that placebo effects mainly reflected report biases. However, Price and colleagues (2007) have recently conducted an fMRI study of IBS patients exposed to clinically relevant pain stimuli under no treatment, rectal placebo and placebo match (where pain stimuli were reduced to match pain ratings in the placebo condition). In this study a large placebo effect was produced by suggestions and accompanied by large reductions in known pain-related areas, such as thalamus, somatosensory areas 1 and 2 (S1, S2), insula and ACC during the period of stimulation, thereby reflecting effects unlikely to results from report biases. Interestingly, in the placebo match condition a reduction in brain activity similar to that observed during the placebo effect was seen, thereby indicating that the pain-relieving effect of placebo was similar to the effect of lowering pain stimuli.

In several of the brain imaging studies changed neural activity has been observed in the ACC and the periaqueductal grey (PAG) (Petrovic et al. 2002;

Wager et al. 2004; Price et al. 2008). These areas are involved in reward/aversion, emotions and the classical descending pain modulatory pathway (Basbaum & Fields 1978). The pain modulatory system involves rACC–PAG–rostroventral medulla–spinal cord connection. Through that pathway pain-related signals are inhibited at the dorsal horn of the spinal cord. It is activated by attentional, expectational and emotional processes, thought to originate in the cingulated cortex, which activate neurons in the midbrain (PAG) containing and releasing endogenous opioids inhibiting pain processes downstream (Reynolds 1969; Watkins & Mayer 1982).

Endogenous opioids

As early as 1978, Levine and colleagues were able to reverse placebo effects in postoperative pain patients by administration of the opiate antagonist naloxone, which blocks opioid receptors. This finding indicated that placebo analgesia effects may be mediated by endogenous opioids. The first study suffered from methodological limitations but subsequent studies added new controls and more sophisticated methods and these studies have basically replicated the initial finding. However, studies have also shown that not all placebo analgesia effects are opioid-mediated (Posner & Burke 1985; Amanzio & Benedetti 1999).

In 2001 Amanzio et al. tested how induction of placebo effects in healthy volunteers exposed to ischaemic arm pain and rating tolerance influenced the activation of the endogenous opioid system. When placebo effects were induced via verbal suggestions for pain relief the placebo effect was completely reversed by naloxone. However, when placebo effects were induced via conditioning, placebo effects were only reversed by naloxone if the conditioning procedure was carried out with an opioid substance, morphine. Interestingly, conditioning with the non-opioid drug, ketorolac, produced an analgesic effect that was not naloxone-reversible, pointing to the fact that other systems apart from the endorphine system play a role in placebo analgesia and can be specifically conditioned.

Zubieta and colleagues (2005) have employed in vivo receptor binding techniques to test the involvement of endogenous opioids in placebo analgesia effects directly. Healthy volunteers were exposed to muscle pain and received saline injections along with verbal suggestions for pain relief. The radiotracer carfentanil, which is a mu-opioid agonist, was applied. Following placebo administration subjects reported lower pain levels and a decrease in negative emotions. At the same time there was an increased mu-opioid neurotransmission in the dorsolateral prefrontal cortex, the ACC, the insula and the nucleus accumbens. These findings directly show that placebo analgesia effects may involve release of endogenous opioids and they furthermore corroborate that placebo effects and emotional feelings are related.

The findings that placebo analgesia effects may involve release of endogenous opioids and that placebo effect may reduce nociceptive input at early pain-processing levels such as the thalamus indicate that placebo analgesia effects constitute true antinociceptive effects. Thus, there is strong evidence against the notion that placebo effects are nothing but response bias.

ANXIETY

The involvement of brain areas implicated in emotional regulation and hence in placebo responses is not restricted to pain modulation. Petrovic et al. (2005) demonstrated a placebo effect related to the reduction of anxiety associated with viewing unpleasant pictures. Reductions in experienced unpleasantness were accompanied by increases in brain areas involved in reward/aversion and previously shown to be involved in placebo analgesia. These areas included those previously implicated in emotional modulation, such as the orbitofrontal cortex, rACC and amygdala. They also included areas involved in treatment expectation, such as ventrolateral prefrontal cortex and rACC.

DEPRESSION

Evidence of significant and increasing rates of placebo responses in antidepressant trials has been documented in several studies (Khan et al. 2000; Andrews 2001; Walsh et al. 2002). In a placebo-controlled study of fluoxetine, a serotonin reuptake inhibitor, Mayberg and colleagues (2002) acquired positron emission tomography (PET) scans before and 1 and 6 weeks after treatment. At 6 weeks patients in both groups reported clinical improvement as compared to baseline. PET changes were associated with clinical response in both the fluoxetine group and the placebo group. There was a clear overlap of active areas in placebo responders and treatment responders. While activation of the thalamus was reduced in both conditions and activation of prefrontal areas was enhanced, fluoxetine showed enhanced activity in the pons, and reduced activity in the hippocampus and striatum, a finding not seen with placebo. Fluoxetine effects were generally more pronounced. But, interestingly, activation of the right prefrontal cortex was more pronounced in placebo responders.

This finding is qualified by another imaging study (Leuchter et al. 2002). Here high-resolution quantitative electroencephalography was used to locate areas of higher or lower electrical activity. In an antidepressant trial, it was found that responders to placebo, responders to pharmacological agents and non-responders had distinctive activation patterns. While placebo responders showed increased activity in the prefrontal cortex, drug responders showed a decreased activity in that area, and non-responders showed no change. This seems to show that meaning effects indeed reflect in altered brain metabolism and activity.

As some of these studies have been using inhibitors of serotonin reuptake, it is plausible that serotonergic mechanisms may be involved in the antidepressant effect produced by placebo. However, more experiments are needed to understand better the possible mechanisms involved (Benedetti 2008).

PARKINSON'S DISEASE

Meaning and expectation seem to play a key role in Parkinson's disease as well. Expectation of either good or bad motor performance has been found to modulate the therapeutic effects of deep brain stimulation in Parkinson's disease patients (Pollo et al. 2002; Mercado et al. 2006) and this effect is independent of previous conditioning (Benedetti et al. 2003). De la Fuente-Fernandez and colleagues (2001) tested the effect of apomorphine and placebo on dopamine release in patients with Parkinson's disease using PET scan. The study utilized the competition of radioactively marked raclopride (RAC) and endogenous dopamine. The authors observed 17% and 19% diminution of RAC in the nucleus caudatus and the putamen, respectively. Both areas contain many dopamine-producing neurons. This finding suggests that patients expecting dopaminergic pharmacological effects will produce dopamine. These findings have been confirmed by a recent study using sham transcranial magnetic stimulation as a placebo (Strafella et al. 2006). Dopamine is an important neurotransmitter which activates the reward system and the endorphine system (Pitchot et al. 2001), and is important in learning (Schultz 1999; Waelti et al. 2001; Rossi 2002). Thus, this finding further illustrates how placebo may produce effects beyond pain relief and influence areas such as affect, learning and motivation. More recently, researchers have started to speculate whether there may be large overlaps between the neurotransmitter systems involved in placebo effects in relation to pain, depression and Parkinson disease so that for instance both opioids and dopamine are involved in placebo effects in relation to Parkinson's disease (Benedetti et al. 2005; Benedetti 2008).

In summary, the way in which patients attribute meaning to a treatment is likely to be influenced by the context, the interaction with the practitioner and the verbal suggestions given in relation to the treatment. These factors seem to influence patients' expectations and emotional feeling and these psychological changes appear to be associated with neural changes at higher cortical levels as well as limbic areas. These changes may in turn elicit release of neurotransmitters such as endogenous opioids, endogenous dopamine and possibly serotonin. These findings support the understanding that meaning responses have real psycho-neuro-physiological underpinnings. Therefore it is important to understand how these meaning responses affect research design and execution and may be elicited in clinical practice.

IMPLICATIONS OF MEANING RESPONSES FOR STUDY DESIGN AND CONDUCT

This evidence, showing the ubiquitous effects of expectation, conditioning, communication, emotional valence and social and cultural context on therapeutic outcome, has profound implications for study design and the conduct of clinical research. First, factors that are considered placebo (incidental) effects to one therapy (e.g. drug therapy), such as listening and positive reinforcement, may be specific (characteristic) factors in another therapy, such as mind–body practices, acupuncture or physiotherapy (Paterson & Dieppe 2005). Failure to distinguish these differences clearly in each trial risks false-negative findings.

Second, information in the informed consent section of clinical trials must be carefully crafted as it may set up expectations that influence trial outcome. For example, Bergmann et al. (1994) explored the effect of informed consent on pain in a randomized placebo-controlled trial of naproxen (a pain drug) in cancer patients. Patients given informed consent reported more pain relief when they knew they might get an active medication than those who were not given this information.

Conditioning also has to be taken into account. In cross-over designs, the order of administration may influence the outcome. Those given an active agent first may be conditioned to respond to the placebo or sham treatment and show a false-positive effect once crossed over (Ader 1997). Even without cross-over design, simple two-arm placebo-controlled RCTs cannot detect the degree that conditioning contributes an active drug's response.

To the extent that a therapeutic effect incorporates learning and feedback into the intervention, blinding may interfere with the therapy. This is important in many conventional and complementary therapies, such as psychotherapy, physiotherapy, biofeedback, mind–body or bioenergy practices, massage and comprehensive lifestyle therapies (Jonas 2005).

Meaning responses can determine what is scientifically provable or not. The therapeutic variability of social and cultural context and meaning is important even if the treatment is known to be efficacious. For example, Moerman (2002) reported that responses in the placebo arms of uniform studies of H_2-blockers in the treatment of ulcer disease vary from 0% to 100%. Effect sizes in Germany were in the 60–70% range and even after six large studies it could not be proven that these drugs worked better than placebo pills for ulcers. In contrast, placebo responses were significantly lower in the Netherlands and their specific efficacy over placebo could be easily proven.

Finally, meaning and context responses show that all treatments, whether they have proven efficacy or not, require full evaluation outside of RCT designs and outside the evidence hierarchy framework (Jonas 2005). Figure 16.1 illustrates why a full evidence framework is needed, especially in complex interventions such as CAM. Treatment A in Figure 16.1 involves a complex intervention that maximizes meaning responses but uses an agent with only a small characteristic (specific) effect. An example of treatment A could be acupuncture in low-back pain. Treatment B in Figure 16.1 shows a treatment with a small meaning effect but uses an agent with a larger characteristic effect. An example might be the use of a non-steroidal anti-inflammatory agent in back pain. While treatment B can be scientifically proven in a placebo-controlled RCT, treatment A may not

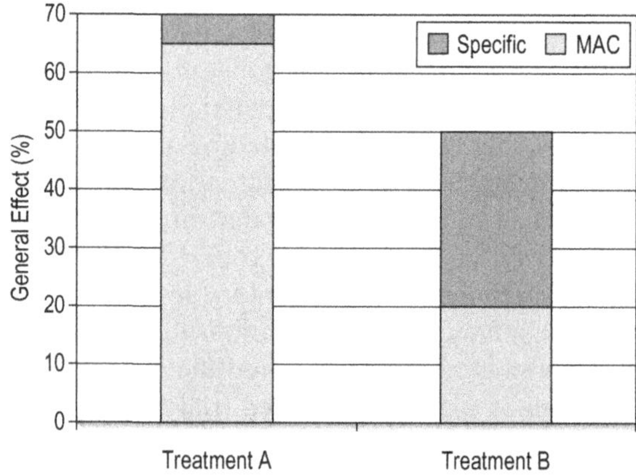

FIGURE 16.1 Hypothetical example showing differential importance of meaning and context (MAC) effects.

be able to be proven in this way. However, most patients and practitioners would prefer treatment A.

The proper evaluation of meaning responses in clinical research requires more than internal and external validity. To address the full implications of placebo effects in clinical research the components of the meaning response need to be considered in validity assessments. This additional type of validity includes assessment of components that make up meaning responses when designing and evaluating clinical research. These factors have been termed 'model validity' and are described in Chapter 1 of this book and in other guides to clinical research (Jonas 2002).

CONCLUDING REMARKS: HARNESSING MEANING RESPONSES

Although this review has been far from exhaustive and has highlighted a rather selective list of findings, it has shown:

- Meaning effects are real and can be quite strong.
- If conceived as an individual response to the meaning of an intervention, many paradoxes inherent in traditional usages of the concept of placebo disappear.
- This latter usage of the concept can also contribute to a broader understanding of healing responses. Meaning effects seem to involve patient–practitioner interactions, conditioning, expectation and emotional feelings and they can involve multiple central mechanisms and neurotransmitter pathways.
- Placebo analgesia may be mediated by endogenous opiate systems, which are similar to those activated by exogenous opiates. Placebo effects in relation to depression and Parkinson disease may involve serotonin and dopaminergic systems respectively.

CAM therapies might be elegant, efficient and comparatively harmless ways to harness these processes (Walach 2001). Acupuncture placebos, for instance, have recently been shown in the largest trials available to be significantly and clinically superior to conventional therapy using guidelines for osteoarthritis and back pain (Haake et al. 2007). It is expected that, depending on the meaning system, what is seen as placebo by some may be more effective in treating other than proven effective interventions. We should view that as a virtue rather than a vice. But CAM is not the proprietor of meaning effects. These responses are ubiquitous and can be used in every healing context. From the literature we can glean the following suggestions on how to harness these processes:

1. In order to elicit meaning effects one need not give placebos like sugar pills. Meaning effects may arise and be optimized in a realistic manner in ordinary conventional or complementary healing settings. Therapeutic rituals are likely to elicit meaning response (Frank 1989; Kaptchuk et al. 2008) and a significant portion of the effects from modern devices used in both conventional and complementary medicine may be caused by such effects. Hence: elaborate your rituals.

2. Listening to and talking with the patient may be an effective step towards cure already. Rapport between doctor and patient is a most important vehicle for suggesting therapeutic effects and enhancing expectations. Jerome Frank went so far as to say that the effects produced by the general ambience of treatment are the most important therapeutic factors (Frank 1961, 1989). Hence find out what patients expect.
3. One of the greatest skills of the doctor, and a topic often left out of the discussion around evidence-based medicine, is individualization. It is in the subtle changes to therapy and how they are delivered by a skilled healer that the meaning response is harnessed to its fullest. Any therapist who individualizes treatment will likely have better results, because he or she can harness the meaning response. Hence: introduce simple ways of individualization or use a therapy that forces you to individualize.
4. Always work with and not against patients' expectations. If patients expect an intervention to be harmful, dangerous, fraught with side-effects and not curative, they are likely to experience just that. Thus every physician and therapist should find out about those expectations and optimize them in a realistic manner. If treatment choices are given, use the one which is most conforming to patients' expectation. For instance, if a patient expects to get better from a 'natural product' or a 'chemical product', it is likely that this preference is clinically significant. Hence: find out, what patients expect.
5. Pay attention to patients' emotional feelings. Raising hope and alleviating anxiety in a credible way is one of the most therapeutic acts in general. It has been shown empirically that giving a clear diagnosis and positive prognosis improves outcome (Thomas 1987). If patients receive clear and positive communications conveyed with trust, credibility and confidence, healing is more likely. This must be mastered in a world in which knowledge is transitory and changes quickly and frequently contradicts previous knowledge. Truth and integrity are integral components of a trusting relationship; however, the patient should not be made the primary target for transferring our insecurity. Hence: establish your patients' trust.

Box 16.1 lists clinical factors to consider when attempting to maximize meaning responses in clinical settings. While all of these factors may not be appropriate for every setting, there is evidence to indicate they could enhance the effect of any therapy, conventional or complementary.

Taken together, we have shown that placebo effects, reframed as meaning responses, can evoke powerful healing and therefore should be utilized and have implications for clinical research design and execution. The meaning response is ubiquitous, and can be used or abused in any therapeutic context. To ignore it is to risk producing random and possibly harmful effects. To understand it and use it intelligently is to increase therapeutic benefit. Placebo research can and should be directed toward providing the evidence base for developing optimal healing environments.

BOX 16.1 Ways to enhance healing responses from the placebo literature

- Use more frequent dosing (de Craen et al. 1999)
- Apply therapies in 'therapeutic' settings (de Craen et al. 2000)
- Match the appearance to the desired effect (de Craen et al. 1996, 1999)
- Attend to the route of administration (de Craen et al. 2000)
- Deliver therapies in a warm and caring way (de Craen et al. 2000)
- Deliver therapies with confidence and in a credible way (Uhlenhuth et al. 1966)
- Determine what treatment your patient believes in or not (Frank 1961; Kirsch 1985; Cassidy 1998)
- Be sure that you believe in the treatment and find it credible (Gracely et al. 1985; Cassidy 1998)
- Align all beliefs congruently (Phillips et al. 1993; Uexküll 1995; Cassidy 1998; Moerman 2000)
- Deliver a benign but frequent conditioned stimulus along with therapy (Ader & Cohen 1975; Ader 1983; Kirsch 1985; Voudouris & Peck 1985; Wickramasekera 1985; Voudouris et al. 1989, 1990; Montgomery & Kirsch 1997)
- Use the newest and most prominent treatment available (Johnson 1994; Lange & Hillis 1999)
- Use a well-known name brand identified with success (Margo 1999)
- Cut or stick the skin or poke into an orifice when believed important (Johnson 1994)
- Inform patients what they can expect (Skovlund 1991; Bergmann et al. 1994)
- Use a light, laser or electronic device to deliver and track the treatment (Lange & Hillis 1999)
- Incorporate reassurance, relaxation, suggestion and anxiety reduction methods (Georgiu et al. 1989; Stefano et al. 2001; Vase et al. 2003)
- Listen and provide empathy and understanding (Thomas 1978; Brody 2000)
- Touch the patient (Cherkin et al. 2001; Moerman & Jonas 2002)

Reprinted from Walach & Jones 2004.

ACKNOWLEDGEMENT

Our work is supported by the Samueli Institute, Alexandria, VA and Corona del Mar, CA.

REFERENCES

Ader, R., 1983. Behavioral conditioning and immunity. In: Fabris, N., Garaci, E., Hadden, J., et al. (Eds.), Immunoregulation. Plenum Press, New York, pp. 283–313.

Ader, R., 1997. The role of conditioning in pharmacotherapy. In: Harrington, A. (Ed.), The Placebo Effect: An Interdisciplinary Exploration. Harvard University Press, Cambridge, pp. 138–165.

Ader, R., Cohen, N., 1975. Behaviorally conditioned immunosuppression. Psychosom. Med. 37 (4), 333–340.

Amanzio, M., Benedetti, F., 1999. Neuropharmacological dissection of placebo analgesia: expectation-activated opioid systems versus conditioning-activated specific subsystems. J. Neurosci. 19 (1), 484–494.

Amanzio, M., Pollo, A., Maggi, G., et al., 2001. Response variability to analgesics: a role for non-specific activation of endogenous opioids. Pain 90 (3), 205–215.

Andersen, L.A., 1997. Placebo – historisk og kulturelt. In: Andersen, L.A., Claësson, M.H., Hròbjartsson, A., et al. (Eds.), Placebo – historie, biologi og effekt. Akademisk Forlag, Lyngby, pp. 69–119.

Andrews, G., 2001. Placebo response in depression: bane of research, boon to therapy. Br. J. Psychiatry 178, 192–194.

Basbaum, A.I., Fields, H.L., 1978. Endogenous pain control mechanisms: review and hypothesis. Ann. Neurol. 4 (5), 451–462.

Beecher, H.K., 1955. The powerful placebo. J. Am. Med. Assoc. 159 (17), 1602–1606.

Benedetti, F., 2008. Mechanisms of placebo and placebo-related effects across diseases and treatments. Annu. Rev. Pharmacol. Toxicol. 48, 33–60.

Benedetti, F., Amanzio, M., 1997. The neurobiology of placebo analgesia: from endogenous opioids to cholecystokinin. Prog. Neurobiol. 52 (2), 109–125.

Benedetti, F., Pollo, A., Lopiano, L., et al., 2003. Conscious expectation and unconscious conditioning in analgesic, motor, and hormonal placebo/nocebo responses. J. Neurosci. 23 (10), 4315–4323.

Benedetti, F., Mayberg, H.S., Wager, T.D., et al., 2005. Neurobiological mechanisms of the placebo effect. J. Neurosci. 25 (45), 10390–10402.

Benedetti, F., Lanotte, M., Lopiano, L., et al., 2007. When words are painful: unraveling the mechanisms of the nocebo effect. Neuroscience 147 (2), 260–271.

Benson, H., 1975. The relaxation response. William Morrow, New York.

Bergmann, J.F., Chassany, O., Gandiol, J., et al., 1994. A randomised clinical trial of the effect of informed consent on the analgesic activity of placebo and naproxen in cancer pain. Clin. Trials Metaanal. 29 (1), 41–47.

Brody, H., 2000. The placebo response. Recent research and implications for family medicine. J. Fam. Pract. 49 (7), 649–654.

Cassidy, C.M., 1998. Chinese medicine users in the United States. Part II: Preferred aspects of care. J. Altern. Complement. Med. 4 (2), 189–202.

Cherkin, D.C., Eisenberg, D., Sherman, K.J., et al., 2001. Randomized trial comparing traditional Chinese medical acupuncture, therapeutic massage, and self-care education for chronic low back pain. Arch. Intern. Med. 161 (8), 1081–1088.

Colloca, L., Benedetti, F., 2004. The placebo in clinical studies and in medical practice. In: Price, D.D., Bushnell, M.C. (Eds.), Psychological methods of pain control: Basic science and clinical perspectives. IASP Press, Seattle, pp. 187–205.

Colloca, L., Benedetti, F., 2007. Nocebo hyperalgesia: how anxiety is turned into pain. Curr. Opin. Anaesthesiol. 20 (5), 435–439.

Colloca, L., Sigaudo, M., Benedetti, F., 2008. The role of learning in nocebo and placebo effects. Pain 136 (1–2), 211–218.

de Craen, A.J., Roos, P.J., Leonard de Vries, A., et al., 1996. Effect of colour of drugs: systematic review of perceived effect of drugs and of their effectiveness. BMJ 313 (7072), 1624–1626.

de Craen, A.J., Moerman, D.E., Heisterkamp, S.H., et al., 1999. Placebo effect in the treatment of duodenal ulcer. Br. J. Clin. Pharmacol. 48 (6), 853–860.

de Craen, A.J., Tijssen, J.G., de Gans, J., et al., 2000. Placebo effect in the acute treatment of migraine: subcutaneous placebos are better than oral placebos. J. Neurol. 247 (3), 183–188.

de la Fuente-Fernandez, R., Ruth, T.J., Sossi, V., et al., 2001. Expectation and dopamine release: mechanism of the placebo effect in Parkinson's disease. Science 293 (5532), 1164–1166.

De Pascalis, V., Chiaradia, C., Carotenuto, E., 2002. The contribution of suggestibility and expectation to placebo analgesia phenomenon in an experimental setting. Pain 96 (3), 393–402.

Dias, R., Robbins, T.W., Roberts, A.C., 1996. Dissociation in prefrontal cortex of affective and attentional shifts. Nature 380 (6569), 69–72.

Diener, H.C., Dowson, A.J., Ferrari, M., et al., 1999. Unbalanced randomization influences placebo response: scientific versus ethical issues around the use of placebo in migraine trials. Cephalalgia 19 (8), 699–700.

Einarson, T.E., Hemels, M., Stolk, P., 2001. Is the placebo powerless? N. Engl. J. Med. 345 (17), 1277; author reply 1278–1279.

Ekeland, T.J., 1999. Meining som medisin: Ein analyse av placebofenomenet og implikasjoner for terapi og terapeutiske teoriar. Institut for Samfunnspsykologi, Psykologisk Fakultet, Universitetet i Bergen, Bergen, NO.

Enck, P., Benedetti, F., Schedlowski, M., 2008. New insights into the placebo and nocebo responses. Neuron 59 (2), 195–206.
Fields, H.L., Price, D.D., 1997. Toward a neurobiology of placebo analgesia. In: Harrington, A. (Ed.), The placebo effect. Harvard University Press, Boston, MA, pp. 93–116.
Frank, J.D., 1961. Persuasion and healing: A comparative study of psychotherapy. John Hopkins University Press, Baltimore.
Frank, J.D., 1989. Non-specific aspects of treatment: The view of a psychotherapist. In: Shepherd, M., Sartorius, N. (Eds.), Non-Specific Aspects of Treatment. Huber, Bern, pp. 95–114.
Gheorghiu, V.A., Netter, P., Eysenck, H.J., et al. (Eds.), 1989. Suggestion and Suggestibility: Theory and Research. Springer, Heidelberg.
Gotzsche, P.C., 1994. Is there logic in the placebo? Lancet 344 (8927), 925–926.
Gracely, R.H., Dubner, R., Deeter, W.R., et al., 1985. Clinicians' expectations influence placebo analgesia. Lancet 1 (8419), 43.
Gryll, S.L., Katahn, M., 1978. Situational factors contributing to the placebo effect. Psychopharmacology (Berl.) 57 (3), 253–261.
Haake, M., Muller, H.H., Schade-Brittinger, C., et al., 2007. German Acupuncture Trials (GERAC) for chronic low back pain: randomized, multicenter, blinded, parallel-group trial with 3 groups. Arch. Intern. Med. 167 (17), 1892–1898.
Hrobjartsson, A., Gøtzsche, P.C., 2001. Is the placebo powerless? An analysis of clinical trials comparing placebo with no treatment. N. Engl. J. Med. 344 (21), 1594–1602.
Hrobjartsson, A., Gøtzsche, P.C., 2004. Is the placebo powerless? Update of a systematic review with 52 new randomized trials comparing placebo with no treatment. J. Intern. Med. 256 (2), 91–100.
Johnson, A.G., 1994. Surgery as a placebo. Lancet 344 (8930), 1140–1142.
Jonas, W.B., 2005. Building an evidence house: challenges and solutions to research in complementary and alternative medicine. Forsch. Komplementarmed. Klass. Naturheilkd. 12 (3), 159–167.
Jonas, W.B., 2002. Evidence, ethics and evaluation of global medicine. In: Callahan, D. (Ed.), The role of complementary and alternative medicine: Accommodating pluralism. Georgetown University Press, Washington DC, pp. 122–147.
Kaptchuk, T.J., 1998a. Powerful placebo: the dark side of the randomised controlled trial. Lancet 351 (9117), 1722–1725.
Kaptchuk, T.J., 1998b. Intentional ignorance: a history of blind assessment and placebo controls in medicine. Bull. Hist. Med. 72 (3), 389–433.
Kaptchuk, T.J., 2001. Is the placebo powerless? N. Engl. J. Med. 345 (17), 1277; author reply 1278–1279.
Kaptchuk, T.J., Kelley, J.M., Conboy, L.A., et al., 2008. Components of placebo effect: randomised controlled trial in patients with irritable bowel syndrome. BMJ 336 (7651), 999–1003.
Khan, A., Warner, H.A., Brown, W.A., 2000. Symptom reduction and suicide risk in patients treated with placebo in antidepressant clinical trials: an analysis of the Food and Drug Administration database. Arch. Gen. Psychiatry 57 (4), 311–317.
Kienle, G.S., Kiene, H., 1996. Placebo effect and placebo concept: a critical methodological and conceptual analysis of reports on the magnitude of the placebo effect. Altern.Ther. Health Med. 2 (6), 39–54.
Kienle, G.S., Kiene, H., 1997. The powerful placebo effect: fact or fiction? J. Clin. Epidemiol. 50 (12), 1311–1318.
Kirsch, I., 1985. Response expectancy as a determinant of experience and behavior. Am. Psychol. 40, 1189–1202.
Kirsch, I., 1990. Changing expectation. A key to effective psychotherapy. Pacific Grove, Brooks/Cole.
Kirsch, I., Sapirstein, G., 1998. Listening to prozac but hearing placebo: A meta-analysis of antidepressant medication. Prevention and Treatment 1, 2a.
Kirsch, I., Deacon, B.J., Huedo-Medina, T.B., et al., 2008. Initial severity and antidepressant benefits: a meta-analysis of data submitted to the Food and Drug Administration. PLoS Med. 5 (2), e45.
Kupers, R., Maeyaert, J., Boly, M., et al., 2007. Naloxone-insensitive epidural placebo analgesia in a chronic pain patient. Anesthesiology 106 (6), 1239–1242.
Kupers, R., 2001. Is the placebo powerless? N. Engl. J. Med. 345 (17), 1278; author reply 1278–1279.
Lancman, M.E., Asconape, J.J., Craven, W.J., et al., 1994. Predictive value of induction

of psychogenic seizures by suggestion. Ann. Neurol. 35 (3), 359–361.

Lange, R.A., Hillis, L.D., 1999. Transmyocardial laser revascularization. N. Engl. J. Med. 341 (14), 1075–1076.

Leuchter, A.F., Cook, I.A., Witte, E.A., et al., 2002. Changes in brain function of depressed subjects during treatment with placebo. Am. J. Psychiatry 159 (1), 122–129.

Levine, J.D., Gordon, N.C., Fields, H.L., 1978. The mechanism of placebo analgesia. Lancet 2 (8091), 654–657.

Lilford, R.J., Braunholtz, D.A., 2001. Is the placebo powerless? N. Engl. J. Med. 345 (17), 1277–1278; author reply 1278–1279.

Margo, C.E., 1999. The placebo effect. Surv. Ophthalmol. 44 (1), 31–44.

Marlatt, G.A., Rohsenow, D.J., 1980. Cognitive processes in alcohol use: Expectancy and the balanced placebo design. In: Mello, N. (Ed.), Advances in Substance Abuse. JAI Press, Greenwich, pp. 159–199.

Mayberg, H.S., Silva, J.A., Brannan, S.K., et al., 2002. The functional neuroanatomy of the placebo effect. Am. J. Psychiatry 159 (5), 728–737.

McRae, C., Cherin, E., Yamazaki, T.G., et al., 2004. Effects of perceived treatment on quality of life and medical outcomes in a double-blind placebo surgery trial. Arch. Gen. Psychiatry 61 (4), 412–420.

Mercado, R., Constantoyannis, C., Mandat, T., et al., 2006. Expectation and the placebo effect in Parkinson's disease patients with subthalamic nucleus deep brain stimulation. Mov. Disord. 21 (9), 1457–1461.

Miller, F.G., 2001. Is the placebo powerless? N. Engl. J. Med. 345 (17), 1277; author reply 1278–1279.

Miller, E.K., Cohen, J.D., 2001. An integrative theory of prefrontal cortex function. Annu. Rev. Neurosci. 24, 167–202.

Moerman, D.E., 2000. Cultural variations in the placebo effect: ulcers, anxiety, and blood pressure. Med. Anthropol. Q. 14 (1), 51–72.

Moerman, D.E., 2002. Meaning, medicine, and the placebo effect. Cambridge University Press, Cambridge, MA.

Moerman, D.E., Jonas, W.B., 2000. Toward a research agenda on placebo. Adv. Mind Body Med. 16 (1), 33–46.

Moerman, D.E., Jonas, W.B., 2002. Deconstructing the placebo effect and finding the meaning response. Ann. Intern. Med. 136 (6), 471–476.

Montgomery, G., Kirsch, I., 1996. Mechanisms of placebo pain reduction: An empirical investigation. Psychol. Sci. 7 (3), 174–176.

Montgomery, G.H., Kirsch, I., 1997. Classical conditioning and the placebo effect. Pain 72 (1–2), 107–113.

Moseley, J.B., O'Malley, K., Petersen, N.J., et al., 2002. A controlled trial of arthroscopic surgery for osteoarthritis of the knee. N. Engl. J. Med. 347 (2), 81–88.

Paterson, C., Dieppe, P., 2005. Characteristic and incidental (placebo) effects in complex interventions such as acupuncture. BMJ 330 (7501), 1202–1205.

Petrovic, P., Kalso, E., Petersson, K.M., et al., 2002. Placebo and opioid analgesia – imaging a shared neuronal network. Science 295 (5560), 1737–1740.

Petrovic, P., Dietrich, T., Fransson, P., et al., 2005. Placebo in emotional processing – induced expectations of anxiety relief activate a generalized modulatory network. Neuron 46 (6), 957–969.

Phillips, D.P., Ruth, T.E., Wagner, L.M., 1993. Psychology and survival. Lancet 342 (8880), 1142–1145.

Pitchot, W., Reggers, J., Pinto, E., et al., 2001. Reduced dopaminergic activity in depressed suicides. Psychoneuroendocrinology 26 (3), 331–335.

Pollo, A., Amanzio, M., Arslanian, A., et al., 2001. Response expectancies in placebo analgesia and their clinical relevance. Pain 93 (1), 77–84.

Pollo, A., Torre, E., Lopiano, L., et al., 2002. Expectation modulates the response to subthalamic nucleus stimulation in Parkinsonian patients. Neuroreport 13 (11), 1383–1386.

Posner, J., Burke, C.A., 1985. The effects of naloxone on opiate and placebo analgesia in healthy volunteers. Psychopharmacology (Berl.) 87 (4), 468–472.

Price, D.D., 2001. Assessing placebo effects without placebo groups: an untapped possibility? Pain 90 (3), 201–203.

Price, D.D., Barrell, J.J., 1984. Some general laws of human emotion: Interrelationships between intensities of desire, expectation, and emotional feeling. J. Pers. 52 (4), 389–409.

Price, D.D., Barrell, J.E., Barrell, J.J., 1985. A quantitative-experiential analysis of human emotions. Motiv. Emotion 9 (1), 19–38.

Price, D.D., Milling, L.S., Kirsch, I., et al., 1999. An analysis of factors that contribute to the magnitude of placebo analgesia in an experimental paradigm. Pain 83 (2), 147–156.

Price, D.D., Craggs, J., Verne, G.N., et al., 2007. Placebo analgesia is accompanied by large reductions in pain-related brain activity in irritable bowel syndrome patients. Pain 127 (1–2), 63–72.

Price, D.D., Finniss, D.G., Benedetti, F., 2008. A comprehensive review of the placebo effect: recent advances and current thought. Annu. Rev. Psychol. 59, 565–590.

Queneau, P., Asmar, R., Safar, M., 2002. L'effet placebo sur les pressions artérielles systolique, diastolique et pulsée. Presse Médicale 31, 1220–1223.

Reynolds, D.V., 1969. Surgery in the rat during electrical analgesia induced by focal brain stimulation. Science 164 (878), 444–445.

Rheims, S., Cucherat, M., Arzimanoglou, A., et al., 2008. Greater response to placebo in children than in adults: a systematic review and meta-analysis in drug-resistant partial epilepsy. PLoS Med. 5 (8), e166.

Rossi, E.L., 2002. A conceptual review of the psychosocial genomics of expectancy and surprise: neuroscience perspectives about the deep psychobiology of therapeutic hypnosis. Am. J. Clin. Hypn. 45 (2), 103–118.

Schultz, W., 1999. The primate basal ganglia and the voluntary control of behaviour. Journal of Consciousness Studies 6 (8–9), 31–45 (Special Issue: The Volitional Brain: Towards a Neuroscience of Free Will).

Shapiro, A.K., Morris, L.A., 1978. The placebo effect in medical and psychological therapies. In: Garfield, S.L., Bergin, A.E. (Eds.), Handbook of psychotherapy and behaviour change: an empirical analysis, second ed. Wiley, New York, pp. 369–409.

Shrier, I., 2001. Is the placebo powerless? N. Engl. J. Med. 345 (17), 1278; author reply 1278–1279.

Sinclair, R., Cassuto, J., Hogstrom, S., et al., 1988. Topical anesthesia with lidocaine aerosol in the control of postoperative pain. Anesthesiology 68 (6), 895–901.

Skovlund, E., 1991. Should we tell trial patients that they might receive placebo? Lancet 337 (8748), 1041.

Skovlund, E., Fyllingen, G., Landre, H., et al., 1991a. Comparison of postpartum pain treatments using a sequential trial design. I. Paracetamol versus placebo. Eur. J. Clin. Pharmacol. 40 (4), 343–347.

Skovlund, E., Fyllingen, G., Landre, H., et al., 1991b. Comparison of postpartum pain treatments using a sequential trial design: II. Naproxen versus paracetamol. Eur. J. Clin. Pharmacol. 40 (6), 539–542.

Stefano, G.B., Fricchione, G.L., Slingsby, B.T., et al., 2001. The placebo effect and relaxation response: neural processes and their coupling to constitutive nitric oxide. Brain Res. Brain Res. Rev. 35 (1), 1–19.

Strafella, A.P., Ko, J.H., Monchi, O., 2006. Therapeutic application of transcranial magnetic stimulation in Parkinson's disease: the contribution of expectation. Neuroimage 31 (4), 1666–1672.

Suchman, A.L., Ader, R., 1992. Classic conditioning and placebo effects in crossover studies. Clin. Pharmacol. Ther. 52, 372–377.

Thomas, K.B., 1987. General practice consultations: is there any point in being positive? Br. Med. J. (Clin. Res. Ed.) 294 (6581), 1200–1202.

Uexküll, T.V., 1995. Biosemiotic research and not further molecular analysis is necessary to describe pathways between cells, personalities, and social systems. Adv. J. Mind-Body Health 11, 24–27.

Uhlenhuth, E.H., Rickels, K., Fisher, S., et al., 1966. Drug, doctor's verbal attitude and clinic setting in the symptomatic response to pharmacotherapy. Psychopharmacologia 9 (5), 392–418.

Vase, L., Riley 3rd, J.L., Price, D.D., 2002. A comparison of placebo effects in clinical analgesic trials versus studies of placebo analgesia. Pain 99 (3), 443–452.

Vase, L., Robinson, M.E., Verne, G.N., et al., 2003. The contributions of suggestion, desire, and expectation to placebo effects in irritable bowel syndrome patients. An empirical investigation. Pain 105 (1–2), 17–25.

Vase, L., Price, D.D., Verne, G.N., et al., 2004. The contribution of changes in expected pain levels and desire for pain relief to placebo analgesia. In: Price, D.D., Bushnell, M.C. (Eds.), Psychological methods of pain control: basic science and clinical perspectives. IAPS Press, Seattle, pp. 207–234.

Vase, L., Robinson, M.E., Verne, G.N., et al., 2005. Increased placebo analgesia over time in irritable bowel syndrome (IBS) patients is associated with desire and expectation but not endogenous opioid mechanisms. Pain 115 (3), 338–347.

Vase, L., Petersen, G.L., Riley 3rd, J.L., et al., 2009. Factors contributing to large analgesic effects in placebo mechanism studies conducted between 2002 and 2007. Pain 145 (1–2), 36–44.

Verne, G.N., Robinson, M.E., Vase, L., et al., 2003. Reversal of visceral and cutaneous hyperalgesia by local rectal anesthesia in irritable bowel syndrome (IBS) patients. Pain 105 (1–2), 223–230.

Voudouris, N.J., Peck, C.L., Coleman, G., 1985. Conditioned placebo responses. J. Pers. Soc. Psychol. 48 (1), 47–53.

Voudouris, N.J., Peck, C.L., Coleman, G., 1989. Conditioned response models of placebo phenomena: further support. Pain 38 (1), 109–116.

Voudouris, N.J., Peck, C.L., Coleman, G., 1990. The role of conditioning and verbal expectancy in the placebo response. Pain 43 (1), 121–128.

Waelti, P., Dickinson, A., Schultz, W., 2001. Dopamine responses comply with basic assumptions of formal learning theory. Nature 412 (6842), 43–48.

Wager, T.D., Rilling, J.K., Smith, E.E., et al., 2004. Placebo-induced changes in fMRI in the anticipation and experience of pain. Science 303 (5661), 1162–1167.

Walach, H., 2001. The effectiveness paradox in complementary medicine. Forsch. Komplementarmed. Klass. Naturheilkd. 8 (4), 193–195.

Walach, H., Jonas, W.B., 2004. Placebo research: the evidence base for harnessing self-healing capacities. J. Altern. Complement. Med. 10 (Suppl.), S109.

Walach, H., Sadaghiani, C., Dehm, C., et al., 2005. The therapeutic effect of clinical trials: understanding placebo response rates in clinical trials – a secondary analysis. BMC Med. Res. Methodol. 5, 26.

Walsh, B.T., Seidman, S.N., Sysko, R., et al., 2002. Placebo response in studies of major depression: variable, substantial, and growing. JAMA 287 (14), 1840–1847.

Watkins, L.R., Mayer, D.J., 1982. Organization of endogenous opiate and nonopiate pain control systems. Science 216 (4551), 1185–1192.

Wickramasekera, I., 1985. A conditioned response model of the placebo effect: predictions from the model. In: White, L., Tursky, B., Schwartz, G.E. (Eds.), Placebo. Theory, research and mechanisms. Guilford Press, New York.

Zubieta, J.K., Bueller, J.A., Jackson, L.R., et al., 2005. Placebo effects mediated by endogenous opioid activity on mu-opioid receptors. J. Neurosci. 25 (34), 7754–7762.

Innovative designs and analyses

17

Mikel Aickin

CHAPTER CONTENTS

INTRODUCTION

Issues of innovative design and analysis present a dilemma for researchers in complementary and alternative medicine (CAM). On the one hand, an enormous amount of experience in biomedical research has led us to a codification of valid designs with their corresponding appropriate analyses. On the other hand, for historical reasons, consensus on these issues has been shaped by a model in which preventive and therapeutic strategies are based on pharmacologic doses of specific chemicals (drugs), or by interventions that are sufficiently similar to drugs, with the intent of producing specific effects. The CAM researcher is then faced with a problem: how to do research that is within the current paradigm, so that it will be accepted as valid, while at the same time capturing the effects of healing methods that are not drugs, do not act like drugs and may not have drug-like specific effects.

The solution that will be offered in this chapter is to go back to the fundamental principles of design and analysis of scientific experiments, irrespective of whether or not they currently enjoy favour among clinical triallists or

DOI: 10.1016/B978-0-443-06956-7.00017-3

epidemiologists. The task is, therefore, to search out designs and analyses that resonate with those special aspects of CAM approaches, while keeping within the bounds of our general philosophy of science.

CONVENTIONAL WISDOM AND NOVEL APPROACHES

One starting place is to consider conventional clinical trial methodology, but to try to see it from a broader perspective. There are several threads here that have been very tightly interwoven into a convincing conventional research paradigm, and so it is challenging to pull each thread back out. But that is what we must do in order to figure out how to fashion CAM-resonant research.

Perhaps the most important thread is the answer to the following question: what is a clinical trial about? Fortunately, it is easy to answer this question. Simply go to any conventional biomedical journal, and look at the tables presenting the results. You will see two things: outcome measures and treatment groups. We can all agree that outcome measures are important. Conventional wisdom says that treatment groups, or the effects of treatments, are the other important component. So, given that outcomes are important, clinical trials are about treatments.

Treatments are very important to the people who promulgate them. If I want to perform treatment *x* on people because it addresses issues of condition *y*, then I would very much like to see clinical trials for *y* in which groups receiving *x* do better than groups receiving something else. So, to a purveyor of a treatment like *x*, conventional clinical trials serve a central purpose. But suppose I am a sufferer of *y*, and I am going to visit a healer who might or might not give me *x*. My interest in *x* is whether it will do better for me than something else. I am not interested in the results of some trial, which probably enrolled many people who are not like me. I want the healer to use his or her expertise, as applied to me, to recommend *x* or not, for me. From my perspective, clinical trials are battles between treatments, where victories and defeats are decided by group-level statistical measures, and where in the end the rewards go to treatments. As a patient, I want the reward to go to me. I wish that clinical trials were about individual patients, but I see they are instead about treatments. This is the first lesson about refocusing on CAM-resonant research: clinical trials should be about people, not just treatments.

The second thread is about what is measured, and when. A paradigm that has been promoted in conventional biomedical research is the 'large, simple trial'. Among the aspects of this approach are two principles; enrol very large numbers of participants, and then measure on each of them the minimum you can get away with to satisfy the aims of the trial. It is perhaps obvious that this strategy follows from the idea that clinical trials are about treatments, not patients. An enormous number of participants is necessary in order to have a decent statistical chance of detecting the miniscule difference between the treatments. The fact that the overlap in outcomes between the two treatment groups may be substantial will be wiped out by the statistical *P*-value that declares the tiny difference between their mean effects to be 'significant'. The organization of the design has everything to do with finding a 'treatment effect', and nothing whatsoever to do with finding any individual effects in any individual patients. The consequence of this strategy is that the amount of information accrued on each patient is designed to be tiny and superficial. The idea is that, by averaging poorly measured results on enormous numbers of people, the winning treatment will be determined, but no one is really interested in the fate of any particular patient. Thus the second lesson about CAM-resonant research is recognition that there needs to be more measurements on each individual, so that participant-level outcomes can be meaningfully included in the report of results.

The third thread involves the question, why should all clinical trials be of the same form, or at least very similar? Given a well-defined research question, reliable measurements that can be made pre- and posttreatment and adequate numbers of participants, the design of a conventional trial is completely prescribed, and its analysis is for the most part quite straightforward. But this describes a programme of research in its mature form. Many – perhaps most – CAM research programmes are inevitably at an earlier stage. After all, it took conventional western biomedical research one or two centuries to go through its development from a primitive and error-prone practical craft to a scientific discipline. Why is it reasonable to expect research on CAM practices to accomplish a similar feat in a few decades, especially when it has become saddled with methods that may not be appropriate?

This leads to the position that most areas of CAM research are currently at an earlier phase in their scientific development than the corresponding areas in conventional biomedical research. This would in turn lead to the notion that most CAM research should employ early-phase research methods, which are substantially different from mature-phase methods. The conception that mature-phase methods are ineluctably appropriate for all biomedical research is perhaps one of the most profound misunderstandings in conventional biomedicine.

Our search for novel CAM research methods might, therefore, be guided by three principles: (1) clinical trials should be about people first, and treatments second; (2) enough measurements should be taken on each person to understand something about that person; and (3) early-phase CAM research should use early-phase research methods. The rest of this chapter is about some places where these ideas might lead us.

EARLY-PHASE RESEARCH: INFERENCE

Research that has an impact on practice generally goes through a sequence of programmatic steps. The first step is to explore aspects of the condition under study, often in conjunction with a pilot study of potential interventions. The purpose of this stage is to learn what to measure, how to measure it and how the condition behaves when untreated or with usual care, if lack of treatment is unethical. It is frequently appropriate not to do any new intervention at this stage, especially when the condition has not been researched before, or the research literature suggests that technical improvement will be necessary before it can be studied well. At some point, however, one will want to try out one or more potential interventions, and here is where the problem of conventional wisdom enters the picture.

When biomedical researchers assess treatments, they invariably compare them with statistical hypothesis tests. The so-called 'null hypothesis' in this case is almost always that two treatments have the same average effect. (There are other types of outcomes than averages, but the issues are the same irrespective of the particular form of the outcome criterion.) One of the numbers that needs to be specified in order to carry out the hypothesis test is the probability of rejecting the null hypothesis when it is true (the 'type I' error). This is an annoying aspect of statistical tests, because there is no objective way to pick the type I error probability. For historical reasons, based on an almost offhand comment by the great statistician RA Fisher, the value 0.05 has been adopted in practice as the standard choice for this probability. This choice determines cutoff points for measures such as the difference between two treatment group means. The second annoyance is that there is another error probability ('type II'), for the error of falsely confirming the null hypothesis when there is in fact some specific difference between the treatment group means. Thus, for every such difference, there is an associated type II error probability, and in effect its value is determined from the amount of variability in the outcomes, the choice of a 0.05 type I error probability and the sample size. The important point is that in most cases the variability in the outcome measurement (along with the choice of 0.05) forces the sample size to be rather large, in order to have a low type II error probability for mean differences that are clinically or practically meaningful. This explains why there is a conventional drive in favour of large trials.

In the small trials that are characteristic of CAM research, this plays out somewhat differently. The sample size is determined by the budget, not by statistical criteria. The resulting probability of type II error is then rather large for the actual mean difference (in the population, not in the sample). This has the consequence that the study has a high probability of being 'negative', which means that the null hypothesis of no treatment difference is confirmed. Thus the typical pattern is that early-phase, small trials will produce an excess of negative studies that prematurely cut off further research on therapies whose true effects (in the population) would be worth realizing.

The solution that I have offered is called the 'separation test' (Aickin 2004). It works for any measurement of treatment effects, not just differences between means. Here are the steps:

1. On the computer output, find the treatment effect estimate (such as the mean difference, or a regression coefficient).
2. Also on the output, find its standard deviation (the SDE). It is usually labelled 'SE' or called 'standard error', or occasionally 'SEM'.
3. Compute $\Delta=1.645 \times \text{SDE}$.
4. If the treatment estimate is in the direction favourable to the treatment and above $\Delta/2$, then recommend further study.
5. If the treatment estimate is in the direction unfavourable to the treatment and below minus $\Delta/2$, recommend against further study.
6. If the treatment estimate lies between $-\Delta/2$ and $\Delta/2$, remain indecisive.

The basis for this modification of conventional procedure is to provide a testing procedure with both type I and type II error probabilities set at about 0.05, without increasing sample size, but instead by changing the null hypothesis to a separation hypothesis. The separation hypothesis tests a treatment effect of $-\Delta/2$ (unfavourable to treatment) against $\Delta/2$ (favourable to treatment), but instead of picking Δ before the study, it is in fact determined by the study data. Thus you need also to look at the value of Δ in order to determine whether the whole approach was reasonable. (Note: this description assumes that 0 is the null hypothesis value for the treatment effect, and that positive values favour the treatment. Also, the value 1.645 comes from the normal distribution, and should often be replaced by values from other distributions, such as a *t* distribution for appropriate degrees of freedom.)

The conventional statistician will complain about this procedure, because it has the effect of increasing the error probabilities, if it were viewed as a null hypothesis test. The whole point is, however, that it is not a null hypothesis test, so interpreting it in that way is a mistake. The null hypothesis test confirms or rejects a null treatment effect. The separation test indicates or contraindicates further research (or it may say nothing).

By using the separation test, the early-phase CAM research literature would contain fewer prematurely negative reports on newly studied approaches. I and a colleague of mine, Elizabeth Sutherland at the National College of Natural Medicine, assembled nearly 100 examples of small (total sample size below 100) CAM early-phase studies in which it would have been appropriate to compare groups using some kind of statistical test. Table 17.1 shows the results for a total of 294 tests.

Over all tests, 112 provided definitive answers using conventional null hypothesis testing, and the separation test would have given exactly the same answers here (this is always true). There were, however, an additional 104 tests in which the separation test made an indication, 51 for and 18 against further research, and the remainder were either unclear or a comparison of two active treatments. Thus, the suggestion from this small study is that the number of continue/discontinue decisions in early-phase CAM research might nearly double by introducing the separation test. Note also the important fact that there were 51 tests in which further research would be recommended by the separation test, but they were indicated against by inappropriate null hypothesis tests. These represent potential losses of valuable CAM approaches.

Table 17.1 ***Results of a literature review of hypothesis tests in complementary and alternative medicine research***

	Qualitative results			
	Positive for treatment	**Negative for treatment**	**Not applicable or not clear**[a]	**Total**
Statistically significant	81	11	20	112
Separation test makes decision	51	18	35	104
No separation test decision	35	17	26	78

[a]Includes cases where treatment/control was not appropriate, such as comparison of two new treatments.

THE CONDITIONAL CHANGE MODEL

There are cases in which the avoidance of a common but weak statistical procedure might be counted as innovative. One of these concerns the ubiquitous pre–post change design. Here all participants contribute baseline measurements at the start of the study, and endpoint measurements at the end of the study, with respect to an outcome variable. The issue is to compare the change scores (post minus pre) in the treated and control groups. By far the most frequent statistical procedure used in these situations is the two-sample *t*-test based on the change scores. This is perhaps because virtually all textbooks recommend this approach.

More than 20 years ago, Ian Plewis (1985) wrote a book in which he gave very clear arguments against this procedure and reasons why one should do something different: see also Frison & Pocock (1992). He proposed to regress change scores on an indicator (a 0/1 variable) of the treated group, and the baseline value. He called this the conditional change model, and clearly it differs from the usual *t*-test only by the inclusion of the baseline values. There are three arguments in favour of Plewis' approach. Firstly, in nearly all cases the SDE of the treatment effect is reduced, making estimation of the treatment effect more precise, or lowering the type II error if one is hypothesis testing. Note that since the separation test is based on the SDE, it will also tend to be favourably affected. Secondly, it tends to adjust for any average imbalance at baseline between the treatment and control groups with respect to the outcome variable. Such imbalances are regularly produced by randomization in small studies. Thirdly, it tends to correct for the regression-to-the-mean phenomenon. This issue relates to the fact that any variable which must remain in some range in order for the organism to remain viable will show a pattern of relatively high values followed shortly by lower values, and relatively low values followed shortly by higher values. This has the statistical effect that changes are negatively related to baseline values. The eugenics movement in early 20th-century Great Britain erroneously interpreted this to be a real biological phenomenon, which would lead to the ultimate dominance of mediocrity in the human species. But in fact it is usually just a numerical result of the existence of a viable range. Since it is so often just an artifact, it seems reasonable to try to remove it from the analysis to the extent possible, and the conditional change models try to do just that.

As a small methodological aside, if one (1) computes the changes, (2) centres the baseline values at their means (just subtract off the mean) and (3) regresses change on treatment indicator and centred baseline, then the intercept term in the regression is the control mean change, and the coefficient of the treatment indicator is the difference between the treated mean change and the control mean change. Thus the intercept, which is often ignored in regression analyses, can be turned into a meaningful parameter.

There is another step that can be taken, in order to feature the results of individual participants. This is to compute adjusted baseline values and adjusted changes, and to use them in tabular, or better, graphical form, in order to show explicitly what happened to individual people in the study. The method for doing this is schematized in Table 17.2. The adjusted baseline values are adjusted for the treatment group, assuring that in the adjusted data

Table 17.2 ***Algorithms for adjusting baseline and change values***	
Adjusting baseline	**Adjusting change**
1. Regress baseline on treatment group indicator 2. Compute fitted values of baseline 3. Compute residuals 4. From the fitted values, subtract the term coefficient × treatment indicator, and add coefficient × average treatment indicator 5. Add residuals to the results of 4. These are the adjusted baselines	1. Regress change on baseline and treatment indicator 2. Compute fitted values of change 3. Compute residuals 4. From the fitted values, subtract the term coefficient × baseline, and add coefficient × average baseline 5. Add residuals to the results of 4. These are the adjusted changes

the groups have the same mean. The change values are adjusted for baseline, removing regression-to-the-mean effects. It is to be emphasized that the adjusted data are to be used for display purposes only, in tables or graphs, but not for analyses. They contain artificially less variability than the original data (an inevitable consequence of adjustment) and would produce specious precision in formal statistical analyses.

TIME-DEPENDENT TREATMENTS

TWO-PERIOD CROSS-OVER

A class of designs that is especially useful for examining individual-level effects, and also for investigating potential mechanisms, involves administering different treatments at different times to the same participant. The simplest of these is the two-period cross-over. Each participant appears in each of two periods, but receives different treatments; the order of the treatments is usually randomized (Figure 17.1).

The point of the design is to compare within all individuals their change while treated, with their change while receiving the control treatment. For half the participants the time order is treated–control and for the other half control–treated, but the comparative measure is always (end treated)–(baseline treated) – ((end control)–(baseline control)), irrespective of the order in which the treatments were received. This gives one outcome for each participant, making it particularly easy to table or graph results.

The cross-over design has both attractive strengths and dangerous weaknesses. The great strength is that it uses each participant as his or her own

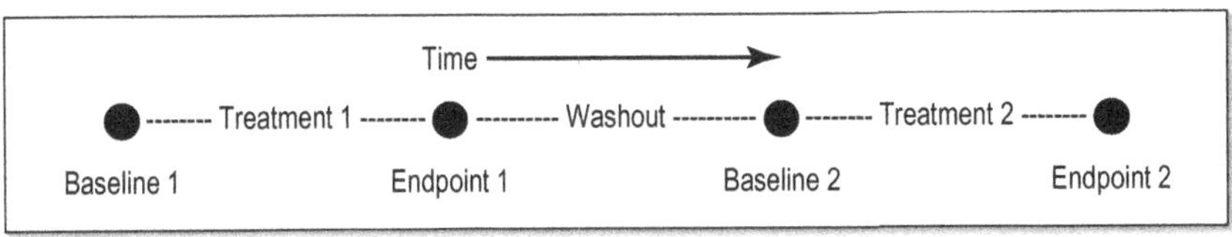

FIGURE 17.1 The two-period cross-over design. Each participant receives one of the treatments, then a washout period with no treatment, and finally the other treatment. Outcomes are measured at the four points indicated by ●.

control. This usually drastically reduces the variability in the outcome comparisons, and thus provides a very desirable statistical benefit. Moreover (and more importantly, as I will argue below) the cross-over design permits a more powerful causal analysis than any other biomedical design.

Most of the weakness comes from the possibility of 'carry-over' effects. To see what this means, refer to Figure 17.1. A participant as shown received 'treatment 1' and then 'treatment 2 following treatment 1', while someone who received them in reverse order would have received 'treatment 2' and then 'treatment 1 following treatment 2'. The analysis implicitly treats 'treatment 1' and 'treatment 1 following treatment 2' as the same, and similarly 'treatment 2' and 'treatment 2 following treatment 1' as the same. But if the presence of a previous treatment influences the effect of the subsequent treatment, then these pairs of treatments are not really the same, and this is called a carry-over effect. Statistically, a carry-over effect appears as an interaction between the treated versus control effect and the order of administration. For many years the conventional statistical procedure was to perform a statistical test for the interaction, and then upon failure to reject, to proceed to the outcome measure given above for each participant. Senn (1994) has pointed out that this is an exceedingly questionable path. Except when the sample size is enormous, the interaction test has low statistical power, which means that the analyst will often be led to the carry-over-free model, when in fact carry-over exists. This means that the analyst will be using the wrong model, which generally has the effect of inducing bias in the effect estimates of interest. Thus, the two-step process (test interaction, then compute participant-level outcome) is biased. The only way out of this offered by Senn is to know that there is no carry-over ahead of time. Clearly this is not very useful advice in early-phase research, but one might take this to mean that an early-phase objective could be to assess whether it is likely that there is carry-over. If not, then the highly efficient cross-over design might be used for subsequent studies, but if so then it should probably be abandoned.

It is worth noting that the length of the washout period may have an influence on whether or not there is carry-over. The term 'washout' comes from drug studies, in which the body is supposed to have metabolized or excreted all of drug 1 before drug 2 is administered. Even in drug studies, however, the disappearance of the drug may not imply the disappearance of its effects, so that the washout period might be long enough technically but not statistically. An example is when the condition is such that once remedied it tends to stay remedied (such as bleeding following trauma). Thus cross-overs, as with other time-dependent designs, tend to be better for chronic conditions without periods of spontaneous remission. Even this may not be enough. If both groups involve doing something that places a burden on the participant, then compliance in the second period may be worse than in the first, a kind of compliance-carry-over effect, which has nothing to do with treatment efficacy and will confound the analysis.

N-OF-1 DESIGNS

Designs for studying individual participants have been in the literature for a considerable time (Aldridge 1991a, b; Johnson & Mills 2004). In some cases they degenerate into a parody of the conventional two-group design. An example is the case in which the participant's time trajectory is divided into intervals, and treatments are assigned at random to each period. In another version the patient receives different treatments in the two halves of each interval, but in random order within the interval. Washout issues are still relevant, which can prolong the study, and it is clear that the response to treatment or control must occur rapidly enough to be seen with the selected interval length. The statistical methods are then evidently almost exactly what they would have been if different participants had been studied in the different intervals. While such designs are patient-focused, by retaining the main feature of a randomized controlled trial (RCT) they lose their relevance to clinical practice, where treatments are generally not assigned at random. Moreover, results on one patient cannot be generalized to the population of patients any more than the results of an RCT can be specialized to an individual patient.

Perhaps the simplest useful N-of-1 design is the one-way cross-over (Brown & Lilford 2006; Brown et al. 2006). In this design, the participant is tracked for a random length of time, then crossed over to treatment and followed to the end of the study. This may be especially relevant in CAM research, since participants often volunteer for such studies because they want the CAM therapy, and with this design everyone gets it at some point. It is important not to be satisfied with simple pre/post measures. Instead the outcome should be measured with some considerable frequency, far more than in traditional RCTs. The reason is that the force of the analysis comes from observing a stabilization during the pretreatment period and then a shift in the outcome trajectory starting at or shortly after the cross-over time. Each participant's data would be analysed separately, estimating parameters capturing the response to treatment, and then the participant-specific parameters could be summarized. It might be possible to make genuine within-person statistical significance tests if the data are dense enough and within-person variability is low enough (Aickin 2003), but this is not an analytic requirement. In the one-way cross-over it will usually be best to report results on the basis of individual participants, usually graphically with some supportive indices or derived summary measures. This design is especially helpful in situations where different therapies will benefit different patients differentially (that is, in most studies). It is also especially indicated for early-phase research.

In general, one can have more elaborate single-participant studies, bringing the science closer to actual clinical practice, but there is a complexity challenge that must be met. The protocol may be difficult to create, since the large number of possible participant trajectories means that one can only specify rules or guidelines rather than strict treatment decisions. One will generally need more sophisticated statistical analyses (Rochon 1990), requiring expert statistical support. Perhaps the most promising direction for these kinds of studies is to make measurements very frequently, and to make measurements on multiple variables at each point. While studies frequently focus on patient outcomes, the decisions and actions of care-givers are also important, because they respond to the patient's past outcomes and have an influence on future outcomes. Thus, part of the protocol should specify how the practitioners will formulate and record what they do. With a rich dataset for each person, dynamic systems analyses can then be applied at the level of the individual participant. These will usually involve regression or regression-like models at each time point, with multiple current outcomes (simultaneous regression) and multiple past explanatory variables. Despite its potential usefulness, there are few examples of these kinds of studies (Collins & Dunn 2005).

STEPPED-CARE MODEL

Like RCTs in general, the cross-over design imposes treatments irrespective of the responses of the participants. Because this activity has virtually no counterpart in clinical medicine, RCTs have been questioned regarding their clinical relevance. Figure 17.2 shows a phase II design that has been employed at the University of Arizona to try to fashion a trial more like the real world.

This trial concerned patients with temporomandibular joint disorder, a debilitating condition involving unprovoked facial pain and reduced joint mobility. The comparison was to be self-care (SC, an enhanced version of usual care), and traditional Chinese medicine (TCM). The clinical model was that a patient would be tried out on SC and kept there so long as his or her pain achieved a low level, but those who did not respond to SC would be referred to TCM. The overall goal was to see whether those who ever got TCM fared no worse than those who stayed in SC. All patients started on SC. At the first division point in Figure 17.2, those who had low enough pain remained on SC, while those not showing enough improvement were randomized to either continuing SC or to TCM. At the second division, this same procedure was repeated, except that everyone referred to TCM stayed there for the remainder of the trial. At the third division, those still not improving enough on SC were automatically referred to TCM.

There were two randomized comparisons of SC and TCM, with short-term outcomes. The fact that some individuals participated in both can be dealt with in the statistical analysis. More importantly, the trial provided the analysis of different trajectories of care, based on the therapeutic response of the patient, just as would be true in actual clinical practice. This allowed the analysis to focus on groups of patients, and ultimately on individual patient histories. An important factor in this (as in all pain studies) is the amount of

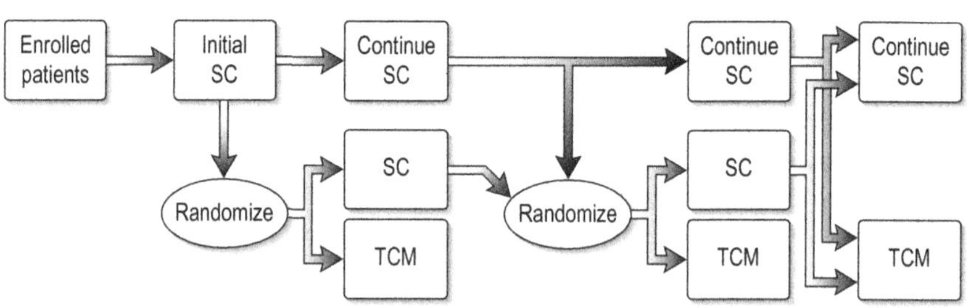

FIGURE 17.2 Stepped-care design: traditional Chinese medicine (TCM) for temporomandibular joint disorder (TMD).
Stage 1: enrolled patients all receive self-care (SC). Those who do well continue; the others are randomized to SC or TCM.
Stage 2: patients doing well on continued SC continue on SC; the others together with all previously randomized SC are randomized to SC or TCM.
Stage 3: SC patients continue if they are doing well; otherwise they receive TCM.
Note: once a patient receives TCM he or she continues with TCM for the remainder of the study.

medication taken by the patient, as it varies over the course of the study, since access to medication was not (indeed, cannot be) controlled. The analytic challenges of a design such as this require some improvisation, but many believe that this is a small price to pay for obtaining information that is actually relevant to clinical practice.

MECHANISM

Perhaps the most promising use of time-dependent treatment designs is for causal analysis in mechanism studies. The idea behind a mechanism study is that a treatment causes a change in a mechanism variable, and then the change in the mechanism variable goes on to cause a change in the outcome. In analysis terms, the mechanism variable acts as a mediator (Aickin 2007). It seems natural to think that evidence in favour of a mechanism would consist of finding participants who showed a change in the mechanism variable and a change in the outcome, as well as participants who showed changes in neither. Those showing either a mechanism change or an outcome change, but not both, would provide evidence against the mechanism. It is clear that one needs to look at individual time trajectories to find the participants in these categories, and this can only occur in a time-dependent treatment design. Mechanism studies are even more valuable when the mechanism is a fundamental causal one, which is prevalent in the patient population, because then it does constitute an argument for generalizing results from a small number of patients to a wider population.

Unaccountably, almost all 'mechanistic' studies carry out two independent analyses in the same study, one looking for mechanistic variable changes in response to treatment, the second looking at outcome responses to treatment, and if both are positive they claim to have evidence for the mechanism. Despite the logical gap in this reasoning, it has been a mainstay in the social sciences for many decades, and it has leaked over into biomedicine, and even into preclinical studies on animals. It is one of the extreme forms of missing the basic question by focusing on groups rather than on individuals.

NOVEL ANALYSES

QUANTILE REGRESSION

Most statistical methods focus on means in groups, or parameters very much like means. An example is linear regression, which relates the mean of an outcome variable to multiple potential explanatory factors, one of which could be a treatment group indicator. This approach inherently focuses on the middle of the distribution of outcomes. In contrast, quantile regression (see Austin et al. (2005) for an example) relates a quantile of an outcome distribution to multiple explanatory factors (which can include treatment group indicators). For example, if one chooses the 80th percentile as the quantile of interest, then quantile regression accounts for the 80th percentile of outcome in terms of explanatory variables. This would be appropriate if one wanted to capture the effect of treatment or other factors on the upper end of the outcome distribution, rather than the middle. For example, in a study to lower blood glucose in participants at risk for diabetes, it would usually be more important to have a treatment impact on those with high values; indeed, one would not expect to be able to lower those whose values were already relatively low. As a special case, one can apply quantile regression to the median (the 50th percentile) if one wants to focus on the centre of the outcome distribution, but without the sensitivity to outliers of ordinary linear regression.

Although quantile regression is still group-oriented, it does focus somewhat on the individual participant through the choice of the quantile to play the role of outcome. There is, of course, no reason why one could not present analyses for a range of quantiles (10%ile, 20%ile ... 90%ile) to give a sense of what part of the outcome distribution is influenced by the explanatory variables.

PARTICIPANT COMPARISONS

An obvious participant-centred analysis would be to compare each treated person with each control person, and then somehow produce a summary measure. I know of only two conventional procedures that do this. First, if one uses the outcome to try to predict treatment group, then the area under the receiver-operator characteristic curve can be interpreted as the probability that the treated person would have a higher value than the control person, if the two were picked at random from their respective groups. Secondly, a simple transformation of the Mann–Whitney U-statistic also equals the above probability.

This leads to the concept of expressing the benefit of treatment as the probability that a treated patient drawn at random would have a better outcome than a control person drawn at random. The estimate of this parameter would be the fraction of such occurrences in the sample. One of the advantages of this measure is that it depends only on how one defines 'had better outcome', which leaves many opportunities. In fact, one can go a step further and allow some comparisons to yield the result that neither patient did better.

In the case where the outcome is either 0 (not better) or 1 (better), this approach can be done quite simply. Let p_1 denote the fraction of 'better' patients in the treatment group, and p_0 denote the corresponding fraction in the control group. Then $p_1(1 - p_0)$ is the sample fraction where the treated patient did better, $p_0(1 - p_1)$ is the fraction where the control did better, and $p_0p_1 + (1 - p_0)(1 - p_1)$ is the fraction where they did the same. The estimates of the variances of these estimates are given in Table 17.3. One would make confidence intervals or do hypothesis tests with these quantities as usual, regarding the estimates as being approximately normally distributed.

DYNAMIC SYSTEMS METHODS

One of the most attractive models for participant-centred analysis looks at each individual participant as a dynamic system. The aim is to measure the right variables on the participant over time, as his/her condition progresses, and especially in relation to the occurrence of intentional interventions or unintended life events. This kind of research is possible when the measurements on the individual can be made frequently relative to the rate of change of their condition.

Table 17.3 *Estimates and their variances for patient comparison probabilities*

Interpretation: probability that...	Estimate	Variance of the estimate
Treated patient does better	$p_1(1-p_0)$	$p_1(1-p_0)\frac{p_0(1-p_1)+n_0(1-p_0)(1-p_1)+n_1p_0p_1}{n_0n_1}$
Control patient does better	$p_0(1-p_1)$	$p_0(1-p_1)\frac{p_1(1-p_0)+n_1(1-p_1)(1-p_0)+n_0p_1p_0}{n_0n_1}$
They do the same	$p_0p_1 +$ $(1-p_0)(1-p_1)$	$\frac{p_0(1-p_0)}{n_0}+\frac{p_1(1-p_1)}{n_1}-4p_0p_1(1-p_0)(1-p_1)\frac{n_0+n_1-1}{n_0n_1}$

n_0, control sample size; n_1, treated sample size; p_0, fraction of controls better; p_1, fraction of treated patients better.

For example, one of the simplest interesting dynamic systems was developed by Rössler (1976), defined by the differential equations for three variables x, y and z as:

$$\frac{dx}{dt} = -y - z$$

$$\frac{dy}{dt} = x + \alpha y$$

$$\frac{dz}{dt} = \beta + z(x - \gamma)$$

The left sides of these equations are the rates at which these variables change. The x, y and z values vary over time, as they satisfy the above equations. The rates of change can be estimated provided that the measurements are made sufficiently frequently, and then estimating the parameters α, β and γ is a simple regression exercise.

The reason that the Roessler system is important is that it exhibits behaviour that seems to mirror what happens with some chronic conditions. The variables carry out periodic cycles which gradually expand in magnitude, until there is a sudden exacerbation – a rapid excursion to a different set of values, which is then quickly extinguished, and the periodic behaviour resumes (Figure 17.3).

There are a number of extensions of the Roessler system. First, one can allow multiple kinds of exacerbations: the Lorenz system is an example (Lorenz 1963). Secondly, given that the analysis is based on regression, one can include (on the right side in the above equations) measures that represent interventions or unintended life events, thus modelling both the internal dynamics of the individual person together with the influences of outside forces. Thirdly, the parameters (α, β, γ in the Roessler system) may themselves change over time. This kind of change is exceedingly important, because it signifies that the internal dynamic process of the person is shifting. An intervention that results in change of parameters has the effect that, when external forces are removed, the

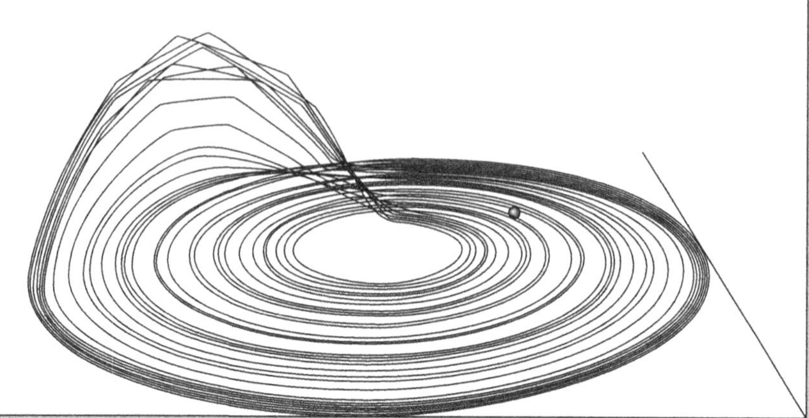

FIGURE 17.3 Trajectory of the Roessler system. The Roessler system involves three variables: here the vertical variable might represent pain. The dot is the current situation of the patient, and the curve traces out the time trajectory the patient has followed up to that point. The patient periodically cycles around the 'floor' in an outward spiral, to be interrupted by upward pain exacerbations that quickly vanish.

individual will show a different pattern of behaviour than he or she had previously. In some ways this can be considered the difference between suppression of symptoms (forcing the x, y, z variables to be different) and cure (changing the parameters so that the natural behaviour of the x, y, z variables is different).

To use a dynamic systems approach, one must make more frequent measurements than is usual in a conventional clinical trial. This problem can, however, be addressed in two steps. In early-phase research the measurements must indeed be frequent, because one wants to plot the trajectories (as in Figure 17.3; Raudenbush 2001), in order to try to understand what kind of model will reflect the underlying system. Once a model is settled on (like the Roessler equations) then much less data is required to estimate the parameters for an individual (α, β and γ in the Roessler system). Intensive measurement is often used in psychophysiology (the electroencephalogram) and cardiology (the electrocardiogram), as well as in neuromuscular disease (the electromyogram). Increasingly, indices that are said to display 'chaos' or 'complexity' are computed from these signals, but instances of parametric modelling remain rare.

One argument against the use of dynamic systems is the considerably increased measurement burden. To a certain extent, however, the magnitude of this burden may have been overestimated, due to a paucity of real-world tests. In psychophysiology, for example, intensive measurement processes appear to be feasible (Fahrenberg & Myrtek 1996), and one suspects that the same is true in other areas in which they are not currently being attempted.

CONCLUSIONS

One of the opportunities that CAM offers to general biomedicine is a re-focus on the patient as the unit of concern in clinical research. Another is the idea that multiple-outcome, whole-systems studies will enrich both our medical science and clinical practice to a greater degree than rigid adherence to a unitary model devised to test drugs. The tension between the RCT and the demands of CAM research can be viewed constructively as an impetus to develop, employ, test and refine novel treatment-oriented designs (Institute of Medicine 2005). The ideas presented in this chapter are on the boundary between what is being done and what could be done. Beyond that, there remain designs we have not thought of, and analyses not yet invented.

In the end, however, we must return to the dilemma that started this chapter. If one conceives of CAM approaches as falling outside the realm of conventional, reductionist, single-cause/single-effect, drug mechanism-oriented biomedical research, then there seem to be powerful arguments for giving serious consideration to novel designs and analyses. On the other hand, we confront significant practical barriers, chief of which may be the desire to attract research funding and publish results that promote one's career (Kuhn 1996). The centripetal force of convention is not to be underestimated, nor are the penalties that Kuhn's 'normal science' imposes on those who prematurely advocate a 'paradigm shift'. Just as there is a tension between research focused on individual patients and research expressed in terms of group averages, it is also true that the CAM researcher needs to weigh the personal necessity of professional survival against the societal need for occasional spurts of progress due to innovation.

REFERENCES

Aickin, M., 2003. Participant-centered analysis in complementary and alternative medicine comparative trials. J. Altern. Complement. Med. 9 (6), 949–957.

Aickin, M., 2004. Separation tests for early-phase CAM research. Evidence-Based Integrative Medicine 1 (4), 225–231.

Aickin, M., 2007. Conceptualization and analysis of mechanistic studies. J. Altern. Complement. Med. 13 (1), 151–158.

Aldridge, D., 1991a. Single-case research designs for the clinician. J. R. Soc. Med. 84 (5), 249–252.

Aldridge, D., 1991b. Single-case research designs: an extended bibliography. Comp. Med. Res. 5 (2), 99–109.

Austin, P.C., Tu, J.V., Daly, P.A., et al., 2005. The use of quantile regression in health care research: a case study examining gender differences in the timeliness of thrombolytic therapy. Stat. Med. 24, 791–816.

Brown, C.A., Lilford, R.J., 2006. The stepped wedge trial design: a systematic review. BMC Med. Res. Methodol. 6, 54.

Brown, C.H., Wyman, P.A., Guo, J., et al., 2006. Dynamic wait-listed designs for randomized trials: new designs for prevention of youth suicide. Clin. Trials 3, 259–271.

Collins, M.P., Dunn, L.F., 2005. The effects of meditation and visual imagery on an immune system disorder: dermatomyositis. J. Altern. Complement. Med. 11 (2), 275–284.

Fahrenberg, J., Myrtek, M. (Eds.), 1996. Ambulatory Assessment. Computer-Assisted Psychological and Psychophysiological Methods in Monitoring and Field Studies. Hogrefe & Huber, Seattle.

Frison, L., Pocock, S.J., 1992. Repeated measures in clinical trials: analysis using mean summary statistics and its implications for designs. Stat. Med. 11, 1685–1704 (comment: Senn, S., 1994. Stat. Med. 13, 197–198).

Institute of Medicine, 2005. Complementary and Alternative Medicine (CAM) in the United States. National Academies Press, Washington DC (Chapter 4).

Johnson, B.C., Mills, E., 2004. n-of-1 randomized controlled trials: an opportunity for complementary and alternative medicine evaluation. J. Altern. Complement. Med. 10 (6), 979–984.

Kuhn, T.S., 1996. The Structure of Scientific Revolutions. third ed. University of Chicago Press, Chicago.

Lorenz, E.N., 1963. Deterministic nonperiodic flow. J. Atmos. Sci. 20, 130–141.

Plewis, I., 1985. Analysing Change: Measurement and Explanation using Longitudinal Data. John Wiley, Chichester UK.

Raudenbush, S.W., 2001. Comparing personal trajectories and drawing causal inferences from longitudinal data. Annu. Rev. Psychol. 52, 501–525.

Rochon, J., 1990. A statistical model for the N-of-1 Study. J. Clin. Epidemiol. 43 (5), 499–508.

Rössler, O.E., 1976. An equation for continuous chaos. Physics Letters 57A, 397–398.

Senn, S., 1994. The AB/BA cross-over: past, present and future? Stat. Methods Med. Res. 3 (4), 303–324.

Questionnaires – development, validation, usage

18

Harald Walach • Niko Kohls • Corina Güthlin

CHAPTER CONTENTS

CONCEPTUAL FOUNDATIONS

THE PROBLEM OF MEASUREMENT

Measurement tries to solve the problem of how to convert something that is basically a quality into a quantity that can be treated numerically, so that its size or type may be expressed in figures which can be compared and gauged. Some things, length for example, are straightforward. With an established gauge length – a foot, a yard, a metre –consistent measurement can begin and, most importantly from a practical point of view, can be compared. But what

DOI: 10.1016/B978-0-443-06956-7.00018-5

about more elusive, intangible constructs, such as happiness, quality of life, 'unstuckness', mindfulness? Let us introduce a couple of relevant distinctions and definitions here.

DESCRIPTION VERSUS MEASUREMENT – SURVEYS AND MEASUREMENT INSTRUMENTS

A basic distinction is the one between description and measurement. Sometimes we only want to describe things: what people think of a medical service, whether or not they find the refurbishment of the clinic appealing. We use survey instruments to do this. When we are interested in surface layers of reality, we observe and describe. When we want to know about a deeper structure and quantify it, then we are entering the domain of measurement. Let us use an example from politics to make this distinction clear: we can ask people about their political opinion. Should the USA bomb Iran? Should Israel be allowed to kill the residents in Gaza and flatten the land to build factories in order to protect its citizens? Should money be abolished? Should everyone just get the same amount of money from the government, whether they work or not? If you collect answers to these sorts of question, you will get a pattern of 'yes', 'undecided', 'no' answers that describe proportions of the people you have surveyed who hold this particular opinion. You could also assume that there are certain political traits that hang together, for instance 'right-wing radicalism', or 'leftist state interventionism'. Then you could view the first two types of questions as illustrating 'right-wing radicalism', the last two as illustrating 'leftist state interventionism'. Your questions are then tokens of a supposed underlying trait or construct. How do we identify this? By combining our historical knowledge of political movements, current theory and certain empirical patterns which we observe in certain leaders and people who we take to be the embodiment of one or the other, we derive the deeper structures of 'right-wing radicalism' and 'leftist state interventionism'. We would even be able to predict similar views, belonging to this set, likely to be held by this type of person. We would then use the tokens of type that hang together to measure the underlying construct. The difference, then, between surveying and measuring is that in the first instance we just describe something; in the second we are using the descriptors to derive information about a more complex, intangible construct from them. So how exactly do we do this?

ISOMORPHIC AND HOMOMORPHIC RELATIONSHIPS

In the case of measuring length, things are simple. Length has one clear attribute; the extensiveness of a certain object, the distance from end to end. Hence we only need to apply one measurement process to capture this parameter. Such relationships between measurement and the measured object are called isomorphic, from the Greek *isos*, same, and *morphe*, figure. However, it is immediately obvious that things like 'right-wing radicalism' are, unlike length, not directly measurable, and additionally far more complex. There are many viewpoints that may be applied to it. Hence, all relationships between descriptors, statements that describe it and the construct itself, can only be more or less similar. This is, then, called a 'homomorphic' description or relationship, stemming from Greek *homoios*, similar, and, again, *morphe*, figure. The more complex a construct is, as a rule, the more descriptions we will have to use in order to capture the facets of its complexity. However, as we can only take a reasonable and practicable amount of criteria into account in the measuring process, we will probably be able to capture only a limited number of facets. For this reason, most instruments are multi-item instruments. They want to capture a complex construct with several homomorphic descriptions, called 'items', hoping that they then reflect the construct more or less completely.

SCALING

Once we have tokens of our construct, the items we take to be descriptions of it, we need to convert answers into numbers to measure it. The easiest way is to formulate statements or questions with which people can simply agree or disagree. Statements like 'Iran should be bombed' can really only be agreed or disagreed with, perhaps with an 'undecided' category. You cannot bomb a country 'just a little', or 'quite a lot'. It is obvious, in this case, that in order to measure the construct 'right-wing radicalism' you would have to use a series of such statements, with the number of times someone has agreed with them then being counted. If you include some very radical statements to which only very few people would agree, for example, 'Iran should be nuked', 'Everyone who falls into debt should be put into prison for as many years as he owes in thousands of dollars' or 'People who have lost their jobs should be put into labour camps', then you have an implicit scaling, as it is likely that only the most radical will agree with such statements. The likelihood of the trait being possessed by one who agrees with a radical statement is called the 'difficulty' of the item (see Box 18.1, below). In that sense, the latter two examples are clearly more 'difficult' to answer, even for right-wing radicalists, than the first one (unless, of course, they are actually Iranian!).

In this type of scaling we devise a series of statements that have to be either agreed or disagreed with. They then translate into '1' and '0'. If we add them up we get a score that expresses the degree to which a respondent possesses a certain trait or is an exemplar of a certain construct. Such a procedure is often used when a large number of comparatively clear items can be devised. The benefit of such an approach is that people are forced to make decisions (this is why it is sometimes referred to as forced-choice technique), and each positive answer can be interpreted as one step towards a full, exhaustive description of the construct.

However, often this is not straightforward. Some responses defy a clear format and there are degrees to which someone would assent. To establish someone's satisfaction with the medical services he or she has received during an inpatient stay, you would have to break that experience down into certain aspects: administration, patient care, medical care and services, paramedical services, food and housing. While patients might, for example, be happy with the food most of the time, they might not have always been happy with the patient service or vice versa. Forcing the respondent to decide either 'yes' or 'no' runs the risk of leaving an item unanswered because your respondent finds the answer format inadequate, or the answer is not precise. Likewise,

BOX 18.1 The methodological framework of psychometric testing: classical test theory versus item response theory

The body of psychometric theory can be divided into two prevailing theories: classical test theory (CTT: Magnusson 1967) and item response theory (IRT: Mokken 1971) (for a more extensive treatment, see Rao (2007)).

Classical test theory (Magnusson 1967)

CTT was influenced by the measurement theory in physics. CTT assumes that an individual's measured score is comprised of the true score (one which could be obtained by an impeccable measurement procedure) and a random measurement error component (occurring as a consequence of an imperfect, blurred measurement procedure that has to utilize a finite number of items). It is generally assumed that the measurement error is uncorrelated with the true score and that it has a mean value of zero. The criterion for reliability of a specific test item is assessed by the amount of variance that can be explained in the total variance in the true scores of the factor it is supposed to contribute to. Cronbach's alpha is a parameter commonly used to predict the reliability or internal consistency of a given scale with regard to assessing the underlying factor (see also reliability).

Item response theory (Mokken 1971)

Since the 1970s IRT has gradually become more popular, and has superseded CTT in several areas of research, such as IQ testing. In contrast to CTT, IRT does not assume that the true score of the item is an absolute characteristic of the test, but, rather, dependent on the context. Correspondingly, the latent ability of a subject to answer an item correctly is considered to be independent of the test. For example, if you ask both a 5-year-old child and a professor of physics whether or not objects have a tendency to fall to the ground, you will probably get similar answers. However, if you invite them to explain the underlying principles of the natural law of gravity, it is probable that only the professor would be able to address this question properly. This example shows that if subjects with different latent ability or knowledge levels are being asked simple or more difficult questions, this will inevitably lead to different results in test scores. In a nutshell, this is the argument brought forward by IRT against CTT. Thus IRT tries to gauge the item difficulty of every item, describing the relationship between the probability of answering an item and the latent ability of the individual.

A pragmatic framework for measurement instruments

Although IRT was developed out of dissatisfaction with several aspects of CTT, it has also taken over distinct assumptions of CCT: To give an example, most proponents of IRT would not dispute the existence of random error in the measurement process. Additionally, in practical terms, IRT assumes unidimensionality. Viewing CTT and IRT as opposing theories is not accurate. These days, aspects of both theories are used together in a pragmatic framework that applies characteristics both of CTT (reliability, Cronbach's alpha) and IRT (item difficulty).

depending on how the question is stated, they may answer the whole question about quality of food in the negative in response to one bad meal. Allowing people to scale these answers themselves captures their degree of agreement: 'never', 'rarely', 'sometimes', 'most of the time', 'always'. By then translating the answers into figures – such as 0, 1, 2, 3, 4 – a scaled answer to each item may be obtained. These can then be added up across all the items tapping into the same dimension, producing a quantitative score. These types of psychometric scales, which are most commonly used for questionnaire research, are know as Likert scales. Depending on the question and the construct, the most frequently used scale dimensions are three-point, five-point or seven-point scales. In the case of odd-number scaling, the respondents are offered a middle ground that usually represents a realm of indecisiveness. Sometimes we want to avoid this and want to force people at least to nudge towards one direction or another. Then even-numbered options can be used, such as a four-point, six-point or even eight-point scale. In practice, though, four- or five-point scales are most widely used, although scales with more options seem to be preferable and give more reliable results (Preston & Colman 2000). This is related to the fact that the capability of respondents and descriptors to differentiate dwindles as more scaling categories are applied. For instance, if you scale with a time frequency descriptor ('never' to 'always'; see above), it is difficult to see how you could convincingly elicit a more fine-grained description. One option is to introduce figures, anchoring only the end points, and leaving it to the respondent to estimate the position on the scale. As you move towards a finer-grained numerical scale, say a 10-point scale, verbal description of the options becomes next to impossible.

Sometimes, however, especially if there are only very few items and a reasonable differentiation is desired, it may make sense to go for the finest-grained measurement possible: a visual analogue scale (Zealley & Aitken 1969; Melzack 1983; Champion et al. 1998). This is a scale that shows the respondent a straight line of defined length which is only anchored at both ends. This is often, but not exclusively, used for pain measurement. Thus the anchors to the question 'How is your pain today?' could read from 'no pain at all' to 'as bad as it could possibly be', with a 10-cm line in between. 10 cm is not essential, but is a handy format. The point where the line is crossed is measured, usually from the left, and expressed in millimetres. Care should be taken to take the cultural convention into account: for example, most languages are read from left to right, with the natural reading and gauging process also running from left to right. However some languages, like Hebrew or Arabic, are written from right to left, with a corresponding change in process, and some vertically. Visual analogue scale design would have to respect such conventions.

DIMENSIONALITY

Often constructs are not simple, and some research and thinking is necessary to find out how a construct might be structured. Let's use our example of 'satisfaction with medical services in an inpatient setting'. As is immediately obvious, from preparation to treatment, we have many different interlinking services which are part of the whole package of care. Some might be excellent, such as the treatment facilities and the skill of the specialist surgeons; some might be bad, such as food or the efficiency of the administration. In order to get a differentiated picture we need to take the construct apart and parcel it out into several dimensions. This can be done conceptually. Sometimes, however, we don't know which dimensions are involved. In such a case we operate empirically: we devise a long list of potential indicators or items, give them to a large number of respondents and analyse the underlying patterns.

The standard way of doing this is exploratory factor analysis. There are three major approaches: (1) principal component analysis; (2) principal axis factor analysis; and (3) maxiumum likelihood factor analysis (Loehlin 1998; Fabrigar et al. 1999). (There are some conceptual differences and different ways of calculation, which we won't cover; for more details, also regarding other approaches, see Fabrigar et al. 1999.) Exploratory factor analysis is a method of exploring data and understanding the underlying structure better. Once such a structure is found, it can be tested with a method that fits a model according to the postulated structure and tests the model fit, so-called confirmatory factor analysis. A good description can be found in Loehlin (1998)].

Exploratory factor analysis takes the covariance or correlation matrix of all items, and asks the simple question: how many underlying components or dimensions can account for this pattern of correlations most satisfactorily? Statistically this problem is solved by laying variates, variables that collect the variance of multiple variables, into the correlation pattern, such that variance of the items captured by these variates becomes maximal; or, geometrically speaking, that the distance between the variate and the data points representing the single measurements becomes minimal.

This is a stepwise, exploratory process. The following questions and steps have to be taken into account, and sometimes revisited in the same sequence, if the first solution is not satisfactory:

How many dimensions?

Normally, a given covariance matrix can be reduced to varying numbers of dimensions. How many, depends on statistical and conceptual decisions. Statistically, only factors with eigenvalues greater than 1 (Kaiser Guttman criterion) are sensible, since they collect the variance of more than one item, and this is the idea of a reduction of items to dimensions, after all. But often, if all factors that have an eigenvalue greater than 1 are extracted, one has too many factors, and when looking at them finds they are difficult to interpret. Hence normally one chooses somewhat fewer factors for extraction. A useful tool is the scree plot. This is a graphical plot of the distribution of the eigenvalues of all possible factors, starting with the one with the highest eigenvalue. The plot normally looks like a mountain, and at some point the curve breaks and tapers out more smoothly, like in a scree at the foot of the mountain. This point, where the smoothness of the curve breaks, can be used as a break-off point for the choice of dimensions. A rule of thumb is that the Kaiser–Guttman criterion extracts too many, and the scree plot procedure often too few factors. Therefore, it is important to inspect the outcome carefully, and revisit the procedure, if the result is not readily interpretable.

Another alternative for determining the number of factors which has become more and more popular among researchers is parallel analysis (Hayton et al. 2004). Parallel analysis is a procedure that, after specifying variables and cases, estimates an average distribution of random eigenvalues based on a reiterative estimation process that is subsequently compared to the empirically observed distribution. The intersection of calculated and estimated distribution marks the cut-off point for the factors to be retained.

Correlated or uncorrelated factors?

Are the dimensions independent or not? This is a difficult question. For instance, would one determine the quality of administrative services in an inpatient treatment completely independently of the quality of food, or medical services? Standard factor extraction procedures normally make the assumption that the dimensions that are extracted are independent or uncorrelated, and technically orthogonal (i.e. geometrically they form a cartesian coordinate system with 90° angles in between). Personality theory, the home ground of factor analysis, operates on the assumption of independent dimensions of personality; hence many researchers implicitly use these procedures for other problems as well. However, orthogonality in a euclidean sense is a very limiting constraint that is rarely found in natural settings and most dimensions in health-related situations are correspondingly more or less correlated. The answer to the question, whether dimensions may be heuristically treated as correlated or not, determines the method of factor extraction: orthogonal (uncorrelated factors) or oblique (correlated factors). Oblique rotation produces a primary factor and a given number of correlated secondary factors, and the result is usually more difficult to interpret. Orthogonal rotation produces the stipulated number of theoretically independent factors, although in reality they are mostly correlated nevertheless. For practical purposes, it is important to inspect the outcome of each method and decide which procedure is not only statistically better, but also yields results that can be readily interpreted.

Factor rotation

After deciding on the number of factors to extract, the stipulated number of factors is 'rotated' in the virtual space of the covariance matrix. In the simple case of two factors one can envisage this process as laying an orthogonal coordinate system into the matrix and then turning it round to a point where the distance of the data points to the vectors becomes minimal. In the case of more factors it is a higher dimensional process, but essentially the same. There are several ways in which this can be done. The most popular orthogonal rotation is the so-called varimax – rotation which maximizes the variance between the factors. It starts with one axis, where the variance of most items is collected, and then adds the other dimensions. Hence it always tends to produce one strong common factor (correspondingly care should be taken that a methodological artefact is not interpreted as an empirical finding). If, for conceptual reasons, this is not warranted, a different rotation procedure could be tried. Practically, one often starts with this simplest method, inspects the result, and if not satisfied, moves to more complex procedures of rotation. If those do not work well either, one starts at step one, extracting more or less factors.

What does it mean?

The decisive point is: can we make sense of the results? The outcome of this procedure is a matrix of so-called factor loadings of each item on each of the factors. Factor loadings can be interpreted as correlations of an item with a factor. High loadings mean that an item is very characteristic of a dimension, and most of the times also mean that cross-loadings on other factors are low. As items become less characteristic for a dimension their loadings are lower, and cross-loadings on other factors increase. Ideally, each item should load only on one factor strongly, and loadings between 0.9 and 0.35 are normally considered sufficient. If too many items load on more than one factor, the factor structure is not well chosen and the process needs to be repeated. Sometimes, one might also drop an item, even though it might be psychometrically sound, because it cannot be easily attributed to one factor only.

If the first solution is not satisfactory, the procedure will need to be repeated, perhaps with either a different number of factors, or a different rotation method, until the factor solution is not only statistically sound, but also makes sense from a conceptual point of view. If the analysis has produced a good set of factors, it is normally easy to find a name for the factor from the items that load on it. If this is not possible, something is wrong.

PRACTICAL SOLUTIONS

There are two major criteria for good measurement instruments: they should be valid and they should be reliable. By validity we mean that an instrument should measure what it says it does. Reliability means that an instrument measures whatever it is supposed to measure well enough. An intelligence test should really measure intelligence, and not verbal fluency; a quality-of-life questionnaire should really measure quality of life, and not, say, resignation to one's fate. Validity has several aspects. One of the most important but sometimes neglected aspects concerning validity is content validity.

FINDING GOOD INDICATORS – CONTENT VALIDITY

This is guaranteed by a solid conceptual basis and by a good set of indicators, based on qualitative research and a sound theoretical basis. How do we identify good descriptors for a construct that we want to measure? The answer to this question depends on how well we know the construct already. Health-related quality of life, for instance, was a comparatively new construct in the 1980s (Guyatt et al. 1986; Staquet et al. 1998). A lot of conceptual work was carried out, experts and patients were questioned and huge item pools were developed. Normally this stage of development, which can be quite time-consuming, is based on a mix of formal or informal qualitative research, literature research, conceptual work and analysis. Our group, for instance, was one of the first to develop a questionnaire of mindfulness (Buchheld et al. 2001; Walach et al. 2006). At the time no appropriate questionnaires existed, and we were interested in measuring it. A graduate student scanned the Buddhist literature on the meaning of mindfulness and produced a long list of potential descriptions and applications. From these she developed a set of items which she then presented to experts in the field. These experts had to decide whether or not these descriptions were good and valid, with the option of improving them. This yielded the first set of items, which was then further investigated empirically. In this example, the construct is well known from a 2500-year-old tradition of Buddhist meditation practice, and the task was to translate this knowledge into a workable, contemporary questionnaire instrument.

At other times, the construct may be hypothetical or quite new, such as 'satisfaction with medical services' or 'meaning of illness'. In that case, it may be necessary first to launch a good qualitative study. This could comprise focus groups with patients and personnel of the hospital. Such qualitative research (see Chapter 2) normally identifies major themes and subthemes, with typical sentences of respondents illustrating such topics. One can then either use typical patient statements, derived from interviews, or use the interview material to devise such statements. Sometimes descriptors will be developed from the top down, stemming from a certain theoretical model. Aaron Antonovsky (1987), for example, developed his theory of salutogenesis over decades of research on how stress does or does not have an impact on people. From this he developed his theory, and from his theory he developed items which he viewed as descriptive of the construct 'sense of coherence' and its subdimensions (Antonovsky 1993). As it turned out, he was only partially right, as the threefold subdimensionality of the construct assumed by Antonovsky could only be partially empirically corroborated. In practice, a mix of a purely bottom-up, empirical approach and a purely top-down theoretical approach is most frequently used.

In fact, whether or not the development of a questionnaire was diligent enough, i.e. its content validity, often decides the overall quality of the instrument. Frequently researchers employ a quick-and-dirty method without scrutinizing the background appropriately. They may take things they find in the literature for granted, or build on previously aborted attempts using existing item pools, or they may not go into the depths of a fully fledged qualitative and conceptual analysis. If the foundation is weak, no amount of empirical work and amassing of data will help at later stages. It is not rare to come across widely used instruments that are not diligently constructed. A typical example is the Medical Outcomes Study (MOS) Short Form (SF) 36, a questionnaire that is widely used for assessing health-related quality of life. Its original item pool was not developed from scratch, but came from a huge database of items from different types of questionnaires measuring varying aspects of illness.

CONSTRUCT VALIDITY

Another type of validity is construct validity. It means that the construct can be empirically differentiated from other similar constructs. Sense of coherence, the construct derived from Antonovsky's theory of salutogenesis, for instance, normally has high negative correlations with different types of depression instruments. So is sense of coherence just an inverse form of depression? Yes and no. Yes, if you adopt correlation measures that show a large construct overlap. No, if you adopt the different conceptual basis. If you consider a correlation of $r = 0.70$ high, which most people do, then you would have to consider that such a correlation describes only 50% common variance between the variables. (The correlation coefficient squared gives us the amount of common variance, and 0.70 squared is 0.49 which, as a percentage, is roughly 50%.) Thus, if sense of coherence and depression are correlated by $r = 0.70$, which empirically is often the case, then we are referring to about 50% overlap. Is that a little or a lot? Is the glass half full or half empty? It's difficult to say. It certainly is a lot, but it is not a complete overlap. In that sense, if we analyse construct validity by correlating new constructs with previously well-known ones, we want to know whether or not there is some overlap with constructs that are similar. Thus we expect at least moderately significant correlations in the range of $r = 0.30$–0.50 if we want to focus on the difference between constructs. This is called 'divergent construct validity'. However, it would be strange if a questionnaire of stress resilience and sense of coherence did not somehow correlate with depression, or a quality-of-life questionnaire with indicators of symptom severity. This is frequently referred to as the convergent aspect of construct validity. Nevertheless if the correlation is near exhaustive ($r > 0.80$), then we would determine that the new construct is in fact not new, but only a new version of a previously existing one.

RELIABILITY

Reliability tells us whether or not the questionnaire measures well enough whatever it is supposed to measure. Reliability is only concerned with the internal properties of an instrument, its statistical coefficients and its quantitative behaviour. It is possible to have a questionnaire which has a near-perfect reliability but is useless, because its validity has never been established, and vice versa. Some instruments may be highly valid but we cannot establish their reliability. This is the case, for instance, for direct measurements through single items or analogue scales. The pain visual analogue scale, for instance, is perfectly valid. For what else other than pain could be measured if you ask a patient: 'How bad is your pain today'? But we will never be able to establish it as a reliable measurement because we do not have the statistical means of testing it. In fact, for formal reasons which we will not go into here, the validity of a test is constrained by its reliability, and vice versa.

Reliability is determined statistically and normally expressed as the average correlation of all items with each other (Box 18.1). The result is a correlation coefficient which is called Cronbach's alpha, and, like a correlation coefficient, it tells us how well the combined items are related to the construct, or how much variance of the construct is being uncovered by the items (by squaring the coefficient). Very good reliability coefficients range around alpha = 0.90 (our long version mindfulness scale, for instance, has an alpha = 0.92). If you square 0.90, you reach an amount of explained variance of 81%, which is quite good, the rest being error variance. The reliability of an instrument is the function of each item's correlation with the total scale, and of the number of items.

Naturally, if you have many indicators of a construct you would expect a more reliable measurement. In our hospital satisfaction example, if you only ask about the quality of the food in general, you have a very crude indicator. But you could ask about the quality of each part, such as soup, main menu, dessert, drinks, coffee, snacks, provision of fresh fruit and vegetables; and also about the state it reaches patients in, whether cold or hot, nicely arranged, whether the range of choices was adequate, and so forth. Remember that classical test theory assumes that the more items there are in a scale, the more reliable the scale will be. However, at a certain point, the amount of items becomes less important to the reliability of a scale than the quality of the items. Hence the challenge is to achieve a substantial reliability with as few items as necessary. Practically, very reliable scales can be diluted down quite a bit before reliability fades. In the example of our mindfulness scale we have developed a 14-item version out of the original very reliable 30-item version, still achieving a reliability of roughly alpha = 0.79, depending on how large and homogeneous the sample is. For research purposes it might even be diluted down to an eight-item version (Kohls et al. 2009). As a rule of thumb, one would normally expect the lower bound of a reasonably reliable instrument to have an alpha > 0.70.

Two other common ways to document reliability are test–retest reliability and split-half reliability.

Test–retest reliability

Test–retest reliability measures a correlation between the scores of a person who has been measured twice with the same instrument. It gives us information about how stable over time the construct being measured is. Depending on whether we are measuring something that we conceive to be a trait, i.e. a construct that is comparatively stable across time, such as intelligence; or a state, such as alertness, we would have to use different time windows for the testing of retest reliability. In the former we might wait for several months to a year, in the latter for hours. Sometimes differences in test–retest reliability can be as important as differences in means. For example, we found in a comparison of two sociodemographically balanced samples of spiritually practising and non-practising individuals that the latter had significantly higher 6-month test–retest reliability in psychological distress. This could be a hint that individuals with regular introspective training perceive distress as a state rather than a trait (Kohls & Walach 2008). In any case, the example shows that the context should be taken into account when interpreting questionnaire scores.

Split-half-reliability

Another way of measuring reliability is to construct a test that has many items, split it in half by randomly allocating items to one of the two forms, give both forms to the same people, and then correlate the two results. If the two test results are highly intercorrelated, identical difficulty can be assumed for both subtests and correspondingly the tests may be used as a substitute for each other. The benefit of this procedure, although rarely done, is that we have two similar but not identical versions of the same test, for instance if we plan to do several follow-ups. This so-called split-half reliability can also be calculated by computer programs by statistically splitting the test, provided the number of items is large enough, i.e. at least eight per construct.

Reliability can be enhanced by dropping items that have unfavourable statistical properties. This is normally done at an early stage of development. Two important statistical parameters here are how well items separate, and how homogeneously they measure the construct. The latter parameter is normally described as the correlation the item has with all other items relevant to the subscale or the whole test, r_{it}, which we want to be reasonably high (normally an item to total scale correlation above $r_{it} = 0.30$ is considered sufficient), but also not so high as to be perfectly correlated, else the item would be redundant with other items. So normally a good item homogeneity should, as a rule of thumb, be between $r_{it} = 0.3$ and $r_{it} = 0.6$.

Another important parameter is the difficulty index (Box 18.1, item response theory). It tells us how many people who in general have endorsed a construct have actually answered an item the same way. Ideally we want to have items that are neither too easy, so that everyone having only a trace of this construct answers it positively, nor too difficult so that hardly anyone would support it. The difficulty of an item is defined as the percentage of respondents answering this item positively in relation to the percentage of respondents being positive on the whole construct. Although the probability of answering an item correctly may be dependent on the population tested, the item difficulty is usually considered to be appropriate between the range of 0.6 and 0.8. This is because items that are too easy are hardly worth including, and those that are too difficult normally don't contribute to the measurement. However, in some cases one might want to include very easy or very difficult items; for instance, if one wants to provide some separability at the ends of a spectrum such as developing a special intelligence test for prodigies.

This is related to floor and ceiling effects. If almost anybody measured is hovering around the lower potential scores of a test, the test cannot clearly differentiate between those who are really low and those who are slightly higher. This can also happen if a well-developed test is given to the wrong population. For instance, if you administer a test that has been validated in severely disabled chronic patients to measure health-related quality of life to comparatively healthy patients almost everyone will have a very high quality of life.

MEASURING CHANGE

This raises the problem of measuring change. Change measurements are, by default, confounded. Our measurement instruments are not perfect. Retest reliabilities are rarely higher than $r_{tt} = 0.70$, and are very often less. That means that if a construct in question is considered stable over time, the error variance, when using the test later again, increases. The tendency is for people with an initial low score subsequently to score higher, and for those with initial high scores to have rather lower scores. This so-called regression to the mean will always confound measurements of the same construct when repeated after a certain time (Ostermann et al. 2008). Normally this regression to the mean mimics an improvement where no improvement has happened. Depending on the initial status of the sample, it may also exaggerate measured improvements, or may help to dampen measured improvements. Several procedures have been proposed to take this into account, for instance by factoring the retest reliability of the measurements into the equation (Jacobson & Truax 1991; Speer 1992).

Apart from this generic problem that befalls all measurement instruments, the problem of sensitivity to change exists. Not all measurement instruments can document change. On the other hand, in clinical settings we are often only interested in change. Hence we want questionnaires that can document this change. This can be tested by comparing change scores of groups that have received an intervention of proven or likely efficacy with those who have not received it, or by using a bona fide intervention and calculating whether the scores before and after the intervention are not only significantly different, but also of a magnitude worth reporting. In practice this is often done by comparing how well a newly established instrument is doing in comparison with standard measures of change in an intervention programme where change has already been shown to happen.

GAUGING

To be meaningful, any observation needs a comparison standard. With questionnaires, we can use a particular sample at a previous time, the data of the original sample or samples of particular patient groups as comparison standards. Really well-developed questionnaires, however, have normative or gauge data that stem from a representative population sample. This is then often used to define clinical cut-offs. For instance, the Centre of the Epidemiologic Study of Depression Scale that measures depression has been studied in various countries and normative data are available, allowing us to define, what score the 'normal, healthy' adult should have (Radloff 1977). It turns out that the average score in the US population US is 9 (Radloff 1977) and in Germany 16 (Hautzinger & Bailer 1993), one standard deviation higher than in the USA, which is a cut-off for depression in the USA (Andresen et al. 1994). Individuals who score average on depression in Germany would thus be diagnosed as depressed in the USA. Thus normative data are not always comparable between countries and cultures, but are useful to make comparisons within one's own culture.

PRACTICAL ISSUES

AVOID REINVENTING WHEELS, BUT ALSO AVOID DRIVING WITH SQUARED WHEELS

Although a plethora of already validated questionnaires exists, there is rarely, alas, a central register. Hence it is always necessary to do good background research before setting out to develop a questionnaire, not only in the published literature, but also in the grey literature – book chapters, dissertations, conference abstracts. For it is here that we find the first indications of work in progress.

Often we find similar instruments, but not one that measures a particular aspect we are interested in. For instance, we also developed a scale to measure exceptional human experiences (Kohls & Walach 2006). Although there were a lot of existing scales that tapped into religious, spiritual or paranormal experiences, there were none that tapped into all those facets. So we decided to construct a new scale. Such a decision should not be taken lightly, as the development of a good scale goes through several cycles of constructions and revisions before it is ready to use, and we are easily talking about one to several years of development work.

Often, foreign-language scales are available, but come out of quite a different cultural context. This will increasingly be the case for countries in Asia and in Africa, where different cultural conditions prevail. It would be inappropriate simply to translate a questionnaire that has been validated in the UK or in the USA, even though all precautions, such as forward and backward translations by two independent native speakers, are being observed. It would rather be warranted to adapt a questionnaire by not only translating, but adapting the content of items to a cultural situation, and more often than not, starting from scratch.

A good rule of thumb is: if you don't want to drive far, a wobbly wheel will do its job. But even if you are not going far, a square wheel will not be good enough. So if your construct is central and there is no adequate instrument around to measure it, consider constructing your own instrument, or team up with those who can do it for you.

The person using a measurement instrument should also know the basics of the theoretical concepts behind it in order to judge whether or not the instrument is adequate. It is not enough to repeat the mantra included in clinical publications that a scale is 'validated' – keep in mind that this is always a relative label. This can mean all and nothing, depending on the job a scale is intended to do or the context in which it is going to be used. Often reasons other than quality alone determine the widespread use of a scale. Some current examples of scales that, from a psychometric point of view, are not really good enough but are used a lot nevertheless – because of the marketing and publication strategy of its authors, its neat fit with a current theory or both – are the SF36 scale (Güthlin & Walach 2007) and the Beck Depression Inventory, to name but two. Always scrutinize the conceptual foundations, the way the construct has been operationalized; only if these foundations are sound does the psychometric ornament really mean anything.

We have given a short and not exhaustive overview of some scales likely to be useful for complementary and alternative medicine researchers in Table 18.1 and a reminder of important benchmarks and steps in developing or using a questionnaire in Table 18.2.

ARTEFACTS: CHANGING STANDARDS, RESPONSE SHIFT, SEMANTIC PROBLEMS AND SOCIAL DESIRABILITY

Imagine you have just had an accident and lost a leg. You will need to adapt to the new situation. If anyone asked you how your general quality of life was shortly after the accident, you would likely compare yourself to your state before the accident and rate many aspects worse than before. Now, imagine you have been the only survivor of a catastrophic coach accident, everyone except you being dead, and you have only lost a leg. You will then likely be comparing yourself to all those you knew and who lost their lives. Questions

Table 18.1 *Comparisons and short descriptions of some questionnaire instruments*

	Name of instrument	Features	References
Generic quality of life measurement instruments	Overview (Coons et al. 2000)		
Examples	Medical Outcomes Study (MOS) Short Form (SF)-36	Eight scales May be condensed into two summary scales for physical and mental health (but handle summary scales with care due to measurement problems) Very robust and not very sensitive to change	http://www.sf-36.org/ McHorney et al. 1993, 1994
	EQ-5D (Euroqol Questionnaire)	Provides a simple descriptive profile and a single index value for health status Value sets for cost computing QUALYs for Belgium, Denmark, Germany, Finland, New Zealand, Slovenia, Spain and the UK Very robust and not very sensitive to change	http://www.euroqol.org/ Euroquol Group 1990; Brooks & Euroquol Group 1996
Symptom checklists	Overview (Schmitz et al. 1999)		
Example	Symptom Checklist-90	Useful tool for measuring psychological status, measuring change in outcome studies or screening for mental disorders	Derogatis 1992
Measurements for specific purposes like depression, anxiety, fatigue in cancer, etc.	Overview of disease-specific quality of life (Bowling 2001) Overview of measuring depression (Nezu & Ronan 2000)		
Examples	Hospital Anxiety Depression Scale	A self-assessment scale for detecting states of depression and anxiety in the setting of a hospital medical outpatient clinic	Zigmond & Snaith 1983
	CES-D	The CES-D scale is a short self-report scale designed to measure depressive symptomatology in the general population	Radloff 1977
	Multidimensional Fatigue Inventory	20-item self-report instrument designed to measure fatigue in cancer patients and in chronic fatigue patients	Smets et al. 1995

Continued

Table 18.1 ***Comparisons and short descriptions of some questionnaire instruments*—Cont'd**

	Name of instrument	Features	References
Particularly appropriate for measuring outcome in CAM research	Overview: Hyland et al. 2008; Thompson et al. 2008.		
	Complementary and integrative medicine outcome scale		Eton et al. 2005
	MYMOP	MYMOP aims to measure the outcomes that the patient considers the most important	http://www.pms.ac.uk/mymop Paterson 1996, 2004; Paterson & Britten 2000;
	CAM Beliefs Inventory	Subscales measure beliefs in natural treatment, participation in treatment and holistic health	Bishop et al. 2005
	Arizona Integrative Outcomes Scale	One-item visual analogue scale, which assesses self-rated global sense of spiritual, social, mental, emotional and physical well-being over the past 24 hours and the past month	Bell et al. 2004
	Holistic Complementary and Alternative Medicine Questionnaire	Six of the HCAMQ items relate to beliefs about the scientific validity of CAM, and five to beliefs about holistic health	Hyland et al. 2003
Internet resources	IN-CAM database	Particularly rich resource listing outcome scales for a variety of purposes within CAM research. Nine outcome domains are covered and could be searched separately: process measures, context measures, holistic measures, quality of life instruments, psychological symptoms, social problems, physical symptoms, spiritual domain and individualized measures	http://www.outcomesdatabase.org/

CAM, complementary and alternative medicine; QALYs, quality-adjusted life-years.

Table 18.2 *Important points to keep in mind when developing or judging a scale*		
Step, problem	**Construction of scale**	**Existing instrument**
Content validity	Good conceptual grounding, qualitative work (focus groups, interviews); develop item pool out of it	Source of items? Check items: do they make sense?
Applicability	Run a first pilot study to check on semantic adequacy of items in a small sample of experts; use to improve clarity	Check original publication
Dimensionality	Factor analysis; sample large enough (at least 4, better 10 cases per item); conduct second study and confirm your factor structure with a structural equation model	Well described? Confirmatory factor analysis available? If enough data, replicate in your own sample
Construct validity	Correlate with scales that measure similar or different constructs	Information available? Satisfactory?
Reliability	Compute Cronbach's alpha; should be at least 0.70, better higher; conduct a longitudinal study with two measurements to establish retest reliability	Check reliability data; calculate Cronbach's alpha in your own sample
Sensitivity to change	Measure in a group that undergoes bona fide treatment; compare effect sizes with those of other measures; measure different groups that are known to be distinct; analyse bottom and ceiling effects: inspect empirical range and compare with possible range	Effect sizes of change measures known? Instrument differentiates between patients with known differences?
Semantic robustness	Analyse missing data: do they cluster around certain items?	Inspect the items; give to your grandmother to fill in and ask her
Population norms	Gauge questionnaire in a random sample of the population or in different patient populations and report age- and gender-specific means and standard deviations	Norm data available?
Response shift	If response shift is likely, conduct then-test	Check data and literature for paradoxically high scores
Social desirability	Establish correlation with a social desirability scale; if available, use objective indicator in parallel and correlate results	If social desirability is a big problem, don't use a questionnaire
Resources	Too small (no time, no manpower, no money): construct a series of visual analogue scales	

regarding your quality of life might then be answered paradoxically high. This, by the way, is a finding that we can see constantly when asking children who are suffering from cancer about their quality of life: they compare favourably with normal, healthy children (Walach & Kohls 2005). So how someone answers a question depends on the internal comparison standards which he or she uses. This can partly be steered by the introduction section that you put in front of your questionnaire, which you should examine carefully for its semantics. If you suggest, for instance, that your respondent should use his or her status before a certain treatment as a (relative) comparison, answers might be different from those using an ideal imagined status as comparison standard.

Once people have adapted to a new situation, their standards shift (Schwartz & Sprangers 1999; Sprangers & Schwartz 1999; Carver & Scheier 2000). As a result, although they have changed, perhaps considerably, you do not see the change in the questionnaire instrument because they are using an altered internal comparison standard. Let's assume someone starts having chronic pain and finds this very irritating. Scores of quality-of-life assessments will likely be much worse than if you ask the very same person after 6 months – pain being equal, let's stipulate for argument's sake – once the person has understood that the pain is changing all the time but is not likely to go away for good. It is difficult to do anything about this. One way of getting to grips with this problem is to tell people not only to estimate their pain after the pain-relieving intervention has happened (and to compare this score with the score you gathered beforehand) but also to let people estimate their pain score how it presumably and in their memory (according to their present internal anchor) was previously. By way of comparing the pre-score with the presumable pre-score (called the then-test) you will learn how the internal standards changed.

We often underestimate the semantic ambiguity that is harboured by seemingly innocent formulations. This often has to do with the culture a questionnaire was devised and piloted in. Translations are especially prone to this problem, but it also exists with native instruments. For instance, in the SF 36 one item asks the respondents whether they could walk 'a block'. Now, this is a typical American thing, walking as far as a block. It makes no sense at all in any other part of the world. Even if you give this English-language questionnaire to respondents who are native speakers but who live in different cultures, in rural Ireland, say, it is unclear what they make of such a formulation (Mallinson 2002).

Questionnaires, and the measurement theory behind them, date back to a behaviourist paradigm in psychology. This stipulates that humans respond to questions as to uniform stimuli. However humans are not automatons, but highly active, creative, contextually and culturally dependent, socially embedded organisms that operate on the basis of their own idiosyncratic theory of mind. That is, they form hypotheses about what someone's intentions and state of mind might be. Hence, they not only respond to questions as we pose them, but also to what they think we want with them. Some patients might surmise that if they get a particularly good or bad score their chances of being taken up into a certain study might increase. We often try to counter this tendency by telling respondents that there are no right or wrong answers and that they should respond as quickly and truthfully as possible. But will they believe us? Only qualitative research accompanying a quantitative study will be able to tell, and this is the reason why the mixed-methods approach combining quantitative and qualitative research has become increasingly popular (Bishop et al. 2005; Kohls et al. 2008).

A similar problem arises if patients are not familiar with concepts that the questionnaire tries to measure, or if they are reluctant to approach them. Indirect indicators of semantic problems are items that have an unusually high percentage of missing data. For that reason a missing data analysis should be conducted by default as part of the descriptive item statistics.

Another important artefact is memory distortion. Most questionnaires ask about some retrospective period: the last week, the last month or even the last quarter. It forces respondents to average mentally. People usually recruit this information from their memory, but in doing so they frequently tend to overestimate. This has clearly been shown by methodological studies that have done both fine-grained measurements every hour or so, followed by retrospective ones daily or weekly (Fahrenberg & Myrtek 1996). The larger the temporal distance, the greater becomes the tendency to exaggerate. Again, this depends on whether something is important to or rather embarrassing for people. If you ask retrospectively for the amount of alcohol consumed over a period of a week or even month, you are likely to get an underestimate. If you ask about the amount of pain over the last 4 weeks in a migraine sufferer, you will likely get an overestimate. There is only one solution: consider a more fine-grained pattern of measurement, daily in a diary, on record cards or on a palmtop for instance (Jamison et al. 2001).

Finally, most questionnaires are prone to bias. If respondents distort questionnaire results consciously, then they cheat. More importantly, such bias occurs automatically, if respondents unconsciously manipulate their answer towards an outcome desired by themselves or the investigator. This is called 'social desirability'. If respondents are in a study of an intervention designed to help them cope with their stress and they have to fill in a stress questionnaire at the end, then they know what you expect. If they like you or the course leader, they will probably nudge their true responses a bit towards the higher extreme. If they dislike the whole thing, they may unconsciously mark you down. In any case, you get a biased response. We try to combat this problem by interspersing the questionnaire with items in a negative formulation; some questionnaires even do this with seemingly important filler items that are not counted to disguise the true target ones. These are manoeuvres that may or may not work. Although introducing negatively worded items is a standard procedure, they also come at a cost, as negative formulations are more difficult to process semantically and thus introduce cognitive errors of simple misunderstandings.

There is only one way out of the conundrum: don't rely solely on questionnaires if you have a chance to collect other data. The sovereignty of quantitative data over the airspace of clinical research is by no means as justified as it may seem at first glance. Questionnaire measurements are not necessarily more powerful tools than their qualitative counterparts. As a matter of fact, mixed-methods research combining the advantages of quantitative and qualitative research has increasingly demonstrated its superior exploratory power.

In the qualitative research tradition 'triangulation' is key. This is a term borrowed from geography, where two different known points are used to gauge the height or the distance of a third. Similarly in research: you could use a different perspective – data from next of kin, significant others, insurance company records, reports from respondents' children – to see whether they match your questionnaire data.

FINAL WORDS

Questionnaire development is interesting and challenging. The theory behind it has allowed us to make many constructs accessible that would otherwise be very nebulous. A huge number of questionnaires exist and are still being constructed. When using one, be sure to be well informed about its properties and do not just mentally tick the boxes of 'validated' checklists. If necessary, adapt it rather than using an unsuitable instrument. If you do not have the time and the resources as well as the competencies for developing a questionnaire and need something measured, be pragmatic. After all, a well-thought-out statement with a visual analogue scale can often produce quite a good, valid measurement result. The problem is, you won't have more than common sense to prove it. The great epidemiologist Alvin Feinstein, at the very end of his career, after a long life of thinking about methodological questions, once said: If we want to know about people's quality of life, why make all the fuss with multiple items and cumbersome questionnaire construction processes? Why not ask people simply: 'How would you rate your quality of life, on a scale from 1 to 10?'(Lara-Munoz & Feinstein 1999). Why instead break a fly on the wheel? We can't see that anything is wrong with that suggestion, apart from the slight irritation that it does not express the mainstream view and has not been taken up widely as yet. This is so because on such an anarchistic statement you can neither build a theory nor run sophisticated statistical analysis. You cannot calculate reliability, it is difficult, really, to gauge; you can only trust common sense and reason. Therefore, it might be wise to use questionnaires, where available and where useful. But especially if the construct to be measured is straightforward in terms of semantics – pain, pleasure in life, happiness with one's remuneration for one's work, kindliness of receptionist – a simple question and a visual analogue or numerical rating scale will also do a fine job. Common sense is vital after all, and no amount of theory will be able to replace it.

REFERENCES

Andresen, E.M., Malmgren, J.A., Carter, W.B., et al., 1994. Screening for depression in well older adults: evaluation of a short form of the CES-D (Center for Epidemiologic Studies Depression Scale). Am. J. Prev. Med. 10 (2), 77–84.

Antonovsky, A., 1987. Unraveling the mystery of health. How People Manage Stress and Stay Well. Jossey-Bass, San Francisco.

Antonovsky, A., 1993. The structure and propeties of the sense of coherence scale. Soc. Sci. Med. 36, 725–733.

Bell, I.R., Cunningham, V., Caspi, O., et al., 2004. Development and validation of a new global well-being outcomes rating scale for integrative medicine research. BMC Complement. Altern. Med. 15 (4), 1.

Bishop, F.L., Yardley, L., Lewith, G., 2005. Developing a measure of treatment beliefs: The complementary and alternative medicine beliefs inventory. Complement. Ther. Med. 13, 144–149.

Bowling, A., 2001. Measuring Disease: A Review of Disease Specific Quality of Life Measurement Scales. Open University Press, Baltimore.

Brooks, R., Euroquol Group, 1996. EuroQol: The current state of play. Health Policy 37, 53–72.

Buchheld, N., Grossman, P., Walach, H., 2001. Measuring mindfulness in insight meditation (vipassana) and meditation-based psychotherapy: The development of the Freiburg Mindfulness Inventory (FMI). Journal for Meditation and Meditation Research 1, 11–34.

Carver, C.S., Scheier, M.F., 2000. Scaling back goals and recalibration of the affect system are processes in normal adaptive self-regulation: understanding 'response shift' phenomena. Soc. Sci. Med. 50, 1715–1722.

Champion, G.D., Goodenough, B., von Baeyer, C.L., et al., 1998. Measurement of pain by self-report. In: Finley, G.A., McGrath, P.J. (Eds.), Progress in Pain Research and Management. International Association for the Study of Pain, Seattle, pp. 123–160.

Coons, S.J., Rao, S., Keininger, D.L., et al., 2000. A comparative review of generic quality-of-life Instruments. Pharmacoeconomics 17 (1), 13–35.

Derogatis, L.R., 1992. The Symptom Checklist-90-revised. NCS Assessments, Minneapolis, MN.

Eton, D.T., Koffler, K., Cella, E., et al., 2005. Developing a self-report outcome measure for complementary and alternative medicine. Explore: The Journal of Science and Healing 1 (3), 177–185.

Euroquol Group, 1990. EuroQol – a new facility for the measurement of health-related quality of life. Health Policy 16 (3), 199–208.

Fabrigar, L.R., Wegener, D.T., MacCallum, R.C., et al., 1999. Evaluating the use of exploratory factor analysis in psychological research. Psychol. Methods 4, 272–299.

Fahrenberg, J., Myrtek, M. (Eds.), 1996. Ambulatory Assessment. Computer-Assisted Psychological and Psychophysiological Methods in Monitoring and Field Studies. Hogrefe & Huber, Seattle.

Güthlin, C., Walach, H., 2007. MOS-SF 36 – Structural equation modeling to test the construct validity of the second-order factor structure. European Journal of Assessment 23, 15–23.

Guyatt, G.H., Bombardier, C., Tugwell, P.X., 1986. Measuring disease-specific quality of life in clinical trials. Can. Med. Assoc. J. 134, 889–895.

Hautzinger, M., Bailer, M., 1993. Allgemeine Depressionsskala (ADS). Die deutsche Version des CES-D. 2. Aufl ed. Beltz, Weinheim.

Hayton, J.C., Allen, D.G., Scarpello, V., 2004. Factor retention decisions in exploratory factor analysis: a tutorial on parallel analysis. Organizational Research Methods 7 (2), 191–205.

Hyland, M.E., Lewith, G., Westoby, C., 2003. Developing a measure of attitudes: the holistic complementary and alternative medicine questionnaire. Complement. Ther. Med. 11, 33–38.

Hyland, M.E., Lewith, G.T., Westoby, C., 2008. Do existing psychologic scales measure the nonspecific benefit associated with CAM treatment? J. Altern. Complement. Med. 14 (2), 185–189.

Jacobson, N.S., Truax, P., 1991. Clinical significance: A statistical approach to defining meaningful change in psychotherapy research. J. Consult. Clin. Psychol. 59, 12–19.

Jamison, R.N., Raymond, S.A., Levine, J.G., et al., 2001. Electronic diaries for monitoring chronic pain: 1-year validation study. Pain 91, 277–285.

Kohls, N., Walach, H., 2006. Exceptional experiences and spiritual practice: A new measurement approach. Spirituality and Health International 7, 125–150.

Kohls, N., Walach, H., 2008. Validating four standard scales in spiritually practicing and non-practicing samples using propensity score matching. European Journal of Assessment 24, 165–173.

Kohls, N., Hack, A., Walach, H., 2008. Measuring the unmeasurable by ticking boxes and opening Pandora's box? Mixed methods research as a useful tool for investigating exceptional and spiritual experiences. Archive for the Psychology of Religion 30, 155–187.

Kohls, N., Sauer, S., Walach, H., 2009. Facets of mindfulness. An online study investigating the Freiburg Mindfulness Inventory. Personality and Individual Differences 46, 224–230.

Lara-Munoz, C., Feinstein, A.R., 1999. How should quality of life be measured? J. Investig. Med. 47, 17–24.

Loehlin, J.C., 1998. Latent Variable Models: Factor, Path and Structural Analysis. third ed. Lawrence Erlbaum, Mahwah, NJ.

Magnusson, D., 1967. Test Theory. Addison-Wesley, Reading, MA.

Mallinson, S., 2002. Listening to respondents: a qualitative assessment of the Short-Form 36 Health Status Questionnaire. Soc. Sci. Med. 54, 11–21.

McHorney, C.A., Ware, J.E., Raczek, A.E., 1993. The MOS 36-item short form health survey (SF-36): II. Psychometric and clinical tests of validity in measuring physical and mental health constructs. Med. Care 31, 247–263.

McHorney, C.A., Ware, J.E., Lu, J.F.R., et al., 1994. The MOS 36-item short form health survey (SF-36): III. Tests of data quality, scaling assumptions and reliability across diverse patient groups. Med. Care 32, 40–66.

Melzack, R. (Ed.), 1983. Pain. Measurement and Assessment. Raven Press, New York.

Mokken, R.J., 1971. A Theory and Procedure of Scale Analysis: With Applications in Political Research. Den Haag, Mouton.

Nezu, A.M., Ronan, G.F., 2000. Practitioner's Guide to Empirically Based Measures of Depression. Kluwer, New York.

Ostermann, T., Willich, S.N., Lüdtke, R., 2008. Regression toward the mean – a detection method for unknown population mean based on Mee and Chua's algorithm. BMC Med. Res. Methodol. 8, 52.

Paterson, C., 1996. Measuring outcomes in primary care: a patient generated measure, MYMOP, compared with the SF-36 health survey. Br. Med. J. 312, 1016–1020.

Paterson, C., Britten, N., 2000. In pursuit of patient-centred outcomes: a qualitative evaluation of the 'Measure Yourself Medical Outcome Profile'. J. Health Serv. Res. Policy 5 (1), 27–36.

Paterson, C., 2004. Seeking the patient's perspective: a qualitative assessment of EuroQol, COOP-WONCA Charts and MYMOP2. Qual. Life Res. 13, 871–881.

Preston, C.C., Colman, A.M., 2000. Optimal number of response categories in rating scales: reliability, validity, discriminating power, and respondent preferences. Acta Psychol. (Amst.) 104, 1–15.

Radloff, L.S., 1977. The CES-D Scale: A self-report depression scale for research in the general population. Applied Psychological Measurement 1 (3), 385–401.

Rao, C.R. (Ed.), 2007. Psychometrics. Elsevier, Amsterdam, Heidelberg.

Schmitz, N., Kruse, J., Heckrath, C., et al., 1999. Diagnosing mental disorders in primary care: The General Health Questionnaire (GHQ) and the Symptom Check List (SCL-90-R) as screening instruments. Soc. Psychiatry Psychiatr. Epidemiol. 34, 360–366.

Schwartz, C.E., Sprangers, M.A.G., 1999. Methodological approaches for assessing response shift in longitudinal health-related quality-of-life research. Soc. Sci. Med. 48, 1531–1548.

Smets, E.M., Garssen, B., Bonke, B., et al., 1995. The Multidimensional Fatigue Inventory (MFI): psychometric qualities of an instrument to assess fatigue. J. Psychosom. Res. 39 (3), 315–325.

Speer, D.C., 1992. Clinically significant change: Jacobson and Truax (1991) revisited. J. Consult. Clin. Psychol. 60, 402–408.

Sprangers, M.A.G., Schwartz, C.E., 1999. Integrating response shift into health-related quality of life research: a theoretical model. Soc. Sci. Med. 48, 1507–1515.

Staquet, M.J., Hays, R.D., Fayers, P.M. (Eds.), 1998. Quality of Life Assessment in Clinical Trials. Methods and Practice. Oxford University Press, Oxford.

Thompson, E.A., Quinn, T., Paterson, C., et al., 2008. Outcome measures for holistic, complex interventions within the palliative care setting. Complement. Ther. Clin. Pract. 14 (1), 25–32.

Walach, H., Kohls, N., 2005. Grade-of-Membership (GoM) – analysis as a sensitive method for evaluating categorical data – introduction and some examples. In: Beauducel, A., Biehl, B., Bosniak, M., et al. (Eds.), Multivariate Research Strategies – Festschrift for Werner W Wittmann. Shaker, Aachen, pp. 151–172.

Walach, H., Buchheld, N., Buttenmüller, V., Kleinknecht, N., Schmidt, S., 2006. Measuring mindfulness - The Freiburg Mindfulness Inventory (FMI). Personality and Individual Differences 40, 1543–1555.

Zealley, A.K., Aitken, R.C.B., 1969. Measurement of mood. Proc. R. Soc. Med. 62, 993–996.

Zigmond, A.S., Snaith, R.P., 1983. The hospital anxiety and depression scale. Acta Psychiatr. Scand. 67 (6), 361–370.

Economic evaluation

David Wonderling • John Brazier • Elisabetta Fenu • Anne Morgan

19

CHAPTER CONTENTS

INTRODUCTION

Complementary and alternative medicine (CAM) is often provided by public health services, such as the UK National Health Service (NHS), and these therapies are therefore competing with conventional medicine for scarce health service resources. It has been suggested that CAM therapies may be cheaper than conventional treatments in many situations or, where there is an extra cost, they offer good value for money. These claims need to be supported by evidence if they are to be accepted by health care providers. Australia and Canada, for example, have long had guidelines on assessing the cost-effectiveness (i.e. value for money) of new technologies. In the UK, the National Institute for Clinical Excellence (NICE) makes recommendations on the use of new and established technologies and prepares guidance for the NHS. Its recommendations are based on a full appraisal of the clinical effectiveness and the cost-effectiveness of interventions. The NHS is expected to use NICE guidelines to ensure that decisions to adopt one medical intervention rather than another will promote an efficient and equitable use of health service resources (Box 19.1). Health economics plays an important role in this process because it is concerned with efficiency and equity and has a set of techniques for assessing relative efficiency by comparing the costs and health benefits of competing alternatives, known as economic evaluation.

DOI: 10.1016/B978-0-443-06956-7.00019-7

BOX 19.1 Key terms

Economic efficiency is achieved when the maximum benefit is obtained from given National Health Service resources
Equity is concerned with how fairly health care costs and benefits are distributed
Opportunity cost is the value of that which must be given up to acquire or achieve something
Quality-adjusted life-year (QALY) is an index of survival that is adjusted to account for the patient's quality of life during this time. It incorporates changes in both quantity (longevity/mortality) and health-related quality of life
Incremental cost-effectiveness ratio (ICER) is the difference in the 'mean cost' and 'mean outcome' for one treatment compared with another

There are a variety of techniques available for conducting economic evaluations in CAM studies. Despite the methodological problems in this area the goal of performing a full economic evaluation is within the reach of most health service researchers. This chapter describes the basic principles of economic evaluation, the different types of evaluation and the circumstances under which the various analytical tools are appropriate. In addition, consideration is given to some of the practical issues in undertaking an economic evaluation. Finally, this chapter summarizes the available economic evidence on CAM.

WHAT IS AN ECONOMIC EVALUATION?

An economic evaluation compares both costs and health outcomes of two or more alternative courses of action. To report costs alone is not an economic evaluation. At the same time, most forms of economic evaluation only make sense where one intervention is compared with the next best option. The purpose is to provide information to aid decision-making about which therapies to adopt within a fixed health care budget.

THE PRINCIPLES OF ECONOMIC EVALUATION

To perform an economic evaluation the following steps are recommended (Drummond et al. 2005). The study or research question needs to be important in terms of resource implications; it should consider both costs and outcomes of the competing alternatives and the perspective of the study should be clearly stated: that is, the viewpoint (health service, patients or society) from which the evaluation is undertaken. The alternative interventions to be included for comparison in the study need to be fully described and the choices justified (e.g. is it really the next best alternative?). Please note that in this chapter we use the term 'alternative intervention' not in the CAM sense but in the more generic sense of two treatments, either of which could be provided for the same patient group.

The type or types of economic evaluation (Box 19.2) to be undertaken must be stated and justified. There are at least four to choose from, though in practice

BOX 19.2 Economic evaluation techniques[a]

Cost minimization analysis seeks to establish which is the least-cost alternative, but is only a technique of economic evaluation if it can be shown that the alternatives achieve identical health outcomes

Cost-effectiveness analysis considers what is the best method of achieving a single health outcome and is usually measured in physical units. Results are presented in terms of cost per unit of effect (e.g. cost per point change in pain intensity score or cost per symptom-free day)

Cost–utility analysis is a special type of cost-effectiveness analysis which requires a single index of health benefit that incorporates quality of life and life expectancy, e.g. the quality-adjusted life-year (QALY)

Cost–benefit analysis compares the benefits with costs of a health care programme, where all the benefits are valued in money terms, including health improvement

Cost–consequences analysis requires a number of different health outcomes to be compared together with costs without establishing a hierarchy among the outcomes

[a]The reader should be aware that these terms are often misused in the literature. In particular, the terms cost-effectiveness and cost–benefit analysis often appear in the title of journal articles that only look at costs and therefore aren't full economic evaluations at all. This is particularly likely to be the case in older studies that were written up before these definitions had been formalized.

it may be necessary to plan for more than one (see below). The techniques of economic evaluation mainly differ in the way in which health benefits are measured and hence the policy questions they are designed to answer. Cost minimization analysis (CMA) and cost-effectiveness analysis (CEA) implicitly assume that a particular health care objective is worthwhile and attempt to answer the question: what is the most efficient way of achieving this goal? Cost–utility analysis (CUA), on the other hand, can be used to inform the question: what is the most efficient way of spending a given health care budget? and hence, whether health service resources should be diverted towards one intervention and if so, how much. Finally, there is cost–benefit analysis (CBA), which in principle can answer the big question: is this programme worthwhile for society as a whole?

Although not recognized as a technique of economic evaluation, there is a more pragmatic approach, known as cost–consequences analysis (CCA), which simply presents various health outcomes for each competing intervention without attempting to combine them in to a single index (see Box 19.2).

Costs need to be described in terms of the resources consumed by each intervention, such as the number of therapy sessions, and the value of those resources such as therapist fees, rental of premises and the price of any prescribed treatment. Quantities of resources used and their unit costs should be reported separately and the methods for estimating each need to be stated clearly. Costing will be discussed in more detail in the section on practical issues, below.

For many reasons individuals prefer receiving benefits earlier rather than later and delaying costs for as long as possible. It is important, therefore, that the time period over which costs and benefits are measured is clearly stated and justified. Costs and benefits often need to be adjusted by a procedure known as discounting when they are spread over a period of years. To illustrate how discounting works, Drummond et al. (2005) use as an example the case where two programmes require different outlays over 3 years, as shown below.

Year	Cost of programme A (£000s)	Cost of programme B (£000s)
1	5	15
2	10	10
3	15	4

Simply adding the two cost streams shows programme B to have a lower cost than A. However, by adjusting for the differential timing of costs by discounting future costs to present values, programme B is shown to be more costly than A. If P = present value, F_n = future cost at year n and r = the discount rate, then

$$P = \frac{F_1}{(1+r)} + \frac{F_2}{(1+r)^2} + \frac{F_3}{(1+r)^3}$$

If the discount rate is 5%, the present value of A = £26.79 and the present value of B = £26.81. For a discussion of choice of discount rate for use in adjusting costs and benefits, see Drummond et al. (2005).

Consideration needs to be given to any uncertainty surrounding data estimates of costs and benefits. For example, if estimates are taken from a sample of the population standard statistical methods can be used. If, on the other hand, cost data have been extrapolated, a sensitivity analysis is more appropriate. This approach examines the impact on the evaluation results of using a range of estimates.

Although a randomized controlled trial is often regarded as the gold standard for producing results on clinical efficacy, it is not always sufficient for conducting an economic evaluation. A trial may not collect results for long enough to assess the full costs or benefits of an intervention or the artificial context of a trial may be unrealistic. In these circumstances, modelling can be used to fill in the gaps and to handle the inevitable uncertainties which exist for many of the key parameters.

The evaluation results should be presented in a clear and generalizable way. A decision-maker is not usually concerned with all or nothing but options for incremental expansion or contraction of programme. In other words, the question is likely to be: what would be the costs (and benefits) of having a little more or a little less of a service in this area? A primary care group, for example, might be considering adding chiropractic, acupuncture or physiotherapy sessions to existing services for patients presenting with low-back pain. The additional costs of introducing these sessions will vary with location depending on local factors such as the supply of relevant practitioners and existing demand for their services. Consequently, the results of an economic evaluation undertaken in one location cannot be universally applied to all settings. It is important therefore that disaggregated data should be presented along with summary measures such as cost-effectiveness ratios.

PRACTICAL ISSUES IN AN ECONOMIC EVALUATION

STUDY QUESTION

Care needs to be given to formulating the study or research question. Once it is established that the resource implications of the new intervention are such that a full economic evaluation is warranted, the alternative therapies for comparison must be selected.

A new treatment, for example, is often compared with the most widely used alternative, although the most cost-effective alternative available is the preferred comparator. CAM therapies are often added to conventional therapies so it may be appropriate to compare a standard therapy, for back pain for example, with and without additional therapy, such as acupuncture. If in practice there is currently no service provided for the condition in question then the comparator should be a 'do nothing' (or best supportive care) option. This may well be the case for certain conditions in many low-income countries. You would also want to compare with a 'do nothing' option if none of the current treatments have been proven to be cost-effective (be that due to 'evidence of absence' or 'absence of evidence'). A comprehensive economic evaluation might compare the new treatment with: (1) a do-nothing option; (2) the standard therapy; and (3) any other strategies that could possibly be more cost-effective than the standard therapy.

Comparison with placebo or its equivalent (e.g. sham acupuncture) is generally not advocated. Instead, pragmatic randomized trials tend to be thought of as the most suitable for economic evaluation (Drummond et al. 2005). Pragmatic trials attempt to replicate the real-world conditions that would exist if the intervention were to be implemented in routine clinical practice. Hence patients should be typical of normal caseload and comparison should be with a relevant alternative with both clinicians and patients unblinded (but investigators blinded). In this way the incremental costs and health gain should closely reflect what will happen if the intervention is rolled out into the wider health service. A study of acupuncture that was based on a sham comparator would not pick up all of the health gain attributable to needling (since both trial arms have needling), nor would it pick up some of the other elements of health gain related to contact, such as the placebo response. (Both of these elements are real health effects which would occur as part of routine practice.) Consequently the cost impact on health services would also not reflect what would happen in routine practice.

CHOOSING THE ECONOMIC EVALUATION TECHNIQUE

Although it is recommended that the type of economic evaluation be chosen at the outset, it is often difficult to decide on the appropriate technique until the results are known. For example, a CEA may change to a CMA if the health outcomes are found to be the same for both interventions. Similarly, if two interventions are found to have similar costs and intervention *A* is more effective than intervention *B*, then intervention *A* is obviously dominant and should be chosen. It is more often the case, however, that the new intervention will be found to be both more effective and more costly and in such situations a CUA or CBA is required.

The possible situations resulting from a CEA or CUA can be explained by means of the cost-effectiveness plane (Figure 19.1), where incremental effectiveness (in this case QALYs gained) is plotted on the horizontal axis and incremental cost is plotted on the vertical axis. The new treatment may lie in one of the four quadrants formed by the intersection of the axes. In the north-west quadrant, intervention *A* is more costly and less effective than its comparator and it is therefore 'dominated'. Conversely, if it lies in the south-east quadrant the new intervention dominates its comparator as it improves the health outcome and reduces costs. More often, a new intervention increases health benefits but at higher costs (the north-east quadrant). However, in one case (point *A*) a substantial additional benefit could be obtained with a small additional cost while in another case (point *B*) a small increase in benefit corresponds to a large increase in costs. The slope of the line from each point to the origin is the intervention's incremental cost-effectiveness ratio (ICER):

$$\text{ICER} = (\text{cost}_a - \text{cost}_x)/(\text{QALYs}_a - \text{QALYs}_x)$$

where x is the current treatment and a is the new treatment

The diagonal line that passes through the origin indicates the maximum the health service is prepared to pay for a QALY. In theory this cost-effectiveness threshold should be set such that if the health service adopted all the interventions with an ICER below the threshold but none of them above the threshold then its budget would be consumed exactly. In practice we don't know the ICERs for every intervention so the threshold must be approximated, essentially by trial and error. For this reason in the UK NICE advocates a range for its threshold between £20 000 and £30 000 per QALY gained. In the hypothetical case in Figure 19.1, we would adopt intervention *A* because its ICER is less than the threshold but not intervention *B*.

For high-income countries, we have some idea of what the cost per QALY threshold is, but rarely do we have an idea for other outcomes that we might

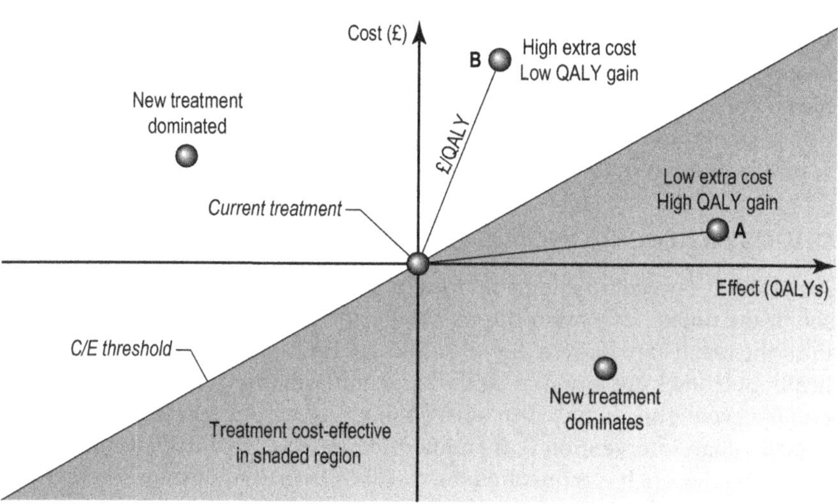

FIGURE 19.1 Cost-effectiveness (C/E) plane. QALY, quality-adjusted life-year.

use in a CEA. So if we want to assess the value for money of an intervention compared with all the other possible interventions across a health service then we will usually require a CUA or CBA.

Conducting CBA, where health benefits are measured in monetary terms, overcomes the need for a cost-effectiveness threshold – one adopts the new treatment if the benefits exceed the costs. However, CBA is beset by its own problems (see below) and is rarely conducted compared with the other techniques.

CCA is more practical than CBA or CUA but it is often unhelpful in decision-making, either because not all the health outcomes move in the same direction or because both health and costs are increased but we can't say whether the intervention is cost-effective or not.

COSTING

Any decision to use resources to satisfy a particular health care demand, such as acupuncture for low-back pain, involves sacrificing the opportunity of using the same resources to satisfy other health care demands, such as primary care counselling services for depression. It is this sacrifice or 'opportunity cost' (Box 19.1) that economic evaluation aims to estimate and compare with treatment benefits.

For all economic evaluations, costs must be identified, measured and valued for each therapy. The identification of costs will be determined by the perspective of the study: that is, the point of view from which the study is undertaken. It is usually recommended to take a societal view but a more limited viewpoint is easier for costing purposes and legitimate provided it is made explicit. In the UK, NICE makes its decisions on the basis of health service costs (rather than societal costs) because its role is to maximize the health gain from a given NHS budget.

All identified resources need to be measured in natural units such as number and length of acupuncture sessions, number of general practitioner surgery visits or number of days taken off work with back pain. Most economic evaluations measure only disease-specific resource use, e.g. treatment costs only for migraine. However, some studies will measure all health care resource use incurred by patients (both disease-specific and non-specific).

Economic evaluations that follow a societal perspective will usually include, in addition to health service costs, both costs directly incurred by patients (e.g. over-the-counter medicines) and 'indirect costs'. Health economists use the term 'indirect costs' to refer to cost of time (paid and non-paid) lost due to illness and treatment. Indirect costs are also known as productivity costs. There are different methods for valuing this time; sometimes time is valued at the patient's weekly wage rate. In the cases of CUA and CBA, there is a risk of double-counting, since it can be argued that both health-related quality of life scores and willingness-to-pay scores could incorporate to some extent the benefits of freeing up the patient's time.

Table 19.1 shows how Thomas et al. (1999) planned to measure and value resources in their study into acupuncture for low-back pain. The first column identifies the resources to be measured. Since this study is taking a societal perspective, the relevant costs are those borne by the health service and by

Table 19.1 ***Measurement and valuation of resources used by patients in the trial***

Resource	Measurement	Data source	Valuation method	Data source
Acupuncture	No. and length of sessions	Records kept by acupuncturists	Standard charges	Practitioners in study, supplemented by data from elsewhere
Primary care				
GP consultation	No. of visits to and by GPs	GP notes	Cost per contact	Netten & Dennett 1996
Drugs	Drugs prescribed	Cost of drugs to NHS		*British National Formulary*
Hospital				
Outpatient clinic attendances	No. of attendances	Patient questionnaire schedule and hospital records	Cost per attendance	Local hospital finance departments
Physiotherapy	No. of sessions	Patient questionnaire schedule and hospital records	Cost per session	Local hospital finance departments
A&E attendances	No. of attendances	Patient questionnaire schedule and hospital records	Cost per attendance	Local hospital finance departments
Admissions	Length of stay	Patient questionnaire schedule and hospital records	Cost per diem by speciality	Local hospital finance departments
Other NHS services				
Physiotherapy	No. of sessions	Patient questionnaire	Cost per session	Netten & Dennett 1996
Non-NHS services				
Chiropractic	No. of sessions	Patient questionnaire	Cost per session	Data from national survey estimates (publication in preparation)
Osteopathy	No. of sessions	Patient questionnaire	Cost per session	
Acupuncture	No. of sessions	Patient questionnaire	Cost per session	
Patient time				
Treatment time	Time spent using services	Patient questionnaire	Cost per minute	Department of Transport
Work time	Time off work	Patient questionnaire	Gross earnings plus employment costs	National average earnings

Reproduced from Thomas et al. (1999).

patients. In the second and third columns the measurement of resources is described. For example, the number and length of acupuncture sessions provided will be quantified using records kept by acupuncturists. Columns four and five describe the valuation method, which in the case of acupuncture sessions will be standard charges, and the data source for these charges will be the practitioners themselves.

MEASURES OF HEALTH BENEFIT

The economic techniques described earlier differ mainly in terms of the way in which benefits are measured.

A simple CMA is required when health outcomes are the same. A North American study, for example, compared outcomes and costs of care for acute low-back pain among patients of primary care practitioners, chiropractors and orthopaedic surgeons (Carey et al. 1995). The authors found that, while clinical outcomes (time to functional recovery, return to work and complete recovery) were similar among the various practitioners, health service costs were lowest for patients seen by primary care practitioners. CMA can only confidently be performed when good evidence of equal effectiveness exists.

A CEA requires one unambiguous objective of treatment alternatives such as reduction in pain intensity score (Niemisto et al. 2003, 2005) or number of migraine attacks (Liguori et al. 2000). Since many of the conditions for which CAM therapies are sought are often chronic and benign rather than life-threatening, measures that incorporate health-related quality of life are therefore often more relevant than biomedical measures.

Economists have attempted to solve this problem by combining quality and quantity of life in a single index of health benefit, such as the quality-adjusted life-year (QALY) to allow CUA to be performed. To estimate QALYs we simply multiply a health-related quality-of-life score (on a 0–1 scale) by the time spent in that health state (in years). Thus a year spent in full health is equal to 1 QALY (1×1) but a year spent at 50% quality of life would be equal to 0.5 QALYs (0.5×1). In theory this is an extremely useful technique for investigating CAM therapies, since it allows them to be compared with other treatments that improve quality of life and with treatments that prolong life (Drummond et al. 2005).

The QALY approach has some conceptual flaws, being based on assumptions that may not always hold true. For example, it assumes utilities can be perfectly added and thus 2 years in a healthy state give twice the utility of 1 year in the same health state. In practice individuals might rate the second year differently if they either adapt or become more intolerant to the condition. Furthermore it assumes a desire to maximize expected utility, but this won't be the case for individuals who are risk-averse. The generic quality-of-life instruments used in QALYs sometimes fail to capture important changes in quality of life when applied to specific conditions. There are alternatives to QALYs, such as the healthy year equivalent, but these methods have their own problems. No health outcome measure is flawless in all situations and a review of the existing economic literature of CAM interventions (see below) shows the QALY to be a popular choice among investigators.

In addition, one of the reasons CUA was developed was to address the problem of having more than one health outcome of interest. To produce QALYs, individuals' preferences or values are used to score health states. Health state values can be elicited directly from patients using one of the three main methods (rating scales, time trade-off and standard gamble – see Drummond et al. (2005) for details). However this requires substantial time and cognitive effort and many clinicians believe it creates an unnecessary burden on patients. Another alternative, and one which requires little effort, is a preference-based measure, which is a standardized health state classification with a pre-existing set of valuations. The system developed by the EuroQol Group is the EQ-5D (http://www.euroqol.org/) which classifies patients according to five dimensions (mobility, self-care, usual activity, pain/discomfort, anxiety/depression). Since each dimension has three possible levels (no problem, some problems, major problems), the total number of possible health states is 245 when death and unconsciousness are added. Health status is usually recorded by the patients themselves by completing the five multiple choice questions. However the value placed on each health state is elicited from a large sample of the general population in the UK and from other populations around the world. There are alternatives to the EQ-5D, such as the SF-6D (Brazier et al. 2002).

In their study of manipulation for back pain, Williams et al. (2004) and the United Kingdom back pain exercise and manipulation (UK BEAM) Trial Team (2004) have used the health utility weights elicited from the EQ-5D questionnaire to calculate QALYs, whereas Niemisto et al. (2003, 2005) have reported only as a secondary outcome the health-related quality of life assessed through the 15D system (Sintonen 2001).

Alternatively, researchers can develop their own descriptions of health states or health experience following an intervention through qualitative patient interviews if questionnaires do not include aspects of the illness or treatment which are thought to be important to patients. This may be useful in investigating CAM therapies where, for example, processes of care may have a considerable influence on patient preferences (Brown & Sculpher 1999).

By using the same unit of account, money, to value both benefits and costs, CBA is conceptually the most powerful technique in economic evaluation because, in theory, one can decide whether a treatment is worthwhile without having to determine the cost-effectiveness threshold. In practice, however, the problem is how to value length and quality of life in money terms. The values individuals place on goods and services are normally indicated by their maximum willingness to pay for them. In health care, however, market values are regarded as inadequate measures of society's values. Economists have therefore either attempted to adjust market values for these imperfections or conducted 'willingness to pay' experiments where individuals are asked what they would be willing to pay for a specified improvement (Drummond et al. 2005). The main criticisms of this approach are the hypothetical nature of the question and that responses will depend in part on existing income distributions, which the NHS may wish to ignore. It could, for example, lead to the 'diseases of affluence' receiving a higher weighting because of the higher incomes of sufferers. CBAs are not common generally and we believe that there has not yet been one conducted for a CAM therapy.

EXISTING ECONOMIC EVALUATIONS OF CAM INTERVENTIONS

We conducted a search of two bibliographic databases: the Health Economics Evaluations Database (HEED) and the NHS Economic Evaluations Database. We used the following selection criteria:

1. Studies had to compare a CAM intervention with one or more other interventions. Given the breadth of CAM and controversy over its definition, we decided to focus on manipulation, acupuncture and homeopathy.
2. Studies could be any type of economic evaluation but had to measure health benefit as well as resource cost.
3. Studies had to derive their measure of health benefit from randomized controlled trials.

We realize that we might have missed some relevant studies by restricting our search to randomized controlled trials and therefore our review is not comprehensive. However, given the potential for bias in non-randomized studies, we believe that we will have found most of the better-quality studies.

ACUPUNCTURE

Ten years ago there were probably no rigorous health economic evaluations of acupuncture in the published literature. Prior to this, economic studies of acupuncture were typically conducted by acupuncture advocates using questionable methods. For example, studies have claimed cost savings on the basis of hypothetical interventions that would have been necessary had acupuncture not been administered (Lindall 1999). Other studies have used before–after comparisons (Myers 1991) or non-randomized controls (Ballegaard et al. 1995, 1996).

We found 11 economic evaluations considering acupuncture based on randomized evidence (Table 19.2). Five of the 11 were from an intensive programme of research into acupuncture conducted in Germany in recent years; three of these trials had more than 2000 patients each. The rest were from Italy, the UK and the USA.

Two of the interventions were not simply acupuncture but instead offered patients a choice of acupuncture or another CAM therapy. Most of the studies evaluated acupuncture as an adjunct to usual care but one compared acupuncture directly with conventional drug treatment. One study compared acupuncture with massage therapy and self-care educational materials. Seven of the studies were CUAs (i.e. they estimated QALYs), three were CCA and one was a CEA. The studies varied in terms of their study cost perspective: five studies (all from Germany) took a societal perspective (including both direct medical costs and indirect costs), another five studies took a health service perspective (including only direct medical costs) and one study included only indirect costs.

The hypothesis that acupuncture will save money does not seem to be supported by the economic evidence, whichever perspective is taken. However, the evidence does seem to show that acupuncture for a variety of pain conditions improves quality of life to an extent that most high-income countries would consider it to be cost-effective (i.e. acupuncture cost less than the £20 000 per QALY, the threshold advocated by NICE).

Table 19.2 ***Economic evaluations based on randomized trials: acupuncture***

Patient group	First author and year	*n*	Intervention	Comparator(s)	Main health outcome(s)	Type	Cost perspective	Result
Acute low-back pain	Eisenberg 2007 USA	444	Choice of acupuncture, chiropractic or massage therapy	Usual care	1. Symptom bothersomeness score 2. Roland disability score 3. Patient satisfaction	CCA	Direct medical	Choice had higher cost but greater satisfaction
Chronic low-back pain	Cherkin 2001 USA	262	Chinese medical acupuncture	1. Therapeutic massage 2. Self-care educational materials	1. Symptom bothersomeness score 2. Roland disability score	CCA	Direct medical	Massage dominates
Chronic low-back pain	Ratcliffe 2006 UK	241	Chinese medical acupuncture	Usual care	QALYs	CUA	Direct medical	£4000 per QALY gained
Chronic low-back pain	Witt 2006a, b Germany	3100	Acupuncture	Usual care	QALYs	CUA	Direct medical (including non-specific) and indirect costs	€11 000 per QALY gained
Chronic neck pain	Willich 2006, Witt 2006b Germany	3451	Acupuncture	Usual care	QALYs	CUA	Direct medical (including non-specific) and indirect costs	€12 000 per QALY gained
Dysmenorrhoea	Witt 2008a Germany	649	Acupuncture	Usual care	QALYs	CUA	Direct medical (including non-specific) and indirect costs	€3000 per QALY gained

Dyspepsia	Paterson 2003 UK	60	Choice of acupuncture or homeopathy	Usual care	1. SF-36 2. MYMOP 3. GWBI	CCA	Direct medical	No differences, but only a pilot study
Migraine or chronic headache	Witt 2006b, 2008b Germany	2682	Acupuncture	Usual care	QALYs	CUA	Direct medical (including non-specific) and indirect costs	€11 000 per QALY gained
Migraine or chronic headache	Wonderling 2004 UK	401	Acupuncture	Usual care	QALYs	CUA	Direct medical	€3000 per QALY gained
Migraine without aura	Liguori 2000 Italy	120	Acupuncture	Conventional drug therapy	Migraine attacks	CEA	Indirect costs	Acupuncture dominates
Osteoarthritis	Witt 2006b, Reinhold 2008 Germany	421	Acupuncture	Usual care	QALYs	CUA	Direct medical (including non-specific) and indirect costs	€18 000 per QALY gained

CCA, cost–consequences analysis; CEA, cost-effectiveness analysis; CUA, cost–utility analysis; QALY, quality-adjusted life-year.

Most of these studies evaluate acupuncture as an adjunct to usual care. Only one study evaluated acupuncture as an alternative to drug therapy but this study did not include direct medical costs so the apparent cost savings should be treated with caution. And there is currently no evidence for the cost-effectiveness of acupuncture for anything other than pain management. One study found that massage therapy was more effective and cost-saving when compared to acupuncture. This particular result may not be conclusive but it highlights the importance of evaluating each CAM intervention against all potential alternatives.

HOMEOPATHY

We only found one eligible economic evaluation of homeopathy (Table 19.2). As this was only a pilot study, it wasn't able to reach any conclusion, due to its small sample size.

SPINAL MANIPULATION

We found eight economic studies evaluating manipulation based on randomized evidence (Table 19.3).

Manipulation was compared with a variety of alternatives, including: GP care, orthopaedic surgeon care, educational materials and physiotherapy. All studies included direct medical costs but only two included indirect costs. Four studies were CCA, two were CUA, and two were CEA. We'll start with the CCAs.

Carey et al. (1995) described the costs and consequences of different interventions for back pain. Outcomes could not be precisely estimated, even though they appeared to be similar for all interventions. This study may be less rigorous than the others in our review as only health care practitioners were randomized whereas patients were those consecutively enrolled by the practitioners.

Neither Cherkin et al. (1998) nor Skargren et al. (1998) could identify significant differences in outcomes at 12 months between manipulation and other interventions. The cost analysis by Cherkin at al. showed that manipulation was less costly than physical therapy but more costly than providing an educational book alone, while Skargren et al. (1998) reported higher direct costs in the manipulation group compared to physiotherapy but similar indirect costs in the two groups.

Manipulation was shown to be cost-saving compared to chemonucleolysis in the treatment of sciatica due to lumbar disc herniation, although the effectiveness is unclear (Burton et al. 2000).

More recently two UK studies have each conducted a CUA alongside a randomized controlled trial on manipulation compared to GP care in back and neck pain patients (Williams et al. 2004; UK BEAM Trial Team 2004), and compared to exercise alone or exercise in combination with manipulation in back pain patients (UK BEAM Trial Team 2004). If we compare the incremental cost-effectiveness ratios obtained in these studies (£3560/QALY and £3800/QALY respectively) with the £20 000/QALY NICE threshold, manipulation is cost-effective for these groups of patients among the interventions considered

Table 19.3 *Economic evaluations based on randomized trials: manipulation*

Patient group	First author and year	*n*	Intervention	Comparator(s)	Main health outcome(s)	Type	Cost perspective	Result
Acute low-back pain	Carey 1995 USA	1633	Manipulation	1. GP care 2. Orthopaedic surgeon's care	1. Time to functional recovery 2. Patients' satisfaction	CCA	Direct medical	No difference in time to recovery but patients more satisfied with manipulation. Manipulation was more costly than GP care and similar to orthopaedic care
Back pain	UK BEAM Trial 2004 UK	1287	Manipulation (for 12 weeks)	1. GP care (+ educational book) 2. Exercise programme (for 12 weeks) 3. Manipulation (for 6 weeks) followed by exercise (for another 6 weeks)	QALYs	CUA	Direct medical	versus (1) £ 4800 per QALY versus (2) £ 2300 per QALY versus (3) £8300 per QALY
Back pain	Cherkin 1998 USA	321	Manipulation	1. Exercise programme (+ educational book) 2. Educational book	Bothersomeness Roland Disability Scale	CCA	Direct medical	Manipulation more effective (not significantly) but more costly than booklet. Manipulation dominates exercise programme
Back pain or neck pain	Skargren 1998 Sweden	323	Manipulation	Physiotherapy	1. Pain intensity (VAS) 2. Disability (Oswestry score) 3. General health (VAS)	CCA	Direct and indirect	No significant difference in health outcomes or costs

Continued

Table 19.3 ***Economic evaluations based on randomized trials: manipulation—Cont'd***

Patient group	First author and year	*n*	Intervention	Comparator(s)	Main health outcome(s)	Type	Cost perspective	Result
Chronic back pain	Niemisto 2005 Finland	204	Combined manipulation/ exercises/ information	GP care (+ educational book)	1. Pain intensity (VAS) 2. Self-rated disability 3. Health-related quality of life 4. Frequency of pain	CEA	Direct and indirect	Only pain intensity was significantly greater in the comparator. Costs were reduced from baseline in comparator while increased in intervention
Chronic back pain	Niemisto 2003 Finland	204	Manipulation	GP care (+ educational book)	1. Pain intensity (VAS) 2. Frequency of pain 3. Self-rated disability 4. Health-related quality of life 5. Degree of mental depression	CEA	Direct and indirect	Outcome (1): $23 per one-point change in VAS scale
Low- or upper-back pain and neck pain	Williams 2004 UK	187	Manipulation	GP care	QALYs	CUA	Direct medical	£3560 per QALY
Sciatica due to lumbar disc herniation	Burton 2000 UK	40	Manipulation	Chemonucleolysis	1. Roland Disability Scale 2. Leg pain intensity (VAS) 3. Back pain (VAS)	CCA	Direct medical	No significant difference in outcomes. Manipulation is cost-saving (£300)

CCA, cost-consequences analysis; CEA, cost-effectiveness analysis; CUA, cost–utility analysis; VAS, visual analogue scale.

in the studies. Williams et al. (2004) and the UK BEAM Trial Team (2004) conducted sensitivity analyses where outliers were excluded from the base case. These analyses confirmed and strengthened the base case findings.

Other economic studies have limited their analysis to a CEA of manipulation alone or in combination with exercise compared to GP care complemented by educational book (Niemisto et al. 2003, 2005). The cost per point change in pain intensity as measured by a visual analogue scale (VAS) was $23 in the manipulation alone group over 1 year and $512 in the combination group over 2 years. In one study (Niemisto et al. 2003), the authors acknowledged that the higher effectiveness in the manipulation group could have been explained by the more numerous contacts that patients had with the health care providers, suggesting that the effect may be due to placebo response.

In summary, the two CUAs seem to show that manipulation is cost-effective compared with either GP care or with an exercise programne. The other studies are harder to interpret, either because the overall impact on quality of life is unclear or, in the case of the CEAs, because we do not know what cost-effectiveness threshold to apply.

CONCLUSION

Health economics has played and will continue to play an important part in evaluating new and existing technologies. Given that many CAM therapies are now being provided by public health services, these therapies must compete with conventional therapies for scarce resources. Economic evaluation in health care is a way of comparing costs and benefits of treatments. The chosen technique will depend on the question posed and the evidence available. CBA measures benefits in monetary units and can be used to compare programmes within the health sector and beyond. Given the difficulty in valuing benefits in such a way, health economists have mostly settled for addressing what are regarded as lower-level efficiency questions. They make an initial assumption that the programme is worthwhile and go on to consider the best means of achieving a given objective. Cost-effectiveness quantifies health outcomes in natural units, which are, for the most part, objective biomedical measures. The limitation of these types of study is that they can only compare interventions with the same clinical outcomes. Cost–utility studies, on the other hand, use a single index measure of health outcome that combines quality and length of life. These allow programmes to be assessed and, in theory, ranked according to their cost per marginal QALY gained. There are practical and methodological difficulties involved in measuring benefits for economic evaluations. However, these difficulties are not insurmountable and should not preclude the researcher from designing and carrying out full economic evaluations of CAM therapies.

The cost-effectiveness of acupuncture and spinal manipulation has already been demonstrated in some patient groups. We would hope to see this evidence base increase to include more CAM interventions (such as homeopathy), more comparator strategies and more patient groups.

Economic evaluation is a framework for systematically examining the costs and benefits of options and explicitly taking account of the necessary value judgements, as well as technical judgements, in choosing between them. This approach would seem particularly relevant to the expanding area of the technology of CAM with its large array of alternative means to help people achieve a better life.

REFERENCES

Ballegaard, M., Johannessen, A., Karpatchof, B., et al., 1995. Addition of acupuncture and self-care education in the treatment of patients with severe angina pectoris may be cost beneficial: an open, prospective study. J. Altern. Complement. Med. 5 (5), 405–413.

Ballegaard, M., Norrelund, S., Smith, D., 1996. Cost-benefit of combined use of acupuncture, shiatsu and lifestyle adjustment for treatment of patients with severe angina pectoris. Acupunct. Electrother. Res. 21 (3–4), 187–197.

Brazier, J., Roberts, J., Deverill, M., 2002. The estimation of a preference-based measure of health from the SF-36. J. Health Econ. 21 (2), 271–292.

Brown, J., Sculpher, M., 1999. Benefit valuation in economic evaluation of cancer therapies: a systematic review of the published literature. Pharmacoeconomics 16 (1), 17–31.

Burton, A.K., Tillotson, K.M., Cleary, J., 2000. Single-blind randomised controlled trial of chemonucleolysis and manipulation in the treatment of symptomatic lumbar disc herniation. Eur. Spine J. 9 (3), 202–207.

Carey, T.S., Garrett, J., Jackman, A., et al., 1995. The outcomes and costs of care for acute low back pain among patients seen by primary care practitioners, chiropractors, and orthopedic surgeons. The North Carolina Back Pain Project. N. Engl. J. Med. 333 (14), 913–917.

Cherkin, D.C., Deyo, R.A., Battie, M., et al., 1998. A comparison of physical therapy, chiropractic manipulation, and provision of an educational booklet for the treatment of patients with low back pain. N. Engl. J. Med. 339 (15), 1021–1029.

Cherkin, D.C., Eisenberg, D., Sherman, K.J., et al., 2001. Randomized trial comparing traditional Chinese medical acupuncture, therapeutic massage, and self-care education for chronic low back pain. Arch. Intern. Med. 161 (8), 1081–1088.

Drummond, M., O'Brien, B., Stoddart, G., et al., 2005. Methods for the economic evaluation of health care programmes. third ed. Oxford University Press, Oxford.

Eisenberg, D.M., Post, D.E., Davis, R.B., et al., 2007. Addition of choice of complementary therapies to usual care for acute low back pain: a randomized controlled trial. Spine 32 (2), 151–158.

Liguori, A., Petti, F., Bangrazi, A., et al., 2000. Comparison of pharmacological treatment versus acupuncture treatment for migraine without aura – analysis of socio-medical parameters. J. Tradit. Chin. Med. 20 (3), 231–240.

Lindall, S., 1999. Is acupuncture for pain relief cost-effective? Acupunct. Med. 17 (2), 97–100.

Myers, C.P., 1991. Acupuncture in general practice: effect on drug expenditure. Acupunct. Med. 9 (2), 71–72.

Netten, A., Dennett, J., 1996. Unit Costs of Health and Social Care 1996. Personal Social Services Research Unit, University of Kent, Canterbury.

Niemisto, L., Lahtinen-Suopanki, T., Rissanen, P., et al., 2003. A randomized trial of combined manipulation, stabilizing exercises, and physician consultation compared to physician consultation alone for chronic low back pain. Spine 28 (19), 2185–2191.

Niemisto, L., Rissanen, P., Sarna, S., et al., 2005. Cost-effectiveness of combined manipulation, stabilizing exercises, and physician consultation compared to physician consultation alone for chronic low back pain: a prospective randomized trial with 2-year follow-up. Spine 30 (10), 1109–1115.

Paterson, C., Ewings, P., Brazier, J.E., et al., 2003. Treating dyspepsia with acupuncture and homeopathy: reflections on a pilot study by researchers, practitioners and participants. Complement. Ther. Med. 11 (2), 78–84.

Ratcliffe, J., Thomas, K.J., MacPherson, H., et al., 2006. A randomised controlled trial of acupuncture care for persistent low back pain: cost effectiveness analysis. Br. Med. J. 333 (7569), 626.

Reinhold, T., Witt, C.M., Jena, S., et al., 2008. Quality of life and cost-effectiveness of acupuncture treatment in patients with osteoarthritis pain. Eur. J. Health. Econ. 9 (3), 209–219.

Sintonen, H., 2001. The 15D instrument of health-related quality of life: properties and applications. Ann. Med. 33 (5), 328–336.

Skargren, E.I., Carlsson, P.G., Oberg, B.E., 1998. One-year follow-up comparison of the cost and effectiveness of chiropractic and physiotherapy as primary management for back pain. Subgroup analysis, recurrence, and additional health care utilization. Spine 23 (17), 1875–1883.

Thomas, K., Fitter, M., Brazier, J., et al., 1999. Longer term clinical and economic benefits of offering acupuncture to patients with chronic low back pain assessed as suitable for primary care management. Complement. Ther. Med. 7, 91–100.

United Kingdom back pain exercise and manipulation (UK BEAM Trial Team) randomised trial, 2004. Cost effectiveness of physical treatments for back pain in primary care. BMJ 329 (7479), 1381.

Williams, N.H., Edwards, R.T., Linck, P., et al., 2004. Cost-utility analysis of osteopathy in primary care: results from a pragmatic randomized controlled trial. Fam. Pract. 21 (6), 643–650.

Willich, S.N., Reinhold, T., Selim, D., et al., 2006. Cost-effectiveness of acupuncture treatment in patients with chronic neck pain. Pain 125 (1–2), 107–113.

Witt, C.M., Jena, S., Selim, D., et al., 2006a. Pragmatic randomized trial evaluating the clinical and economic effectiveness of acupuncture for chronic low back pain. Am. J. Epidemiol. 164 (5), 487–496.

Witt, C.M., Brinkhaus, B., Reinhold, T., et al., 2006b. Efficacy, effectiveness, safety and costs of acupuncture for chronic pain – results of a large research initiative. Acupunct. Med. 24, 33–39.

Witt, C.M., Reinhold, T., Brinkhaus, B., et al., 2008a. Acupuncture in patients with dysmenorrhea: a randomized study on clinical effectiveness and cost-effectiveness in usual care. Am. J. Obstet. Gynecol. 198 (2), 166.

Witt, C.M., Reinhold, T., Jena, S., et al., 2008b. Cost-effectiveness of acupuncture treatment in patients with headache. Cephalalgia 28 (4), 334–345.

Wonderling, D., Vickers, A.J., Grieve, R., et al., 2004. Cost effectiveness analysis of a randomised trial of acupuncture for chronic headache in primary care. Br. Med. J. 328 (7442), 747.

Evidence-based practice: more than research needed!

20

Andrée le May • John Gabbay

CHAPTER CONTENTS

INTRODUCTION

Health care workers have always based their practice on a variety of sources of evidence. Over the last two decades, however, they have been urged to work within a paradigm of evidence-based medicine (EBM) (or perhaps more correctly, evidence-based practice: EBP) in an effort to make clinical care more effective, standardized and efficient through the implementation of research findings (le May 1999). Often described as a social movement – a 'collective enterprise to establish a new order of life' (Blumer 1995; Trinder 2000; Pope 2003), the EBM process has crept insidiously through the borders of medicine to all other groups providing health care and on to social care, to education, to resource management and many others (Trinder 2000). In this chapter we consider the essence of this 'new' order of health care and how it might be better crafted to enable the more fluid movement of research findings into practice.

DOI: 10.1016/B978-0-443-06956-7.00020-3

Several reasons, which extend beyond the obvious desire to move research into practice, have also been put forward for the undoubted success of the movement of EBP into the everyday language and practice of health and social care practitioners, managers, researchers, policy-makers, educators and service users. The most persuasive revolve around the emergence of a heightened awareness of risk and associated emphasis on managerialism and audit within western society (Trinder 2000). The resultant attention placed on risk and accountability has necessitated a search for greater certainty in practice – EBP supplies a way to provide this.

Despite debate surrounding the breadth of evidence that supports practice in reality (which includes theory, research findings, personal experience, expert opinion and guidance from professional bodies, expert committees and government policies), the EBP paradigm gives prominence to evidence generated through high-quality research. Whilst this approach is promulgated by governments, educators and some EBP practitioners, many health care workers find it, for a variety of reasons, difficult, if not unworkable (Dopson et al. 2002, 2003). Some continue to practise ritualistically without questioning the appropriateness of their knowledge base and/or assessing its impact, others practise using outdated research evidence that fails to provide the best available care, whilst some who do practise 'good health care' would not describe themselves as practising EBP. This variation has fuelled division among health care professions and researchers, educationalists, managers and policy-makers. Segmentation, as this suggests (Pope 2003), may stimulate the development of vying factions and power struggles associated with social movements, thereby causing uncertainty and unrest. This, in turn, may be further complicated by competition when different factions compete for resources or clients, as may be the case within and between practitioners of conventional and complementary and alternative medicine (CAM).

Some of the problems associated with the uptake of EBP are undoubtedly linked to the existence of slightly different definitions of EBP, uncertainty around the importance and value of different types of evidence to different professional groups involved in providing care and different individual preferences for the use of particular types of evidence. These are all important factors in the success (or not) of EBP since health care, whether conventional or complementary and alternative, is a multidisciplinary undertaking and therefore some shared understanding of what it comprises is important if we are to implement EBP and deliver care that is of the highest quality. The challenge then appears to be to find a more relevant model for practice – one that pragmatically blends evidence from different sources and encourages health care workers, regardless of specialism, to integrate research evidence into established health care systems, whether conventional or complementary and alternative. This in turn should be based on a clearer understanding of the way in which clinicians currently use evidence in practice.

Recent research focusing on medical and nursing practitioners (Gabbay & le May 2004, 2009) suggests that in reality they rarely, when practising, use research findings in isolation from other sources of evidence or in its purest form as a research paper. We discuss this in more detail below, but in brief our observations suggested that clinicians practise according to complex internalized guidelines that they have built up and refined – often through discussion with their peers – throughout their careers. Such 'mindlines', as we have called them, are based on their training and subsequent general reading and educational opportunities, but tend to give prominence to an accretion of their own and others' experiences. Clinicians also seek out or rely on expert opinion to filter important research findings to them, and use information from audit and from their day-to-day interactions with patients to support or guide decisions. Reference to research evidence is confined to very brief readings of journals, and guidelines are only infrequently used. Yet these latter two sources of reliable research findings are most commonly referred to as being gold-standard ways to disseminate evidence to practitioners.

In order for practitioners to be able to understand some of the problems surrounding the implementation of EBP and propose solutions to them we will, in the first part of this chapter, focus on defining EBP and discussing various types of evidence. In addition we will highlight recent research which supports the view that health care workers use multiple sources of evidence, often simultaneously, to guide their practice. Finally, we will consider mechanisms that are known to help or hinder the movement of evidence into practice so that readers may determine their usefulness to their own approach to using an evidence base for practice.

EVIDENCE-BASED PRACTICE: TOWARDS A DEFINITION

Probably the most well-known and useful definition of EBP originates from medicine, where Sackett et al. (1996) stated that EBM is 'the conscientious, explicit and judicious use of current best evidence in making decisions about the care of individual patients' (p. 71). Later this was refined to suggest that EBM could be defined as the integration of best research evidence with clinical expertise and patient values (Sackett et al. 2004).

Both of these definitions suggest a stepwise, linear process for EBP – firstly a conscious recognition that evidence is needed in decision-making, secondly that that evidence should be the 'best' available at the time and therefore requires some kind of appraisal performed on it to determine its worth, and finally that the use of evidence is linked to individual patient/client care (and, one could assume, the evaluation of that) and therefore is relevant to care (Box 20.1). This latter point is particularly relevant when considering EBP and CAM since clients often seek out and use CAM because of the centrality of the client to the treatment process when compared to conventional medicine.

BOX 20.1 The process of evidence-based medicine (Sackett et al. 2004)

Converting information into clear questions
Seeking evidence to answer those questions
Evaluating (critically appraising) the evidence for its validity (truthfulness) and usefulness
Integrating findings with clinical expertise, patient needs, patient preferences and, if appropriate, applying these findings
Evaluating performance (and the outcome of our decision/practice)

BOX 20.2 Examples of hierarchies of evidence

Example 1: Long (1996)*

1. Evidence obtained from at least one properly designed randomized controlled trial
2a. Evidence obtained from well-designed controlled trials without randomization
2b. Evidence obtained from well-designed cohort or case-control analytical studies, preferably from more than one centre or research group
2c. Evidence from comparisons between times or places with or without the intervention. Dramatic results in uncontrolled experiments could be included in this section
3. Opinions of respected authorities, based on clinical experience, descriptive studies or reports of expert committees

Example 2: Muir Gray (1998)

I. Strong evidence from at least one systematic review of multiple well-designed randomized controlled trials
II. Strong evidence from at least one properly designed randomized controlled trial of appropriate size
III. Evidence from well-designed trials without randomization, single group pre- post-, cohort, time series or matched case-control studies
IV. Evidence from well-designed non-experimental studies from more than one centre or research group
V. Opinions of respected authorities, based on clinical evidence, descriptive studies or reports of expert committees

*Based on Canadian Task Force on the Periodic Health Examination (1979)

Although others have presented more simplistic definitions, for instance that evidence-based health care (EBHC) is about 'doing the right things right' (Muir Gray 1998), it appears that defining EBP is relatively unproblematic so long as one remembers that EBP is a dynamic process that needs to be sufficiently versatile to reflect the varying demands of practice and the uniqueness of patients'/clients' needs (le May 1999). One of the underlying reasons for the growth of the EBM movement was to promote the integration of research findings into practice and this led to the creation of early hierarchies of evidence (Box 20.2), which were designed to help practitioners determine 'best' evidence and present options for decision-making if the 'best' evidence was not available.

However, despite the clear view that practice should be based primarily on research findings and the creation of hierarchies of evidence, there is debate amongst the users of EBP as to what, for each faction/segment, forms the most appropriate research for practice (see Chapter 1 for some of the issues and solutions put forward for CAM and also for examples: Verhoef et al. 2002; Schmidt 2004).

HIERARCHIES OF EVIDENCE

As with any hierarchy, the best option is presented at the top. If that is unavailable then the next layer down becomes acceptable and so on; the health care worker simply works down the hierarchy until sound evidence is found in one of the subsequent layers. Yet even this is problematic: might not an indepth qualitative study be more valuable than a small, well-conducted RCT? Leaving that question aside, the two hierarchies presented in Box 20.2 are very similar in putting evidence from the randomized controlled trial firmly at the pinnacle. However, for many practitioners the main problem is that evidence from the more conventional formats that top the hierarchy may not exist to support many of the practical decisions that actually have to be made. (Two obvious examples: most drug trials exclude patients who are over 75 and/or have multiple pathologies; few drugs that are used for children have been adequately trialled in that age group.) Clinicians therefore often find themselves relying on the lower layers of the hierarchy for 'best' evidence. Of course this raises many questions and concerns about the effectiveness and quality of care since by moving away from the pinnacle of any hierarchy it is easy to assume that care is not best but 'second best'; this has become one of the many dilemmas associated with the movement towards EBP.

In addition other notable concerns associated with the ownership and the construction of the hierarchies also need to be addressed. For instance:

- Whose hierarchy is it? Which disciplines own it? Which disciplines cannot work within it?
- Is it relevant to the practice arena or the individual(s) within it?

It is also worth bearing in mind that the varying values that different disciplines working in health care put on different types of evidence may cause friction within multidisciplinary teams. Some members will want to use different evidence from others and this diversity, whilst often being beneficial for patients/clients, may also be detrimental to their care if consensus cannot be reached (Box 20.3).

Perhaps two solutions are available. The first is explicitly to consider evidence more broadly; the second is to accept that we may use several elements of a hierarchy when making judgements and not just one, since in

BOX 20.3 Vignette

Consider the care of an older person with multiple pathology who is taking many different types of drug treatments. The team of doctors looking after this person will rely on the best evidence from clinical trials to support their decisions to prescribe treatments. However these trials may not have included people from this age group with comorbidity; the research evidence is therefore based on a trial that excludes patients like this. So it may fail to give a true picture of the effectiveness and drug interactions which may accompany complex treatment. On the other hand, the nurses and occupational therapists may not draw on this sort of trial-based evidence but be drawing on other sources of evidence such as their experiences when providing day-to-day care for the person or the findings from qualitative research studies which emphasize the experiences of older people with similar complaints. The complementary and alternative medicine practitioner who provides acupuncture to relieve pain in the ward will again have a different source of evidence privileging a different type of research to draw on.

Combining all of this evidence will provide a rich and appropriate package of care for the patient, as indeed many multidisciplinary teams do; using only one source of evidence will impoverish rather than improve care.

reality practice is complex and is therefore informed by many sources of evidence. The reliance on multiple sources of evidence may, in fact, strengthen our ability to provide a confident rationale for care. The challenge then is to be able to fit together many pieces of evidence, collected from a variety of different sources, in order to find the most appropriate approach to care within each situation – perhaps through multidisciplinary team meetings or other forms of case conferencing or, as we discuss below, through the use of communities of practice.

That being so, we could widen the notion of evidence to encompass:

- evidence from a variety of research designs (either our own or others)
- evidence based on our experiences (professional and general)
- evidence based on theory which is not grounded in research
- evidence gathered from our clients/patients and/or their carers
- evidence passed on to us by role models/experts
- evidence based on policy directives (from le May 1999)

and accept that many, if not all of these sources of evidence, can influence practice simultaneously.

Doing this, however, does not mean just taking all the evidence and using it haphazardly; we still need to make a judgement about 'best' or sound evidence for the situation and link it to decisions made with individual, or groups of, patients/clients within the process outlined in Box 20.1.

The next section of this chapter elaborates on this.

WHAT IS SOUND EVIDENCE?

In all instances knowing whether or not the evidence is sound relies on a series of judgements associated with:

knowing the question you want to answer
finding the evidence
assessing the quality of the evidence
determining which evidence provides a basis for the best approach to care is relevant to the clinical and social context of the patient/client, and can be provided by the organization within which care is given.

FINDING EVIDENCE

For many people finding evidence centres on searching both published and unpublished literature. Several writers/organizations (NHS Centre for Reviews and Dissemination 1996) have proposed strategies for doing this. However, if we accept the breadth of evidence available to support practice, an enlarged repertoire for finding evidence, using some of the approaches listed below, may be more suitable (le May 1999).

EVIDENCE FROM RESEARCH

- Searching the literature (published and unpublished) using electronic and manual databases, the internet and browsing through library shelves for:
  - meta-analyses of research studies

- reviews of literature (systematic and narrative: secondary sources)
    - original research papers (primary sources)
    - cited references in others' original research papers (secondary sources) that focus on each specific area of concern.
- Making personal contacts with experts/researchers in the area to establish areas of new research, research in progress or discuss issues in relation to research already completed.
- Reviewing clinical guidelines or research-based standards of care.

EVIDENCE BASED ON OUR EXPERIENCES

- Reflecting on practice and explicitly articulating these reflections, preferably with colleagues.
- Facilitating appraisal and evaluation of practice, either formally through audit or informally through discussion with peers, clients/patients, carers.
- Searching the literature and websites (DIPEx 2008) for narratives, patient stories and case studies which may inform practice and enhance understanding (non-research-based papers).

EVIDENCE BASED ON THEORY WHICH IS NOT RESEARCH-BASED

- Searching the literature (published and unpublished).
- Learning from others (e.g. through formal education).
- Facilitating discussion and debate.

EVIDENCE GATHERED FROM CLIENTS/PATIENTS AND THEIR CARERS

- Searching the literature for experiential writings and/or research findings.
- Using audit data: analysing levels of satisfaction and/or complaint.
- Facilitating discussion and collaborative decision-making.

EVIDENCE PASSED ON TO US BY ROLE MODELS/EXPERTS

- Facilitating discussion and observation with individuals.
- Forming/consulting panels with expert opinions.
- Reviewing policy directives based on expert opinion using recognized experts.
- Searching the literature for findings from consensus-reaching techniques:
    - Delphi surveys
    - Nominal group techniques
    - Consensus conferences.

EVIDENCE PASSED ON THROUGH POLICY DIRECTIVES

- Searching the literature.
- Searching the internet.
- Reviewing clinical guidelines or published research-based standards of care.
- Analysing local community plans and profiles.

Each of the above sources has its place and in the field of CAM and medicine in general some of them will tend to come more naturally than others. For example, many CAM practitioners will naturally gravitate towards basing their practice on theory and experience; there will be few appropriate trials (although the availability of research evidence will, of course, be much improved as a result of this book!); the economic nature of the CAM marketplace may discourage collaborative reflective practice and audit; policy directives may be few and far between. Nevertheless, the key point that we wish to stress here is the importance of maximizing the sources one uses. The good practitioner tries to triangulate the evidence since the more sources of evidence that can be found to suggest a particular course of action, the more likely will it be that that action is the best one available. Conversely, reliance on just one of these sources – be it an excellent piece of research, an apparently watertight theory or years of experience – is likely to mislead.

ASSESSING THE QUALITY OF THE EVIDENCE AND DETERMINING THE BEST APPROACH TO CARE

Once the sources of evidence have been found a decision needs to be made about their usefulness and appropriateness in practice and much has already been written on assessing the quality of research evidence (Crombie 1996; Haines & Donald 1998; Muir Gray 1998; Cullum & Droogan 1999; CASP 2008). The key points to remember when assessing any evidence centre on establishing the rigour of the evidence and its clinical relevance.

Rigour is associated with the ways in which the evidence was gathered and is important regardless of the type of evidence. Much of the literature surrounding critical appraisal does focus entirely on appraising evidence from research, both quantitative and qualitative primary research studies (Forchuk & Roberts 1993; Crombie 1996; CASP 2008) or syntheses of research studies such as systematic reviews or meta-analyses (Oxman 1995; Cullum & Droogan 1999). But if we are to rely on other sources of evidence such as theory, experience or expert opinion, it is important to judge their rigour too. Some initial questions that may help to determine this for a variety of sources of evidence are presented in Table 20.1.

Clinical relevance centres on several factors ranging from appropriateness to the client to the ability of the organization to facilitate the implementation of the evidence; some points for consideration can be found in Box 20.4.

MECHANISMS FOR APPLYING EVIDENCE TO PRACTICE

Using the best and most up-to-date evidence appropriately for each situation is one of the central tenets of effective practice. This is a complex process that involves:

- selling the evidence to others (colleagues, clients, managers) and convincing them of its usefulness
- finding the resources, enthusiasm and commitment needed to apply it
- minimizing barriers to the application of evidence and capitalizing on opportunities (Table 20.2)

Table 20.1 *Assessing the rigour of evidence – some initial elements for consideration*

Research-based evidence	Own experiences	Theoretical perspectives (non-research-based)	Clients'/patients'/carers' experiences	Role models'/experts' opinions	Policy directives
Link between research and clinical situation Strengths and weaknesses of design in relation to aims of research Reliability and validity/credibility Appropriateness of findings to clinical issue Appropriateness of recommendations for practice How this research fits in with other findings Likelihood of transferability to practice setting Evidence of use elsewhere or evaluation of impact	Relevance to the clinical situation Frequency/uniqueness of experience Extent to which experience has been rigorously subjected to critical reflection/audit Extent to which experiences have been shared by others Extent to which other sources of evidence support experiences Extent of transferability of experiences to current situation	Link between theory and clinical situation Strengths and weaknesses of argument being presented What sources of evidence are used? Credibility/face validity How this theory measures up to other theories Appropriateness of theory to clinical issue Appropriateness of recommendations for practice Likelihood of transferability to practice setting Evidence of successful use elsewhere or evaluation of impact	Relevance to the current situation Frequency/uniqueness of experience Extent to which experiences have been shared by others Extent to which other sources of evidence support experiences Richness of the description Extent of transferability of experiences to current situation	Depth and breadth of expertise Credibility/reputation Face validity of advice Reason for choice – what defines expertise? What sources of evidence are drawn upon to support knowledge? Relevance of advice to current situation Likelihood of transferability of evidence to practice setting Evidence of use elsewhere or evaluation of impact	Possible conflict of interest of policy-makers vis à vis this clinical situation Type and strength of evidence used to support directive(s) Relevance to current situation or clinical issue Currency – date when last reviewed Likelihood of transferability to practice setting Evidence of use elsewhere or evaluation of impact

BOX 20.4 Establishing clinical relevance – useful questions to ask

Could this evidence be used within my practice arena? (And if not, why not?)
What benefits will the implementation of this evidence have for patients/carers/other health care workers?
What risks and costs are associated with implementing this evidence?
What risks are associated with not implementing this evidence?
What are the opportunities for and constraints to implementing this evidence?

Table 20.2 *Barriers to and opportunities for the application of evidence to practice*

Barriers to the implementation of evidence	Opportunities for the implementation of evidence
Mistrust of evidence or its source	Organizational support
Attitudes	New structures for sharing evidence (e.g. communities of practice or knowledge networks)
Beliefs	Multiprofessional/multiagency team working
Colleagues' resistance	Changing individuals in teams or positions of influence
Patient/client wishes or non-compliance	Reorganized services
Dissemination failures	New policies
Organizational constraints	Implementing new techniques
Lack of resources/competition for resources	Recommendation by others
Educational or skills deficits in accessing or using evidence	

- negotiating what changes need to be made to practice (and perhaps to the organization of practice) in order to promote the application of evidence
- considering ways in which any evidence-based change can be sustained
- determining how the impact of the change, for all involved, will be assessed and by whom – how will quality be assured?
- deciding how to tell other people about the use of this evidence in practice and its impact on health care.

MINDLINES

In addition to government initiatives associated with the implementation of EBP, researchers are also trying to understand, sometimes by observing practice, the sorts of evidence that practitioners use every day and how they get evidence in order to deliver high-quality care. This type of research is useful because it allows us to understand what really happens in practice and as a result of this to plan better ways for disseminating and applying research evidence.

Some recent ethnographic research by Gabbay & le May (2004, 2009) suggests that medical and nursing practitioners in primary care rarely access and use explicit knowledge from research or other sources directly, but rely on individual 'mindlines'. Mindlines are collectively reinforced, internalized, tacit sources of knowledge – or personal guidelines that are built up over a lifetime of learning from many sources. Whilst mindlines are informed by brief reading they are also affected by the participants' own and their colleagues' experience, their interactions with each other and with opinion leaders, patients and pharmaceutical representatives, and other sources of largely tacit knowledge. Influenced by organizational demands and constraints and the role that the practitioner is playing at the time (e.g. clinical, managerial, educational, advocacy), mindlines are continuously negotiated socially with a variety of key people – predominantly patients and colleagues –resulting in knowledge appropriate for their practice. And such practice always needs to be much more flexibly adapted to individual circumstances than most guidelines and other EBP sources allow. This may be particularly pertinent for CAM practitioners where the relationship between the practitioner and the patient/client is often described as a 'vital component of effective health care' (Little 2007). Gabbay & le May's research emphasizes the value of interaction in the process of applying evidence to practice – testing out evidence with trusted colleagues and using their knowledge as well as one's own to inform practice; it also emphasizes the importance of merging evidence from different sources for both individual and collective decision-making.

As a result of this and other works (see Pawson's (2006) and Nutley and colleagues' (2008) contributions to the evidence base on how research can inform public services), recognition is growing that the effective transfer of evidence takes time. Moreover it involves people and not simply the dissemination and reading of printed media such as systematic reviews, guidelines, care pathways, policies and research papers. This means that more emphasis should be placed on finding ways through which people can get together to share, shape and evaluate knowledge for their practice; for instance, by working in communities of practice or belonging to knowledge networks. These interactions naturally facilitate the transformation of tacit knowledge into explicit knowledge and discussions related to the application of evidence to practice. This model of knowledge exchange, however, may prove to be difficult in CAM where there remains a predominance of single-handed practices and where knowledge-sharing might be problematic when income relies on maintaining a competitive advantage. Nevertheless it remains an important route to improved and genuinely EBP.

COMMUNITIES OF PRACTICE

Communities of practice are hubs of learning and knowledge transfer and can be defined as:

> *groups of people who share a concern, a set of problems, or a passion about a topic, and who deepen their understanding and knowledge of this area by interacting on an ongoing basis ... These people don't necessarily work together on a day-to-day basis, but they get together because they find value in their interactions. As they spend time together, they typically share information, insight, and advice. They solve problems. They help each other. They discuss their situation, their aspirations, their needs. They think about common issues. They explore ideas and act as sounding boards to each other. They may create tools, standards, generic designs, manuals, and other documents; or they may just keep what they know as a tacit understanding they share ... Over time, they develop a unique perspective on their topic as well as*

a body of common knowledge, practices, and approaches. They also develop personal relationships and established ways of interacting. They may even develop a common sense of identity. They become a community of practice

(Wenger et al. 2001).

Increasingly communities of practice are forming in health and social care settings, either naturally, or deliberately created as a mechanism for getting people together in order to discuss the best ways to implement evidence to suit the needs and context of their area of practice or particular patients/clients and therefore improve the quality of care that they give. As such:

Communities of Practice can positively impact on:
the standard of care delivered to patients/clients
the working environments and job satisfaction of the participants in the community
the ways in which people exchange knowledge and learn
the ways in which problems are solved
the speed with which knowledge and innovation move into practice
the generation of knowledge from practice
the creation of a unified team which may be uni- or multiprofessional
the ownership and sustainability of changes to practice

(le May 2009).

CONTINUING CHALLENGES FOR THE TRADITIONAL MODEL OF EBP

CURRENT INITIATIVES

In order to promote the uptake of EBP in the 1990s in the UK, considerable effort was spent constructing ways to help health care workers to apply evidence in practice. Most of these mechanisms focused on packaging research evidence in different ways and presenting it to practitioners with the expectation that they would then simply implement it: little attention was spent on trying to understand how people actually used different types of evidence in their practice and how therefore research evidence should be integrated with other sources of evidence to make implementation easier. Many of these mechanisms are still used in the UK, and indeed across the world, to encourage the application of evidence to practice today, albeit with varying success (Box 20.5).

Despite a great deal of attention and resource having been spent on these interventions during the last decade in western health care systems, there still remains a notable gap between the availability of research evidence and its application. The existence of this gap has led to the creation of several initiatives to raise the profile of EBP and the implementation of knowledge: the most ambitious one in the UK is probably the creation of the Modernization Agency under the NHS Plan (Department of Health 2000a). The Modernization Agency, established in order to provide the NHS with a centre focusing on how knowledge and 'knowhow' about best practice could be spread (Department of Health 2000b), has now been subsumed by the NHS Institute for Innovation and Improvement. The Institute still continues to offer opportunities for the enhancement of practice through:

BOX 20.5 Some current mechanisms for introducing evidence-based practice (EBP)

- Initial prequalification education that emphasizes the value of EBP
- Ongoing educational opportunities following qualification
- The introduction of compulsory continuing professional development
- The use of guidelines and care pathways/bundles to guide and change practice
- The use of policy directives that push practice forward
- The use of local opinion leaders or knowledge champions/managers
- Audit and feedback, including inspection by monitoring bodies
- Electronic reminder systems often linked to treatment decisions

- working closely with clinicians, NHS organizations, patients, the public, academia and industry in the UK and worldwide to identify best practice
- developing the NHS's capability for service transformation, technology and product innovation, leadership development and learning
- supporting the rapid adoption and spread of new ideas by providing guidance on practical change ideas and ways to facilitate local, safe implementation
- promoting a culture of innovation and lifelong learning for all NHS staff (NHS Institute for Innovation and Improvement 2008).

THE CHALLENGE FOR CAM PRACTITIONERS

Although there is a general consensus that EBP is here to stay, the traditional model of EBP that most of us have been working with needs to be broadened to encompass the variety of sources of evidence that practitioners use and the ways in which they find out about them. And this is especially true for CAM. Several challenges still remain if we are to move practice forward more confidently. These centre on:

- valuing the breadth of evidence which underpins practice
- balancing the need to provide standardized care (e.g. through the use of clinical guidelines) with the need to individualize care
- balancing standardization with innovation
- considering what EBP means to various stakeholders (e.g. managers, clients, other professionals)
- developing supportive organizational cultures, which facilitate corporate and individual commitment to EBP
- being more in tune with the ways in which health care workers, from all disciplines, find out about the evidence that they need to underpin their practice
- encouraging the role of communities of practice and knowledge networks to share and evaluate new evidence.

Alongside these, perhaps the greatest challenge is to integrate our broadened notion of EBP within appropriate quality systems so that care remains dynamic and in tune with individual patients' or clients' needs.

REFERENCES

Blumer, H., 1995. social movements. In: Lee, A.M. (Ed.), New outline of the principles of sociology. Barnes and Noble, New York.

Canadian Task Force on the Periodic Health Examination, 1979. The periodic health examination. Can. Med. Assoc. J. 121 (9), 1193–1254.

CASP, 2008. www.phru.nhs.uk/Pages/PHD/resources.htm accessed 31st October.

Crombie, I., 1996. The Pocket Guide to Critical Appraisal. BMJ Publishing Group, London.

Cullum, N., Droogan, J., 1999. Using research and the role of systematic reviews of the literature. In: Mulhall, A., le May, A. (Eds.), Nursing Research: Dissemination and Implementation. Churchill Livingstone, Edinburgh.

Department of Health, 2000aa. The NHS Plan: a plan for investment, a plan for reform. Department of Health, London.

Department of Health, 2000bb. The NHS Plan: implementing the performance improvement agenda. A policy position statement and consultation document. Department of Health, London.

DIPEx, 2008. www.dipex.org/ accessed 31st October.

Dopson, S., Fitzgerald, L., Ferlie, E., et al., 2002. No magic targets! Changing clinical practice to become more evidence based. Health Care Manage. Rev. 27, 35–47.

Dopson, S., Locock, L., Gabbay, J., et al., 2003. Evidence-based medicine and the implementation gap. Health: An Interdisciplinary Journal for the Social Study of Health Illness and Medicine 7 (3), 311–330.

Forchuk, C., Roberts, J., 1993. How to critique qualitative research articles. Can. J. Nurs. Res. 25 (4), 47–56.

Gabbay, J., le May, A., 2004. Evidence-based guidelines or collectively constructed 'mind-lines'? An ethnographic study of knowledge management in primary care. Br. Med. J. 329, 1013–1016.

Gabbay, J., le May, A., 2009. Practice made perfect? Discovering the roles of a community of general practice. In: le May, A. (Ed.), Communities of Practice in Health and Social Care. Wiley-Blackwell, Oxford.

Haines, A., Donald, A., 1998. Getting research findings into practice. BMJ Publishing, London.

le May, A., 1999. Evidence Based Practice. NT Books, EMAP Healthcare, London Nursing Times Clinical Monographs 1.

le May, A., (Ed.), 2009. Communities of Practice in Health and Social Care. Wiley-Blackwell, Oxford.

Little, C., 2007. Searching for effective health care: a hermeneutic study of traditional herbalism in contemporary British health care. University of Southampton Unpublished PhD.

Long, A., 1996. Health services research – a radical approach to cross the research and development divide? In: Baker, M., Kirk, S. (Eds.), Research and Development for the NHS: evidence, evaluation and effectiveness. Radcliffe Medical Press, Oxford.

Muir Gray, J., 1998. Evidence-based Healthcare: how to make health policy and management decisions. Churchill Livingstone, Edinburgh.

NHS Centre for Reviews and Dissemination, 1996. Undertaking systematic reviews of research on effectiveness: CRD guidelines for those carrying out or commissioning reviews. NHS Centre for Reviews and Dissemination, York CRD Report 4.

NHS Institute for Innovation and Improvement, 2008. www.institute.nhs.uk accessed 31st October.

Nutley, S., Walter, I., Davies, H., 2008. Using Evidence: How research can inform public services. The Policy Press, Bristol.

Oxman, A., 1995. Checklist for Review Articles. In: Chalmers, I., Altman, D. (Eds.), Systematic Reviews. BMJ Publishing Group, London.

Pawson, R., 2006. Evidence-based Policy: A realist perspective. Sage, London.

Pope, C., 2003. Resisting evidence: the study of evidence-based medicine as a contemporary social movement. Health: An Interdisciplinary Journal for the Social Study of Health Illness and Medicine 7 (3), 267–282.

Sackett, D., Rosenberg, W., Gray, J.A., et al., 1996. Evidence-Based Medicine: what it is and what it isn't. Br. Med. J. 312, 71–72.

Sackett, D., Strauss, S., Richardson, W., et al., 2004. Evidence based medicine: how to practice and teach EBM. Churchill Livingstone, London.

Schmidt, S., 2004. Mindfulness and healing intention: concepts, practice and research evaluation. J. Altern. Complement. Med. 10 (1), S7–S14.

Trinder, L., 2000. Introduction: the Context of Evidence-Based Practice. In: Trinder, L., Reynolds, S. (Eds.), Evidence-Based Practice: A Critical Appraisal. Blackwell, Oxford.

Verhoef, M., Casebeer, A., Hilsden, R., 2002. Assessing efficacy of complementary medicine: adding qualitative research methods to the 'gold standard'. J. Altern. Complement. Med. 8 (3), 275–281.

Wenger, E., McDermott, R., Snyder, W., 2001. Cultivating Communities of Practice. Harvard Business School, Harvard.

FURTHER READING

Gabbay, J., le May, A., 2004. Evidence-based guidelines or collectively constructed 'mind-lines'? An ethnographic study of knowledge management in primary care. Br. Med. J. 329, 1013–1016.

le May, A., (Ed.), 2009. Communities of Practice in Health and Social Care. Wiley-Blackwell, Oxford.

Nutley, S., Walter, I., Davies, H., 2008. Using Evidence: How research can inform public services. The Policy Press, Bristol.

Trinder, L., Reynolds, S. (Eds.), 2000. Evidence-Based Practice: A Critical Appraisal. Blackwell, Oxford.

Wenger, E., McDermott, R., Snyder, W., 2001. Cultivating Communities of Practice. Harvard Business School, Harvard.

INDEX

Note: Page numbers followed by *b* indicate boxes; *f* figures; *t* tables.

D

E

F

G

H

I

K

L

M

N

O

P

Q

R

S

T

U

V

W

Y